An illustrated guide
MEDICINAL
PLANTS
OF EAST AFRICA

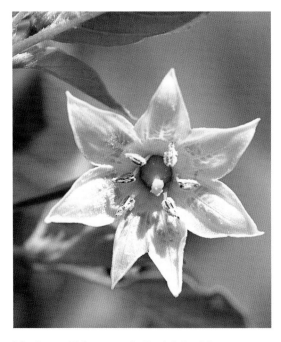

Najma Dharani & Abiy Yenesew

Dedicated to the
indigenous people of Africa

Published by Struik Nature (an imprint of
Penguin Random House South Africa (Pty) Ltd)
Reg. No. 1953/000441/07
The Estuaries No. 4, Oxbow Crescent,
Century Avenue, Century City, 7441
PO Box 1144, Cape Town, 8000 South Africa

Visit **www.penguinrandomhouse.co.za**
and join the Struik Nature Club for updates,
news, events and special offers.

First published by Najma Dharani
in association with Drongo Editing &
Publishing in Kenya, 2010

This edition first published by Struik Nature in
South Africa, 2022

10 9 8 7 6 5 4 3 2 1

Publisher: Pippa Parker
Managing editor: Roelien Theron
Editor: Emsie du Plessis
Project manager: Natalie Bell
Designer: Dom Robson
Concept designer: Janice Evans
Proofreader: Thea Grobbelaar

Reproduction by Studio Repro
Printed and bound in China by
1010 Printing International Ltd.

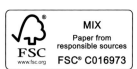

MIX
Paper from
responsible sources
FSC® C016973
www.fsc.org

ISBN 978 1 77584 787 8 (Print)
ISBN 978 177584 788 5 (ePub)

The authors welcome feedback** on the
content of this book. Readers' suggestions
and criticisms will help to ensure that
amendments and additional information
can be included in future editions.
Email comments to: ndbonsai@gmail.com

Photographs
Front cover: *Leonotis* sp., Nick Kurzenko,
Adobe stock
Back cover: Flower of *Gloriosa superba*
Title page: Flower of hot red chili
Capsicum frutescens
Contents page: Flower of tamarind
Tamarindus indica

Contents

ACKNOWLEDGEMENTS

This book would not have been possible without the professional collaboration and friendship of contributing author Professor Abiy Yenesew, whose detailed and wide-ranging knowledge of the chemistry and pharmacology of medicinal plants is amply demonstrated on these pages.

In compiling this book, I have been indebted to the World Agroforestry Centre (ICRAF) in Nairobi, the National Museums of Kenya, the University of Nairobi and the headquarters of the United Nations in Gigiri, Nairobi, for their kindness in allowing me unrestricted use of their respective libraries and resources.

To all my close friends and relatives, who have given me the support, encouragement and strength I needed to complete this book, I owe a particular debt of gratitude.

My work on this, as with my earlier published books, has been very much a family affair. My loving, caring husband and best friend, Firoz, has as usual been a pillar of strength to me, and I have benefitted enormously from his ideas and suggestions, to say nothing of his unflagging support and encouragement. For the company of my wonderful sons, Farhaan and Rizwan, who joined me on many of my long trips around East Africa, I am especially grateful. And to my late mother, my father, my sisters Yasmeen and Naseem, and my late mother-in-law, who all shared with me their vast knowledge of traditional Indian medicine and Indian recipes, I am deeply thankful.

This publication owes much to the dedicated work of the many traditional herbalists – far too many to name individually here – whom I met in local markets, in villages and on shambas (farms) throughout East Africa, and who all went out of their way to share with me their considerable local knowledge of plants and their many medicinal uses and curative properties, while providing invaluable insights into the preparation, dosage and administration of age-old herbal remedies.

I was fortunate as well to meet patients of many of these traditional herbalists and to discuss with them their ailments, past and present, and the results of some of the herbal treatments they have received. Without the vast store of oral knowledge on herbal remedies preserved in the memories of village elders, grandmothers and mothers in these diverse local communities, this book would not have been possible. With these living custodians of an important healing tradition, now sadly vanishing, I have had the singular privilege of being able to share aspects of my own ancestral and family knowledge of medicinal plants.

With this book, I hope only that I have repaid the trust of today's guardians of healing knowledge – and that this compilation will go some way towards helping to safeguard the important tradition they uphold.

The subject matter of this book comes from, and belongs to, the developing world. Attempts to exploit this store of local knowledge for commercial gain, through expropriating under 'patents' the intellectual property of the developing world, must be strenuously resisted. The underlying aim of this book is to ensure that as much as possible of this priceless local knowledge can survive, and that in doing so, it will remain freely accessible to all.

Najma Dharani
Nairobi, Kenya

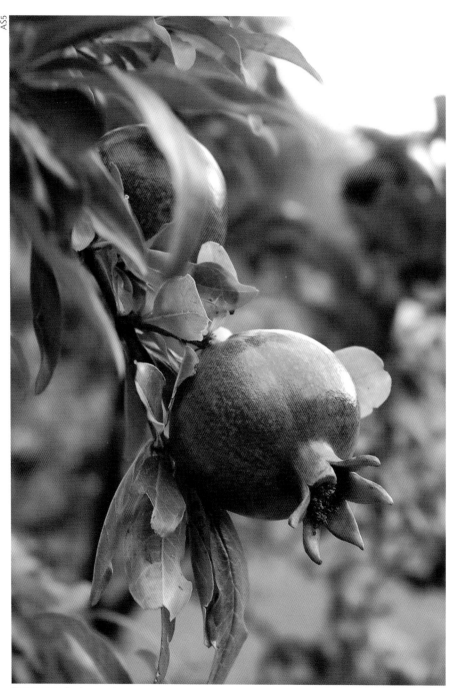

Pomegranate *Punica granatum*

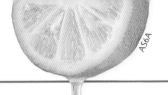

INTRODUCTION

The medicinal virtues of plants

The use of plants and plant derivatives for preventing and treating human diseases and afflictions is as old as civilisation itself. History shows that every culture on Earth has benefitted from the medicinal virtues of plants. Indeed, plants are still the backbone of most medical and health care systems around the world.

Western medicine depends on plants for the active compounds in many of today's most successful and widely used drugs. Where natural products and their derivatives provide the basis for more than half of all the drugs now in clinical use globally, higher plants contribute no less than 25 per cent of the active ingredients. There is, in addition, a thriving global health care market extending to many hundreds of plant-based formulations, which are sold as health foods, herbal teas and nutritional and health supplements.

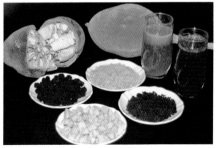

Top Fresh lemon juice helps to relieve severe nausea, vomiting and indigestion. **Above** A refreshing drink prepared from fruit pulp of the baobab *Adansonia digitata* is used to treat fever and diarrhoea.

Estimates put the number of plant taxa in everyday medicinal use around the world at anywhere between 50,000 and 75,000. Yet, despite the ever-growing number of plant-based drugs, fewer than 20 per cent of Earth's plant species have hitherto been

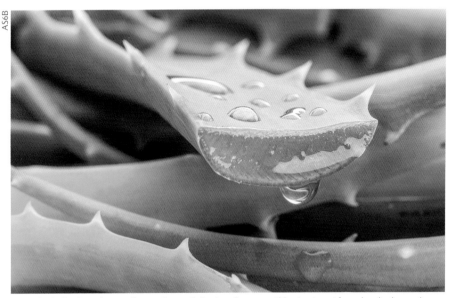

The leaf gel of various aloe species may be applied externally as a soothing treatment for rashes, bruises and fungal infections.

examined for potential healing properties. Well in excess of 200,000 plant species are still awaiting scientific investigation.

Modern science has validated many of the healing attributes for which individual plant species have long been used traditionally. A recent example is the endorsement of antimalarial drugs based on artemisinin, a compound first isolated in 1965 from the Chinese herb *Artemisia annua*, commonly known as sweet wormwood – a plant that traditional healers in China and elsewhere have long been prescribing as a cure for malaria. In trials carried out during a malaria epidemic in Vietnam in the early 1990s, Chinese military researchers found that artemisinin-based drugs reduced the death rate from malaria by no less than 97 per cent. Global health authorities, including the United Nations Children's Fund (UNICEF) and the World Health Organization (WHO), have since embraced the use of artemisinin-based combination therapy (ACT) drugs in the fight against *Plasmodium falciparum* malaria around the world.

The transition of artemisinin from traditional to mainstream medicine follows that of other plant derivatives, including quinine, morphine, aspirin, codeine and reserpine, most of which are household names. More recently, development of the drug vincristine from Madagascar periwinkle, *Catharanthus roseus*, has given scientists new hope in the battle to find effective treatments for cancer. The bark of red stinkwood, *Prunus africana*, has since the early 1970s been used in the formulation of no fewer than 19 different commercial drugs – all in common use today in both North America and Europe for the treatment of benign prostatic hyperplasia (BPH).

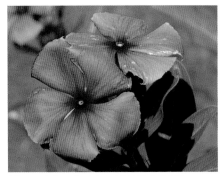

A tea made from the leaves of the Madagascar periwinkle *Catharanthus roseus* is used in the treatment of leukaemia in children.

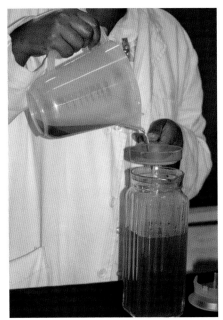

A tea made from leaves of sweet wormwood *Artemisia annua* is widely used as a remedy for cerebral malaria.

Across much of Africa, and elsewhere in the developing world, where access to clinics dispensing modern medicine is either limited or prohibitively costly, traditional herbal remedies are still the primary means of meeting the health and medical needs of most rural communities. Recent figures of the WHO and other sources show that only about 240 million people in sub-Saharan Africa (that is around 21 per cent of a population of 1.4 billion) can be said to have good access to modern health care and pharmaceuticals. Most of the remaining 900 million people still depend entirely on traditional herbal remedies. The ratio of traditional healers to the population in sub-Saharan Africa is 1:500 compared to 1:40,000 medical doctors. Various reports indicate that some 10,000 'highly valued' medicinal plant species are in everyday use on the African continent.

The stalls of traditional healers and herbalists are a familiar sight in rural villages and outdoor markets throughout sub-Saharan Africa. With their stashes of plant materials, powders and potions, the stalls have changed little over hundreds of years, and are still as heavily patronised as ever, despite encroaching modernity. Day after day, thousands of doses of simple, affordable herbal remedies – for stomach ailments, diarrhoea, skin conditions, infected wounds and sores, fevers and a host of other common afflictions – are dispensed to children and adults. For the vast majority of the people in most African countries, the local herbalist remains the principal ally in the continuing battle against perennial diseases such as malaria, bilharzia and trypanosomiasis. And it is the local herbalist to whom people are obliged to turn as well for the treatment of sexually transmitted diseases and for relief from tuberculosis, pneumonia and other devastating afflictions whose resurgence over recent decades is associated with HIV/AIDS.

The dominance of traditional healers is reflected in recent research findings showing how in rural Kenya there is one practitioner of traditional herbal medicine for about 833 people, and in the urban areas one practitioner for every 378 residents. Countrywide, the ratio of practising, university-trained medical doctor to patient is close to 1:7,142. It is estimated that the number of traditional practitioners in Tanzania is between 30,000 and 40,000 in comparison to about 600 medical doctors. In Uganda there are 200–400 patients per traditional healer and 20,000 patients for each qualified medical doctor.

It is estimated that, in all, there are 650,000 traditional healers and herbalists at work in East Africa and that as many as 65 per cent of all East Africans are in the habit of consulting such healers regularly, despite having access to modern clinics and medicines as well. The rural herbalist, or *daktari wa miti shamba*, is invariably a highly respected figure within the local community. In most cases, herbalists are from families that have been practising traditional medicine for generations. Their *miti wa dawa* knowledge has been passed on orally from one generation to the next. Over the course

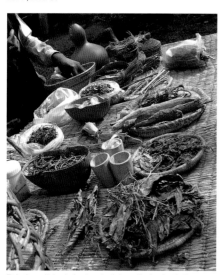

Dried medicinal plant material on display includes roots, leaves and stem bark.

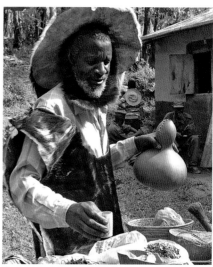

The local herbalist, or *daktari wa miti shamba*, is a highly respected figure within East African communities.

of the 20th century in Africa, influences from abroad were assimilated, as more and more of the region's traditional herbalists became acquainted with the healing properties of exotic or alien plant species introduced by European settlers, or with the enduring and highly developed traditions of herbal medicine espoused by immigrant communities from the Indian subcontinent.

What is relatively new, however, is the proliferation in the region's cities and towns of retail outlets and counters selling herbal teas and therapeutic plant-based products to an affluent and increasingly health-conscious urban population. Both in specialist health shops and on the shelves of most large supermarkets and drug stores in the Kenyan capital of Nairobi, for example, there are rows of beautifully packaged herbal teas made from the leaves of *Artemisia, Ajuga, Prunus, Hypericum, Azadirachta* and *Hibiscus*, among other plants. And there is a rapidly growing selection of other plant-based products, ranging from creams, lotions and ointments incorporating essential oils from genera such as *Allium,*

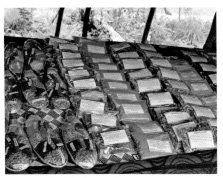

Pre-packed herbal spices such as turmeric powder, red chillies, cloves, ginger powder and cinnamon sticks are sold at a spice farm in Zanzibar.

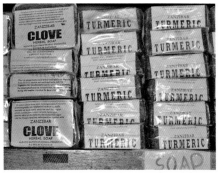

Locally made soaps incorporating turmeric and cloves are used extensively as antiseptics in treating a wide range of skin afflictions.

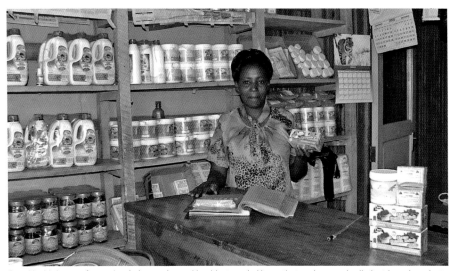

Pure Health is one of many local pharmacies and health stores in Kenya that package and sell plant-based products such as essential oils, tinctures, lotions, ointments, syrups and tea bags.

Eucalyptus, Foeniculum, Zingiber, Citrus and *Trigonella*, to toothpastes containing *Aloe, Azadirachta* and other plant extracts.

This trend is in keeping with a burgeoning global market for health supplements among city dwellers faced with a raft of what, for Africa, are relatively new ailments (including diabetes, high blood pressure and obesity) that are related to the stresses and demands of modern urban life, and to the unbalanced diets and lack of exercise that often go hand in hand with such a lifestyle. Not surprisingly, there now exists a huge export market for plant-based supplements from Africa. The growing popularity of health supplements is adding to the soaring demand for traditional herbal medicines among Africa's rapidly expanding rural populations, and this in turn is fuelling a dramatic surge in popular and commercial interest in medicinal plants.

For a sector that is so well established and which boasts such a long history, traditional herbal medicine in Africa remains surprisingly unheralded. In East Africa, the role that traditional healers and herbalists play has never been formally recognised as an integral part of any of the region's overall health care systems. With no registration procedures or codes of practice, traditional herbal medicine remains almost wholly unregulated. Cut off from the mainstream economy, the field receives little development support and is roundly ignored by donors and development agencies. In both China and India, by contrast, which are by far the world's largest per capita users of medicinal plants, having traditions going back 7,000 years, the fields of Chinese homeopathic and Indian Ayurvedic medicine are today jealously guarded, highly regulated national industries grounded in years of well-documented scientific enquiry, with quality controls and rigorous training programmes and courses of study.

The paucity of information about Africa's medicinal plants, coupled with the headlong rush to exploit their healing properties, presents a number of challenges. Quite apart from the enormous conservation challenges that lie ahead, there is the danger of conflicts arising between bioprospecting companies and local communities over ownership of the rights to exploit what diminishing natural resources are still available. In India, for example, it has taken the collective might of the phytomedical industry as a whole to resist attempts made by some foreign organisations to patent, for their own commercial gain, a number of herbal extracts that have been in traditional use locally for centuries. Governments in Africa have a role to play in ensuring that the intellectual property rights of their citizens are respected and that local communities are given a stake in ventures seeking to make use of their knowledge and traditions. Steps, too, must be taken to ensure that all use of local plants is sustainable and does not threaten local biodiversity.

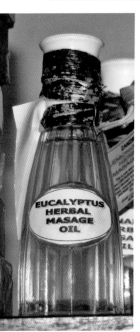 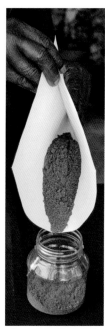

Left Many medicinal plants are the source of essential oils that are key ingredients in preparations used for massage and steam baths. **Right** Dried pounded powder from different parts of medicinal plants is best stored in airtight plastic bottles and kept in a cool place.

Conservation of medicinal plants

By far the most pressing concern is the alarming rate at which the forests of sub-Saharan Africa are being destroyed, as elsewhere in the tropics, to make way for cultivation and settlement. Catastrophic habitat loss, coupled with the wholesale plunder of remaining forests, is threatening the survival of many plants, including such medicinally important endemic species as the camphor tree *Ocotea usambarensis* and *Prunus africana*, along with several species of *Aloe*.

plant species, in the interests of creating a sustainable supply, while at the same time alleviating the pressure on wild specimens. Clearly, there is an urgent need for programmes under which endangered medicinal plants, propagated in special nurseries, can be grown, managed and harvested commercially.

Medicinal plants are an integral part of both the daily lives and the cultural heritage of rural communities throughout Africa. As such, their value is inestimable. It is our responsibility to ensure that this living legacy remains intact for the future.

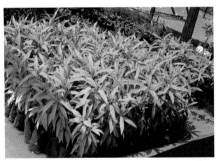

AS11

Seedlings of *Warburgia ugandensis* in the nursery of the World Agroforestry Centre (ICRAF) in Nairobi, Kenya.

Already, the disappearance and depletion of medicinal plants from forests across East Africa is having a severe impact on the livelihoods of traditional herbalists, curtailing their ability not only to administer to the health needs of their own local communities, but also to trade among themselves, as has long been their custom. The traditional taboos that once governed collecting and storage of wild plants are no longer an effective safeguard against overharvesting. There are too few of the plants left and those that remain are increasingly being targeted by the minions of unscrupulous dealers who often have no connection with either the communities or their healing traditions.

In the face of this unprecedented assault on the region's wild medicinal plants, there are still depressingly few examples of projects involving managed domestication and cultivation of threatened

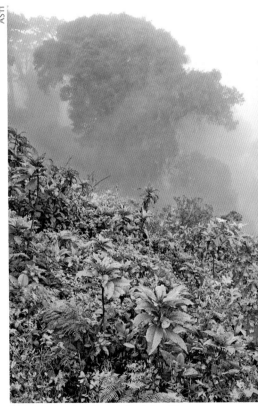

Foggy morning along the lush forest rim of the Ngorongoro Crater, Tanzania. Decisive conservation steps and protective interventions must be taken so that these plants continue to thrive for generations to come.

Phytochemistry – the active principles of plants

Contributed by Abiy Yenesew

Plants, unlike animals, cannot run away or hide when they are threatened or subjected to physical attack. Instead, they have evolved other ways of protecting themselves – they do this by producing chemical compounds called secondary metabolites.

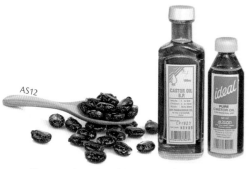

AS12

The purgative action of the seed oil of the castor oil plant *Ricinus communis* is ascribed to ricinoleic acid and its stereoisomer, produced through hydrolysis in the duodenum. Users are cautioned that castor oil seeds contain ricin, one of the most toxic of all compounds. Intake of just two seeds can kill a child; 10–15 seeds may kill a human adult.

The secondary metabolites produced by any given plant species are usually unique to that plant or to closely related plants. On the other hand, primary metabolites are shared by all plants and by all living organisms. These are essential compounds such as sugars, amino acids, common fatty acids, nucleotides and the various polymers derived from these compounds (including polysaccharides, proteins, lipids, and both RNA and DNA).

The secondary metabolites of a plant are the active compounds that play a role in giving the plant an effective and multifaceted defensive armoury. The chemical weapons deployed in such armouries have evolved over millions of years in a bid to stay one step ahead of that plant's principal threats, and they are simultaneously engaged in evolving new and more effective lines of attack.

Throughout history, human beings have found ways of exploiting the diverse array of active compounds arising from the ingenuity of plants. More than 25 per cent of all drugs that are currently at the disposal of modern medicine are either derived directly from plants or are synthetic analogues of the secondary metabolites of plants. The essential role of plants and of their active compounds in medicine, both modern and traditional, will not diminish at any time in the foreseeable future.

The secondary metabolites of plants are classified according to the way plants synthesise them from simple molecules. The most important groups of secondary metabolites and their active principles, from a medicinal standpoint, are described here.

Cardenolides

These include steroidal glycosides (e.g. gigitoxigenin), which have sugar units attached at C-3 and a five-membered ring attached to ring D of a steroid skeleton. Bufadienolides differ from cardenolides in having a six-membered lactone attached to ring D. These compounds are known for their cardiac activities and are found mainly in the plant families Apocynaceae and Asclepiadaceae. On account of their cardiac activities, plants containing such compounds are used as arrow poisons.

Terpenoids

Also known as isoprenoids or terpenes, they are naturally occurring organic compounds formed by a joining of two or more units of a five-carbon precursor. They have C10, C15, C20, C25, C30, C40 or Cn (where n>40) skeletals and are subdivided according to their number of C-5 units into monoterpenes (C10), sesquiterpenes (C15), diterpenes (C20), sesterpenes (C25), triterpenes (C30), tetraterpenes (C40) and polyterpenes (Cn). Terpenoids are widely distributed in higher plants, where they are thought to play a vital ecological role in plant survival. Humans have found various uses for terpenoids – the volatile lower terpenoids (monoterpenes, sesquiterpenes) are used in the perfume industry and as flavouring agents in the food industry. Due to their antimicrobial activities against oral pathogens, terpenoids obtained from essential oils of eucalyptus, mint and lemon are added to toothpaste as an alternative to fluoride. The diterpenes and triterpenes yield a wide range of biologically active compounds. The adrenal hormones and vitamins A, D and E are steroids, which are degraded triterpenes.

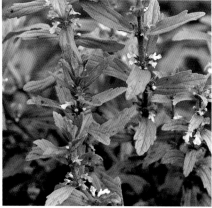

Diterpenes such as *ajugarin B* have been isolated from the leaves of *Ajuga integrifolia* and can help to treat malaria caused by *Plasmodium falciparum*.

Quinones
These compounds are similar to phenolic compounds but are oxidised and possess two carbonyl (C=O) groups in their ring structure rather than hydroxyl (-OH) groups. Various types can be distinguished according to the number of aromatic rings they contain. Benzoquinones (one aromatic ring), naphthoquinones (two aromatic rings) and anthraquinones (three aromatic rings in a linear arrangement) are the best-known examples. Quinones are found in plants from several different families. Benzoquinones occur in the genera *Myrsine* and *Rapanea*, naphthoquinones in the genus *Plumbago*, and anthraquinones in the genera *Cassia*, *Aloe* and *Rumex*. The antimalarial, anticancer, antibacterial and antifungal activities of quinones are well documented.

Alkaloids
These are basic compounds incorporating a nitrogen atom (N) as a member of the ring system. Various classes of alkaloids are distinguished, depending on the ring system (or skeleton) or on the amino acid from which this is formed. The best-known examples are the 'tropane alkaloids' (e.g. atropine) from *Datura stramonium* and the 'pyrrolizidine alkaloids', particularly common in the genus *Senecio*. Most alkaloids are physiologically active, with wide-ranging pharmaceutical effects. The toxic alkaloids, exemplified by *D. stramonium*, affect the nervous system. The less toxic alkaloids, such as caffeine and sparteine, increase renal secretion and are used as diuretics and in the treatment of oedema.

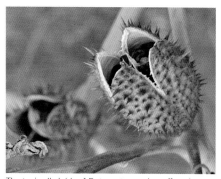

The toxic alkaloids of *Datura stramonium* affect the nervous system, producing symptoms of restlessness, irritability, disorientation, hallucinations and delirium.

Flavonoids
These phenolic compounds (that is, having one or more hydroxyl groups attached to the aromatic ring in their structure) are found almost universally as water-soluble pigments in plants. Some flavonoids lack many free phenolic groups and are not water soluble. Flavonoids have three rings (A, B and C) arranged in a C6-C3-C6 basic skeleton. Different flavonoid types are distinguished according to the levels of oxidation in ring C, giving rise to different subclasses including flavones, flavonols, flavanones and chalcones. Another group, the anthocyanidins, is usually present as water-soluble pigments, having one or more sugar molecules bonded

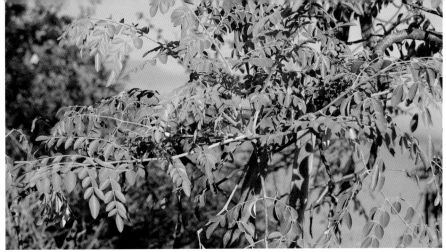

Flavonoids such as rutin have been found in the leaves of *Moringa stenopetala*, a medicinal plant known for its anti-inflammatory and antimicrobial activities.

onto them. An example is cyanidin, which contributes to the red or purple colours of flowers and is also a medicinally important constituent of many rhizomes and roots. Flavonoids are well known medicinally for the anti-inflammatory, antioxidant, antibacterial, antiviral and anti-allergic effects they produce.

Tannins

These phenolic compounds coagulate gelatine and other proteins. The two basic tannin groups occurring in higher plants are hydrolysable and condensed tannins. Hydrolysable tannins are compounds in which one or more sugars (usually

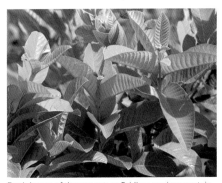

Fresh leaves of the guava tree *Psidium guajava* contain tannins and ellagic acid (with a protective effect on mucous membranes), explaining this plant's enduring use for treating diabetes, diarrhoea and dysentery.

glucose) are bonded to phenolic acid molecules. The phenolic acids are either gallic or ellagic acid. Condensed tannins (also called proanthocyanidins) are quite different. They are made up of two or more flavonoid units, which break down into anthocyanidins when treated with acids at high temperatures. Tannins are among the most abundant compounds in trees and shrubs (e.g. *Acacia*, *Diospyros* and *Kigelia*), where they are found mainly in stems and bark. Tannins have antiseptic, astringent, haemostatic and invigorating effects.

Phenylpropanoids

These compounds possess the basic C6-C3 arrangement of an aromatic ring (C6) and an aliphatic (C3) chain. When the C3 portion is cyclised into lactone, coumarins are formed. Coumarins are found in many plant families, including Umbelliferae (or Apiaceae) and Rutaceae. Dimerisation of phenylpropanoids produces lignans, while extensive polymerisation produces lignins. Some lignans are known for their antitumour properties, while lignins, in being part of cell walls, provide a matrix for cellulose microfibres. Degradation of the side chain of phenylpropanoids produces biologically active compounds such as salicylic acid. Several of the amino acids from which aromatic alkaloids are formed are synthesised from phenylpropanoids.

Herbal medicine preparations

The chemical compounds found in different parts of a woody perennial plant – in the roots, bark, leaves, fruits and seeds of any shrub or tree – often differ markedly from one another. The varied make-up of these compounds, known as the active ingredients of a plant, makes perfect sense in terms of giving a plant the appeal it needs to attract its pollinators and seed dispersers, while at the same time equipping it with a defensive strategy for self-preservation. In this delicate balance of evolutionary give and take, it stands to reason that, whereas one part of a plant may be highly toxic, another part of the same plant may be altogether harmless. Cases where an entire tree or shrub can be used for herbal medicine are therefore very rare.

In most instances, it is only the bark or the roots (or sometimes both) that are used in plant medicine. In general, less use is made of the leaves, while the flowers and fruits of shrubs and trees are seldom utilised. In the case of herbaceous plants of genera such as *Artemisia, Allium* and *Ajuga*, the tendency is to uproot the whole plant, although it is usually the leaves and twigs that are used, more than the roots. The medicinal use of grasses is rare. With cacti and succulent plants such as species of *Aloe* and *Bulbine*, it is the juicy leaves and whole stems that are typically used – in preparing treatments for external application, say, to fungal infections of the skin or as poultices. The gum, exudate and nectar

of some plants are used medicinally, but in most cases medicinal use is limited to roots, bulbs, rhizomes, tubers, bark, leaves, flowers or fruits.

There are various ways of preparing medicine from plants. Each method seeks to make the release and subsequent absorption of a plant's active ingredient, or ingredients, as easy and as effective as possible. A list of the most common methods of preparing medicines from plant materials follows.

Infusions (herbal brews or 'teas')

Making an infusion is a simple and effective way of extracting nearly all active compounds from the delicate parts of plants (e.g. leaves or flowers), with minimal chemical alteration or loss. Typically, a handful of pounded fresh plant material is steeped in a litre of boiled water for 15–20 minutes. The mixture is filtered or sieved/'strained' for drinking as a 'herbal tea' during the day. Powdered dry plant material

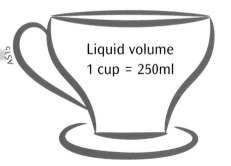

Liquid volume
1 cup = 250ml

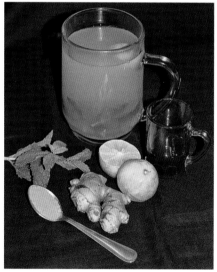

A decoction for treating coughs, sore throat, bronchitis, flu and pneumonia is made with cloves, cinnamon sticks, a pinch of turmeric powder, one teaspoon of dry or fresh ginger, a few crushed mint leaves and one tablespoon of honey in 500ml water. Boil for 10 minutes and drink this tea hot, three times a day.

can also be used, generally in measures of 20–30g per litre of water, which is the equivalent of about a teaspoon per cup. If taken over several days, it is important to prepare a fresh infusion daily.

Decoctions ('herbal teas')

A decoction is usually a brew made from the hard parts of plants (roots, bark, rhizomes or seeds), which must first be boiled to release their active ingredients. Leaf decoctions can be prepared in this way but a disadvantage is that the prolonged heat may cause some of the active plant compounds to become degraded. Typically, a handful (30–50g) of the plant material is boiled in a litre of water for 15–20 minutes. Adults may then drink 3 or 4 cups of this 'tea' at intervals during the day. Half the adult dose is recommended for children aged 6–12, a third for those aged 2–6, and a sixth or less for infants. Decoctions should be prepared afresh every day.

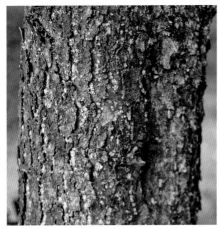

A warm decoction of pounded fresh bark of the African Wild Olive *Olea europaea* subsp. *cuspidata* is a remedy for malaria and intestinal worms.

Cold-water extracts

Cold-water extracts are prepared by soaking pounded or pulped plant material in cold water, generally overnight (in the case of leaves or flowers), but often for 24 hours (in the case of roots or bark). Most such mixtures need to be stirred intermittently.

After straining, adults may drink 3 or 4 cups of extract at intervals during the day. Doses for children are the same as for decoctions (see left). Some cold extracts are prepared using other solvents, usually either oil or alcohol.

Syrups

Some medicinal plant materials have an off-putting taste. Syrups are one way of making such materials more palatable, especially for children. In syrups, the active ingredients often keep longer as well, with the sugar acting as a preservative. Typically, either brown sugar, jaggery or honey is added to a filtered decoction or infusion of the plant material, which is then allowed to simmer over low heat and with continual stirring until the sugars dissolve and the sweetened mixture thickens.

Juices

The squeezed juices of mostly the fresh fruits but also the fleshy leaves of some herbaceous plants are extremely effective in that all active ingredients, especially vitamins, are retained. The concentrated juices should be ingested in small doses only (of teaspoons) and can also be used as bases for syrup.

Tinctures

A tincture is a solution in alcohol of the cold extract of dried plant material. Typically, 100g of the dried plant material is soaked at room temperature in a litre of an alcohol–water mixture (typically 45 per cent or 70 per cent alcohol) for two or three days, but sometimes for a week or longer. In tinctures, it is possible to retain high concentrations of some of the active principles of plants.

Chewing

Juice from the leaves, roots or bark of some medicinal plants can very easily – and quickly – be extracted and swallowed simply by the act of chewing mouthfuls of these materials and spitting out the debris. Chewing is particularly effective in treating a cough, sore throat, mouth ulcers and stomach ailments.

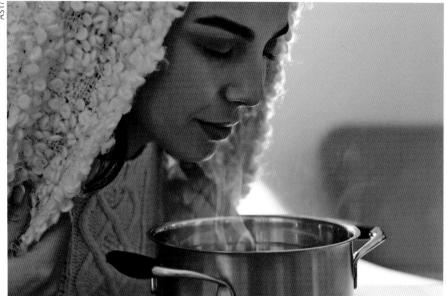

Inhalation of the steam from *Eucalyptus* leaves and drops of the essential oil in boiling water alleviates lung congestion, providing welcome relief from bronchial coughs.

Steam inhalation and steam baths

The use of herbal steaming is very effective in allowing the volatile components and essential oils of some medicinal plants to pass directly into the lungs. Inhalation of the steam vapour from such plants is ideal for the relief and treatment of respiratory conditions such as sinusitis, bronchitis and asthma as well as for throat infections, colds and headaches. For maximum penetration of the active ingredients, a towel should be placed over the head while breathing in the steam. Steam baths can also be applied to the head or even to the whole body. Some herbal preparations, added to warm bathwater, are effective in relieving skin rashes, eczema and measles.

Liniments

Pastes or emulsions of medicinal herb extracts in oil or alcohol, liniments have a soft consistency. Their application to the skin by gentle rubbing allows the active compounds to penetrate underlying tissues for relief from arthritis, rheumatism, backache, joint pains and muscle sprains.

Powder snuffs

The inhalation of finely ground powders made from the dried parts of some medicinal plants is still a common expedient for clearing blocked nasal passages and for combatting the symptoms of respiratory and chest infections. Through inducing sneezing, snuffing can hasten the expulsion of mucus and phlegm.

Enemas

Oily or aqueous solutions that are administered by rectal injection, enemas are used primarily for their purgative, anthelmintic and sedative effects. Some infusions and decoctions are administered in syringes or tubes as enemas. All such mixtures should be freshly prepared and of uniform consistency.

Poultices

Moist, often warm applications used for dressing inflamed areas of the skin, poultices accelerate the healing process through boosting circulation to, and facilitating drainage from, wounds,

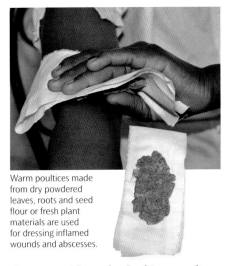

Warm poultices made from dry powdered leaves, roots and seed flour or fresh plant materials are used for dressing inflamed wounds and abscesses.

of the mouth, throat and tonsils. They remove mucus, germs, dead cells and toxins from these areas in the case of irritation, inflammation or infection. They have emollient, antiseptic and astringent effects. Most warm 'herbal tea' infusions can also be used for this purpose. Gargles are not supposed to be swallowed and very hot or highly concentrated liquids are unsuitable for gargling.

Lotions

Infusions, decoctions or cold extracts of medicinal plant materials, or in some cases the raw juices of such plants, can – as lotions – be gently massaged into the skin. Friction lotions, generally containing essential plant oils, are applied in the same way, but require more vigorous massaging. Lotions are commonly used for the treatment of skin afflictions, itching and rheumatism, as a mosquito repellent and as a cosmetic for beautifying the skin.

abscesses and furuncles. Poultices are often prepared from seed flour, mashed fruits or powdered leaves or roots of fresh or dried plants. Bandages are sometimes used over a poultice. Ideally, poultice applications should be renewed at regular intervals rather than left in place for long periods. The ash residues produced after burning dried parts of some medicinal plants are often incorporated in traditional poultices.

Gargles

As medical preparations for washing and treating the mouth and throat, gargles act on the mucus covering the rear part

Ointments

In the preparation of ointments, active ingredients of a plant are dissolved in fatty substances. The substrates most often used are Vaseline®, lanolin and vegetable or animal oils. Ointments are solid at room temperature, but soften when rubbed onto the skin. They are used cosmetically to cover the skin, to treat skin ailments such as fungal infection or to treat rheumatism through penetration into the deeper tissues.

Nasal and eyedrops

Drops of plant liquid, introduced with a dropper into the nostrils, can be very effective in clearing blocked nasal passages during a cold or influenza. Eyedrops can be used to heal soreness or irritation of the eyes or inflammation of the eyelids. The eyes are extremely sensitive, however, and particular care must therefore be taken to ensure that all decoctions to be used as drops or for washing the eyes are properly sterilised (through prior boiling). Eyedrops made from plant extracts should never be highly concentrated and are best administered warm, not hot.

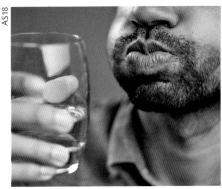

Gargling is a simple and effective way of disinfecting the throat and mouth for soothing relief from irritation or inflammation.

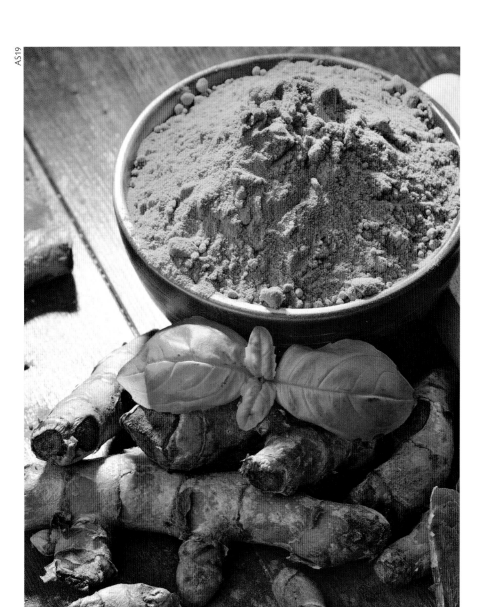

An application of a warmed turmeric paste may relieve swelling and bruising, and pains suffered after accidents. Turmeric is also said to act as an astringent in arresting haemorrhages and bleeding from wounds. Turmeric powder mixed with hot milk is used in the treatment of rheumatic arthritis.

ABOUT THIS BOOK

Most of the 136 plant species described in this book belong to East Africa's indigenous flora. However, some of the more widely cultivated exotic species found in the region have been included, given that their medicinal use has long since been assimilated into the canon of the local herbalist.

It is impossible to describe and depict *all* of the medicinal plant species, indigenous or exotic, that are routinely used in herbal medicine across East Africa. This book, then, is limited to a selection of the best-known and-understood medicinal plants and how they are used.

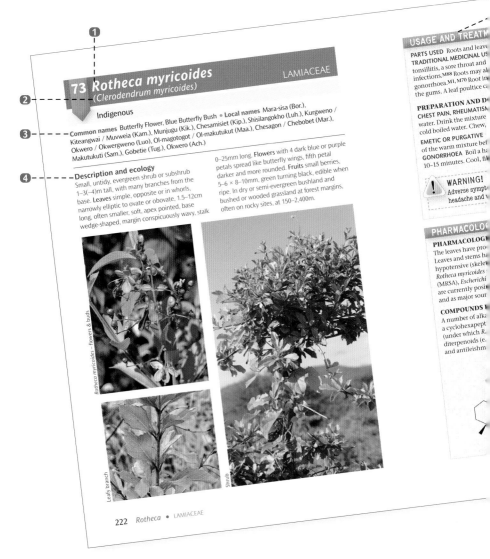

❶

❷

❸

❹

USAGE AND TREATM

PARTS USED Roots and leave
TRADITIONAL MEDICINAL US
tonsillitis, a sore throat and
infections.M88 Roots may al
gonorrhoea.M1, M70 Root in
the gums. A leaf poultice ca

PREPARATION AND D
CHEST PAIN, RHEUMATISM
water. Drink the mixture
cold boiled water. Chew,

EMETIC OR PURGATIVE
of the warm mixture bef
GONORRHOEA Boil a ha
10–15 minutes. Cool, fi

⚠ **WARNING!**
Adverse sympt
headache and v

PHARMACOLO

PHARMACOLOG
The leaves have pro
Leaves and stems ha
hypotensive (skele
Rotheca myricoides
(MRSA), *Escherichi
are currently posi
and as major sour

COMPOUNDS I
A number of alka
a cyclohexapept
(under which *R.*
diterpenoids (e.
and antileishm

73 *Rotheca myricoides*
(*Clerodendrum myricoides*)   LAMIACEAE

Indigenous

Common names Butterfly Flower, Blue Butterfly Bush • **Local names** Mara-sisa (Bor.), Kiteangwai / Muvweia (Kam.), Munjugu (Kik.), Chesamisiet (Kip.), Shisilangokho (Luh.), Kurgweno / Okwero / Okwergweno (Luo), Ol-magotogot / Ol-makutukut (Maa.), Chesagon / Chebobet (Mar.), Makutukuti (Sam.), Gobetie (Tug.), Okwero (Ach.)

Description and ecology
Small, untidy, evergreen shrub or subshrub 1–3(–4)m tall, with many branches from the base. **Leaves** simple, opposite or in whorls, narrowly elliptic to ovate or obovate, 1.5–12cm long, often smaller, soft, apex pointed, base wedge-shaped, margin conspicuously wavy, stalk 0–25mm long. **Flowers** with 4 dark blue or purple petals spread like butterfly wings, fifth petal darker and more rounded. **Fruits** small berries, 5–6 × 8–10mm, green turning black, edible when ripe. In dry or semi-evergreen bushland and bushed or wooded grassland at forest margins, often on rocky sites, at 150–2,400m.

Rotheca myricoides – flowers & buds

Leafy branch

Shrub

222 *Rotheca* • LAMIACEAE

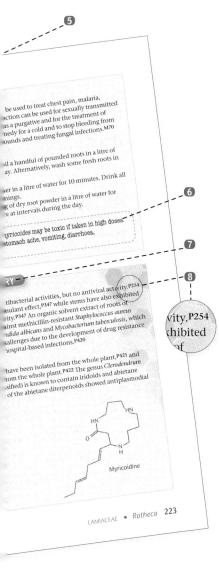

5

be used to treat chest pain, malaria,
...ction can be used for sexually transmitted
...as a purgative and for the treatment of
...nedy for a cold and to stop bleeding from
...ounds and treating fungal infections.M70

...il a handful of pounded roots in a litre of
...ay. Alternatively, wash some fresh roots in

...er in a litre of water for 10 minutes. Drink all
...nings.
...g of dry root powder in a litre of water for
...e at intervals during the day.

...yriooides may be toxic if taken in high doses.
...tomach ache, vomiting, diarrhoea,

6

7

8

...RY

...tibacterial activities, but no antiviral activity.P254
...mulant effect,P347 while stems have also exhibited
...vity.P347 An organic solvent extract of roots of
...inst methicillin-resistant *Staphylococcus aureus*
...idida albicans and *Mycobacterium tuberculosis*, which
...allenges due to the development of drug resistance
...hospital-based infections.P420

...have been isolated from the whole plant,P421 and
...rom the whole plant.P422 The genus *Clerodendrum*
...sified) is known to contain iridoids and abietane
...of the abietane diterpenoids showed antiplasmodial

Myricoidine

...vity.P254
...chibited
...of

LAMIACEAE • *Rotheca* 223

Features of species accounts

1 Accounts, presented at species or genus level, are given in alphabetical order of the scientific names of the plants. The headings are numbered for quick reference. In the case of genera, individual species are labelled with letters, starting with **a**.

2 Some scientific names are followed by an alternative in brackets – such an alternative could be a synonym recognised by the wider botanical fraternity or a reflection of another classification followed by the authors.

3 English common names for plant species are followed by the names commonly used in multiple East African languages, abbreviated for space reasons. A list of the abbreviations used is given on page **301**.

4 All the main features of the plant (growth form, bark, leaves, flowers and fruit) are described, along with key aspects of the distribution and ecology. Extreme sizes have sometimes been given in parentheses, indicating maximum or minimum recorded heights. Colour photographs illustrate each species.

5 The uses of each species in traditional medicine and primary health care are summarised, followed by details about which parts of the plant are used, and how and in what dosages the traditional remedies are prepared and administered. Also included is information gleaned from the oral tradition and from the authors' personal observations and experience, some of which is published here for the first time.

6 Warning boxes caution users about plant-specific risks and symptoms.

7 Current scientific understanding of the active chemical compounds found in different parts of each plant species, and of the biological activities these compounds engender, is reported. In many cases, it is seen that modern scientific research and analysis have been validated, whereas in other cases further research is required.

8 Wherever possible, references are given, acknowledging the published sources that have been consulted while compiling this book. References are abbreviated in the accounts and detailed on page **266** onwards.

Additional material at the back of the book includes: **Glossaries** of medical and botanical terms (pages **294–300**) and a useful **Checklist** that groups ailments and the specific plants that are recommended for their treatment (pages **302–307**).

a. *Acacia nilotica (Vachellia nilotica)*   Indigenous

Common names Egyptian Thorn, Scented-pod Acacia • **Local names** Burguge (Bor.), Chigundigundi (Dig.), Msemeri / Munga (Gir.), Mgunga (Swa.), Musemei (Kam.), Chepitet (Kip.), Ol'kiloriti (Maa.), Sertwet (Nan.), Chalabdo (Orm.), Kopkwo (Pok.), Gilorit / Mirgi (Ren.), Eldekeci (Sam.), Tugerr (Som.), Chebiwa (Tug.), Ekapiliment (Tur.), Ol-giloriti (Aru.), Mfuku (Gogo), Mdubilo / Mgunga (Nyam.), Muhinko (Nyat.), Kihungawisu / Kihungawiswa (Ran.), Mgelegele / Muela (Samb.), Mdubilo (Suk.), Mgungankundu (Zig.), Ekapelimen (Ate.), Goond / Kaloabaval (Guj.), Kikar / Goand (Hind., Urd., Punj.)

Description and ecology

Large, thorny shrub or small tree 2–6m tall but can reach 20m, often branched from the base, with a rounded crown. **Bark** brown-black, rough, fissured, resin or gum exuding from the trunk, young shoots red-brown, hairy, thorns grey-white, straight, 6–10cm long or shorter. **Leaves** bipinnate, each pinna with 10–30 pairs of smaller leaflets. **Flowers** bright golden yellow, fragrant, in round heads 1.2–1.5cm in diameter, axillary or terminal. **Fruits** long, straight or curved pods, up to 17 × 2cm, green and fleshy when young but purple-brown and softly hairy with fruity smell when mature, deeply constricted between seeds, exuding gum when squeezed. A highly variable species, common in arid and semi-arid regions of Africa, in wooded grassland, woodland and open bushland, at 0–2,300m.

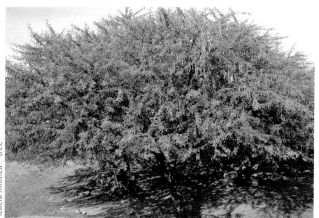

Acacia nilotica – tree

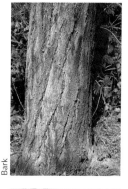

Bark

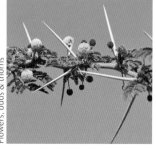

Flowers, buds & thorns

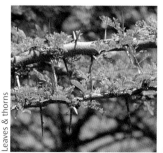

Leaves & thorns

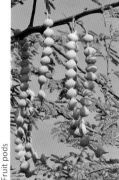

Fruit pods

PARTS USED Roots, bark, leaves, twigs, gum and fruits.
TRADITIONAL MEDICINAL USES Infusions or decoctions of fresh bark are used to treat a cough and sore throat[M16] and as a stimulant to improve digestion. Leaf decoctions are used as a remedy for chest pain and pneumonia. Crushed leaves are used as a poultice on skin ulcers and leprosy. The root has been used to treat tuberculosis and is also said to alleviate impotence.[M112] Both the gum and bark have been used for treating cancers and/or tumours (of ear, eye or testicles),[M112] for chest problems such as colds, congestion, coughs and tuberculosis, for indurations of the liver and spleen, and for fever, gall bladder problems, haemorrhage, haemorrhoids, leucorrhoea, ophthalmia and sclerosis.[M112] Root decoctions are taken for indigestion and stomach ailments, as an emetic,[M3, M4, M70] and to treat gonorrhoea, chest diseases and impotence.[M16] Juice from the twigs and squeezed fruit is used as an eye medicine.[M3] Tender twigs, used as toothbrushes, help to strengthen the gums and prevent gum bleeding.[M70] Bark, young leaves or pods are used to treat spermatorrhoea, premature ejaculation, leucorrhoea and tenuity of semen.[M7, M70] The gum is used to treat coughs, asthma and dryness of the throat, as well as in treatments for dysentery, for relieving backache and for boosting recovery after childbirth.[M7]

PREPARATION AND DOSAGE
COUGHS, ASTHMA, SORE THROAT Peel off fresh bark and remove its soft inner lining. Fold this into little balls and chew, swallowing the juice. Alternatively, chew a piece of the gum at intervals during the day.
PNEUMONIA Boil a handful of fresh leaves in a litre of water with some regular tea leaves for 15 minutes. Add honey and drink 3 cups of the hot mixture a day.
INDIGESTION AND STOMACH DISORDERS Boil a handful of fresh roots or 5g of root powder in a litre of water. Drink a cup of this decoction after every meal.
SPERMATORRHOEA AND PREMATURE EJACULATION Dry fresh sprouting leaves in the sun and then crush into a powder. Add 3g of the leaf powder (or powdered bark) to a cup of cold boiled water, stir and leave for 15–20 minutes. Filter the infusion and drink every morning before breakfast for 3 or 4 days. Alternatively, tender pods (in which seeds have not formed) can be dried in the sun, pounded and sieved, and 5g of this powder added to a glass of milk or water, with a little sugar. This mixture can be taken on an empty stomach every morning for 3 or 4 days.
BACKACHE AFTER CHILDBIRTH Fry 10g of the gum in ghee, with an equal quantity of jaggery or brown sugar. Add a few pistachio or almond nuts and take before breakfast in the mornings for a month.

b. *Acacia senegal* *(Senegalia senegal)*   Indigenous

Common names Sudan Gum Arabic, Gum Arabic Tree, Gum Acacia • **Local names** Iddaado / Baabido (Bor.), Chikwata (Dig.), Idaado (Gab.), Mung'ole / King'ole (Kam.), Chepkomon (Kip.), Otiep / Kiluor (Luo), Olterkeso / Oderekesi (Maa.), Bura diima (Orm.), Chemangayan / Chemanga (Pok.), Hadhaadh / Mirgi (Ren.), Ikerdedi / Loleriberi (Sam.), Adad / Edad (Som.), Kikwata (Swa.), Mung'oora / Mung'ora (Mbe., Tha.), Ekunoit (Tur.), Mirgi (Ren.), Mzasa (Gogo), Igwata / Mkwat (Suk.), Mgwata / Mgwatu (Nyam.), Muhunga (Ran.), Mukhubo (Nyat.), Ekodokodwa (Ate.), Bwara / Mkoto (Zin.), Ekonoit (Ate.T.), Bina (Lugb.), Lakido / Achika (Luo-A), Alal / Okutoketch (Luo-L)

Description and ecology
Low-branching, deciduous, multi-stemmed shrub or small, single-stemmed tree, usually less than 5–8m high but occasionally reaching 15m, with a rounded crown. **Bark** yellow to brown, smooth in young trees but papery and peeling in older trees, becoming dark brown, rough and longitudinally fissured,

armed with recurved prickles just below the nodes, in pairs or in groups of 3, dark grey to blackish brown, 2 curving upwards, central hook curving down, 3–7mm long. **Leaves** have 3–6 pairs of pinnae, each with 8–18 pairs of tiny green leaflets. **Flowers** white or cream, borne in spikes 3–8.5cm long. **Fruits** yellow or dark brown to grey pods, oblong to linear, flattened, papery, 4–20cm long, with permanent veins, straight or curved, tapered at both ends, non-hairy or velvety, deeply constricted between the 6–17 seeds. **Seeds** elliptical to circular, flattened, 6–9 × 5–8mm, dark brown to brownish black. Widespread in dry grassland, deciduous bushland, dry scrub and woodland, at 0–1,900m.

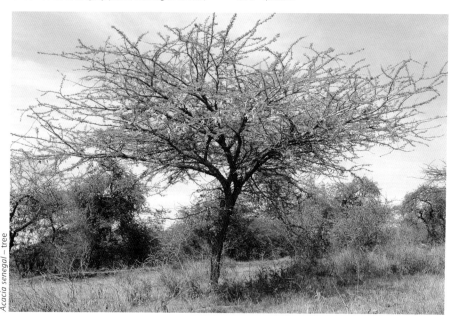

Acacia senegal – tree

USAGE AND TREATMENT

PARTS USED Roots, bark and gum.
TRADITIONAL MEDICINAL USES A decoction of bark is taken as a remedy for diarrhoea, dysentery and stomach disorders. A root decoction is used as a mild purgative and in treatments for stomach ache and gonorrhoea.[M4, M16, M70] Freshly squeezed juice from the fruit is used to soothe eye infections.[M3] Bark infusions are used to treat diarrhoea and malaria. Gum arabic is used in the global food, confectionery, beverage and pharmaceutical industries[M16, M70] as well as in local medicine, where its applications are the same as for the gum of *Acacia nilotica* (Egyptian thorn).

PREPARATION AND DOSAGE
DIARRHOEA AND DYSENTERY Boil 2–3g of powdered bark in a cup of water for 10 minutes. Cool, filter and drink twice a day.
PURGATIVE Boil 3g of powdered roots in a cup of water and drink warm on an empty stomach in the early morning.
BACKACHE AFTER CHILDBIRTH As with *A. nilotica*, fry 10g of gum in ghee, with an equal quantity of jaggery or brown sugar. Add a few pistachio or almond nuts and take before breakfast in the mornings for a month.

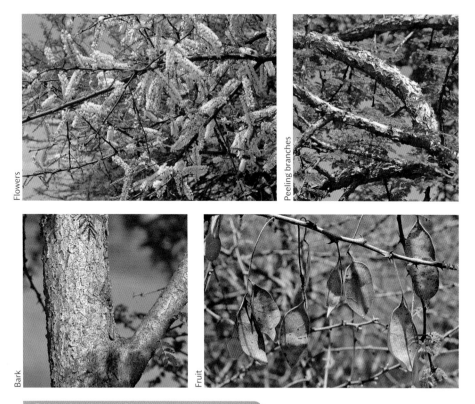

Flowers

Peeling branches

Bark

Fruit

PHARMACOLOGY AND CHEMISTRY

PHARMACOLOGICAL PROPERTIES

A great many pharmacological activities – including antibacterial,[P1] antifungal,[P2] anti-yeast,[P3] antiviral (against HIV),[P2] antipyretic,[P4] antimalarial,[P5] anti-inflammatory, antispasmodic[P6] and antioxidant[P7] effects – have been reported for *Acacia* species.

COMPOUNDS REPORTED

Compounds of different classes – including the flavonoids catechin,[P8] epigallocatechin-5-7-digallate[P9] and kaempferol[P10] as well as epigallocatechin-5-7-digallate – have been isolated from fruits of some acacias. *Acacia* bark and leaves contain tannins. The bark also contains benzenoids (e.g. catechol),[P8] alkanols (e.g. octacosan-1-ol)[P9] and triterpenes (e.g. α-amyrin).[P11]

Catechin

Catechol

α-Amyrin

a. *Acokanthera oppositifolia* — Indigenous

Common names Arrow-poison Tree, Bushman's Poison • **Local names** Muva-wa-ngo / Mukweu (Kam.), Kiururu (Kik.), Olmorijoi (Maa.), Mururu (Mer.), Rumbara (Tav.), Usungu / Musungusungu (Tai.)

Description and ecology

Attractive small, evergreen tree 2–7m tall or sometimes a multi-stemmed, woody shrub. **Bark** rough brown becoming deeply fissured with age, young branches reddish, glabrous, angled and ribbed. **Leaves** simple, opposite, entire, tough, shiny above, larger than those of *A. schimperi*, 4–10(–13)cm long, obovate to elliptical, with rounded base and pointed apex. **Flowers** white with pink tube, longer than in *A. schimperi*, fragrant, in dense, many-flowered, axillary cymes. **Fruits** ellipsoid or plum-shaped berries, larger than those of *A. schimperi*, 1.5–3(–4)cm long, green to purple when ripe, edible, pulp green to deep red, 1- or 2-seeded. **Seeds** ellipsoid, 6–10mm long, glabrous. Found in dry forest margins, often on termite mounds, in riverine forest, riparian forest edges and open woodland, at 1,000–2,300m.

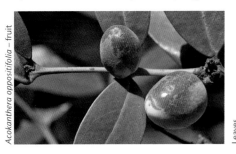

Acokanthera oppositifolia – fruit

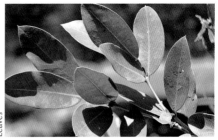

Leaves

USAGE AND TREATMENT

PARTS USED Leaves and roots.

TRADITIONAL MEDICINAL USES Decoctions or infusions of the roots are used in the treatment of syphilis.[M4, M70, M112] Small pieces of stem are chewed to soothe toothache.[M115] A leaf infusion is used to treat abdominal pain, colds, measles and blood poisoning. A root infusion is taken to expel tapeworm and to treat excessive and irregular menstruation.[M112, M115] Powdered dried leaves and roots are used to treat snakebite.[M1, M115] Leaf infusions are taken for stomach pain.[M70, M112] To treat snakebites and spider bites, a small amount of the leaves is eaten, a leaf or root decoction is drunk and the leaf or root pulp is rubbed into the wound.[M112] In South Africa, the leaves and roots of *Acokanthera oppositifolia* are used to treat toothache, colds, anthrax and tapeworm, and dried leaves and roots are used for snakebite and headache.[M2, M70]

PREPARATION AND DOSAGE

COLDS AND HEADACHES Soak dried leaves or dry leaf powder in water. Filter the solution and use as nasal drops.

SNAKEBITES AND SPIDER BITES Apply dried leaf or root powder or a paste thereof directly to the bite.

⚠ **WARNING!** All parts of *Acokanthera* plants are highly toxic and treatment should therefore be administered with caution.

b. *Acokanthera schimperi*

Common names Arrow-poison Tree, Common Poison Bush • **Local names** Karraru (Bor.), K'arraaru (Gab.), Chungu / Utungu (Gir.), Kivai (Kam.), Muricu / Murichu (Kik.), Olmorijoi (Maa.-Ken.), Mururu (Mer.), Keliot / Kelyo (Nan., Kip.), Kolion / Kolyon (Pok.), Ilmorijoi (Sam.), Get mariid (Som.), Kelyon / Kelwon (Tug.), Msungu (Hehe), Mshunguti (Samb.), Msungu / Msunguti (Swa.), Kelyo (Sebei)

Description and ecology

Much-branched, evergreen shrub 2–5m tall or a small tree reaching 8–10m, with a dense, rounded crown and a short bole. **Bark** dark brown, corky, deeply fissured. **Leaves** simple, opposite, elliptical to ovate or broadly ovate, 2–10 × 1.5–6cm, dark glossy green above, paler and dull below, base rounded, apex often pointed, margin entire. **Flowers** white with pink tube, 8–12mm long, fragrant, in dense axillary clusters. **Fruits** oval berries, 1–2(–2.5)cm long, green-red becoming purple when ripe, with pulp green to deep red, 1- or 2-seeded. **Seeds** oval, 6–12mm long, smooth, non-hairy. Widespread in East Africa in dry highland forest margins, in thickets, wooded grassland and rocky bushland, especially in red or black rocky soils, at 1,100–2,400m.

USAGE AND TREATMENT

PARTS USED Roots, bark and leaves.
TRADITIONAL MEDICINAL USES A warm infusion of pounded root is drunk in small quantities to treat sexually transmitted diseases such as syphilis, and it is also consumed as an aphrodisiac.[M1, M4, M112, M115] A decoction of bark has been used succesfully during heavy menstruation.[M112, M115] Externally, leaves and bark are applied to treat skin disorders and infections.[M112, M115] A warm infusion of leaves is gargled to treat tonsillitis. Dried leaf powder is taken with honey as a contraceptive (for birth control).[M112, M115]

PREPARATION AND DOSAGE
SKIN PROBLEMS (RASHES, BOILS, ECZEMA, FUNGAL INFECTIONS) Make a paste from dried bark or leaf powder, and apply directly to the affected areas.

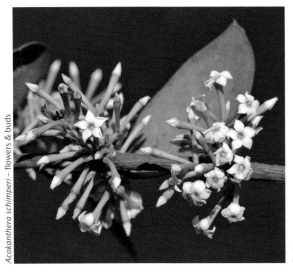

Acokanthera schimperi – flowers & buds

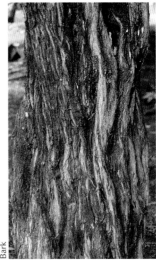

Bark

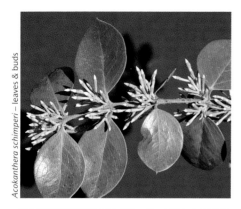

Acokanthera schimperi – leaves & buds

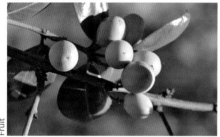

Fruit

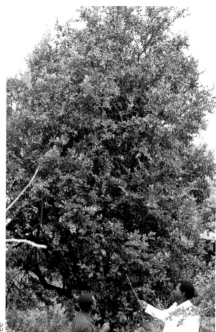

Tree

PHARMACOLOGICAL PROPERTIES

Leaves and stems are toxic to humans and animals, causing death in 3–21 days.[P12] Strong antibacterial activity against various organisms has also been reported.[P13] In congestive heart failure, ouabain (strophanthin-G) is administered as an injection.[P14] Leaves of *Acokanthera schimperi* showed in vivo antimalarial[P15] and antiproliferative[P16] activities.

COMPOUNDS REPORTED

Species of *Acokanthera* are very poisonous owing to the presence of cardioactive glycosides.[P17] Several cardenolides, such as acolongifloroside G,[P14, P18] have been reported from various parts of *A. schimperi*. Such compounds are acknowledged to have cardiac effects.[P14, P17] *A. oppositifolia* contains many heart glycosides (e.g. acovenoside A) among its major compounds, along with minor amounts of acolongifloroside K.[P19] Triterpenoids, including alagidiol, have been reported from leaves of *A. schimperi*.[P20]

Acolongifloroside K

Alagidiol

Indigenous

Common names Baobab, Upside-down Tree • **Local names** Muyu / Muuyu (Baj., Chon., Dig.), Jah (Bon.), Musemba (Emb.), Namba / Muamba (Kam.), Ol-imisera / Ol-mesera (Maa.Ken.), Muramba (Mbe., Mer., Tha.), Yak / Yaaq (Orm., Som.), Mbuyu / Muuyu (Swa., Dig.), Lamai (Sam.), Mulamba (Tai.), Mesera (Aru.), Mpele (Gogo, Lugu.), Mkondo (Hehe, San.), Ol-mesera (Maa.Tan.), Mramba (Pare), Mwiwi (Ran.), Mwanda / Mwandu / Ngwandu (Suk.)

Description and ecology

Large, deciduous tree, 10–20m tall. Trunk enormously thick and swollen, bottle-shaped, reaching a diameter of 5–10(–14)m. **Bark** smooth, shiny, reddish brown to greyish brown, with thick, wide and very stout branches. **Leaves** alternate, large, digitately compound (like fingers of a hand), divided into 5–7 leaflets, leaf stalk 10–12cm long. **Flowers** large, solitary, up to 20cm in diameter, pendulous, white, scented, on long hanging stalk, very short-lived, unpleasantly scented. **Fruit** a large, egg-shaped, hard-shelled capsule, often longer than 12cm, covered with velvety greyish hairs, hanging on a stalk. A sour-tasting, powdery white pulp, which is edible, surrounds the seeds. One of the longest-lived of all trees, the baobab is commonly found in coastal and inland bush and woodland. Deep rooted and drought resistant, it grows in well-drained soils, at 0–1,250m.

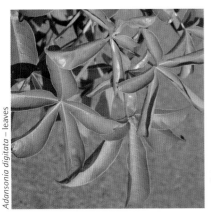

Adansonia digitata – leaves

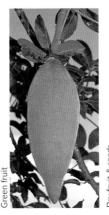

Green fruit

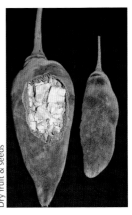

Dry fruit & seeds

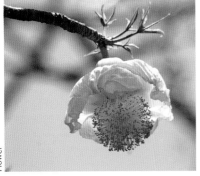

Flower

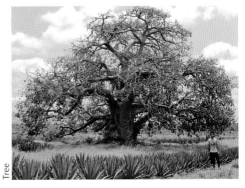

Tree

PARTS USED Dried whitish fruit pulp, seeds, gum, bark, roots, leaves and flowers.
TRADITIONAL MEDICINAL USES Infusions or decoctions of fresh leaves are used to treat kidney and bladder diseases, asthma, general fatigue, diarrhoea and insect bites.[M111] Bark decoctions are used for steam-bathing infants or adults with high fever,[M3] as a diaphoretic and as a general remedy for pain and fever. Gum from the bark is used for cleansing sores and wounds.[M111] A decoction of roots is taken as a remedy for exhaustion/weariness.[M1, M4, M70] A refreshing drink, prepared from the whitish fruit pulp, is used to treat fever and diarrhoea.[M4, M70] Bark and leaves are used as an anti-inflammatory and for treating urinary disorders and diarrhoea.[M5, M70] Leaf and flower infusions are taken for respiratory problems, digestive disorders and eye inflammation.[M111] Seed oil is used to treat a variety of skin conditions like eczema, psoriasis, dermatitis and scaly skin disorder. The oil is also used for massage and as a moisturiser. In South Africa, the leaves are used to treat fever, reduce perspiration and as an astringent; powdered seeds are given to children as a remedy for hiccups[M2] and to manage gastric, kidney and joint problems.[M111] A bark infusion is used for colds, fever and influenza.[M111]

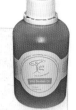

Dried seed oil is used to treat skin conditions.

PREPARATION AND DOSAGE
DIARRHOEA Boil 10g of fruit pulp in a cup of water. Add some honey or brown sugar. For children, use 5g of pulp boiled in a cup of water. Drink twice a day.
BODY PAIN, FEVER AND WEAKNESS Boil a handful of fresh bark or fresh fruit pulp in half a litre of water for a few minutes. Strain and take a cup of the decoction 2 or 3 times a day.

PHARMACOLOGICAL PROPERTIES
Anti-sickling activity has been recorded in studies of the roots and bark.[P21] Weak analgesic and anti-inflammatory activities have been recorded for dried fruit pulp.[P22] Leaves have shown antioxidant activity. Dried stem bark has shown antimalarial activity.[P23] This species showed antioxidant,[P24] antipyretic,[P25] antitumour,[P25] antidiabetic[P25] and cardioprotective[P25] activities.

COMPOUNDS REPORTED
The white fruit pulp contains both citric and tartaric acid.[P26] Flavonoid glycosides, such as quercetin-7-O-D-xylopyranoside and 3,3',4'-trihydroxyflavan-4-one-7-O-α-L-rhamnopyranoside, have been reported from roots of this plant.[P27] The plant also produces sterols, triterpenes, saponins and tannins in the pulp.[P28] Alkaloids, glycosides, fatty acid derivatives, carbohydrates and dimeric flavonoids (e.g. epicatechin-(4 ß, 6)-epicatechin)[P29, P30] have also been reported.

R=α-L-rhamnose

3,3',4'-Trihydroxyflavan-4-one-7-O-α-L-rhamnopyranoside

Epicatechin-(4 ß, 6)-epicatechin

Indigenous

Common names Ajuga, Bugleweed • **Local names** Mataliha (Luh.), Chemogong / Cheborus (Tug., Kip.)

Description and ecology

Low-growing, erect, hairy, perennial herb, much branched and spreading at the base, often rhizomatous, with ascending hairy stems 5–20(–30)cm high. Leaves usually in many pairs, lance-shaped to elliptic, 3–10 × 0.5–4cm, without a stalk, coarsely toothed, tip pointed to rounded, base wedge-shaped, hairy, with very bitter taste. Flowers small, axillary, pale blue-and-white, with short pedicels. Fruits brown, obovoid nutlets 2–3mm long, hairless. Found mostly in moist and damp places, in upland grassland and mountainous areas throughout East Africa, at 1,100–2,600m.

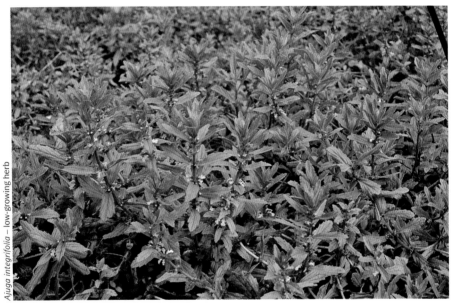

Ajuga integrifolia – low-growing herb

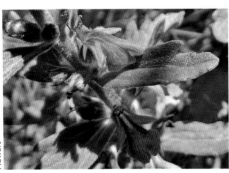

Flowers

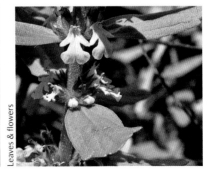

Leaves & flowers

PARTS USED Dried or fresh parts from above ground (mainly leaves).
TRADITIONAL MEDICINAL USES Infusions of fresh leaves are taken as a remedy for fever, toothache and dysentery, and are used to treat high blood pressure.[M1, M70] Mixed with extracts from other plants, powdered dried leaves are taken as medication for malaria.[M70, M71] The paste of fresh or powdered leaves is used externally to treat burns, cuts and boils.[M112] Juice of the root and leaves mixed in water is used to help combat diarrhoea and dysentery.[M112]

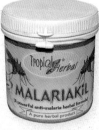

Powdered dried leaves are used to treat malaria.

PREPARATION AND DOSAGE
MALARIA, FEVER AND DYSENTERY Dry 5g of fresh leaves along with 5g each of fresh leaves of *Artemisia annua* and *Azadirachta indica*. Combine and crush to form a powder and mix a tablespoon of it in water or make a 'tea' in a cup of hot water. Drink twice a day until symptoms disappear. Alternatively, pound a handful of fresh leaves, add to a litre of cold water and stir. Drink the infusion or gargle it for relief from toothache.
BURNS, CUTS AND BOILS Pound a few fresh leaves and apply them externally on the affected areas of the skin.

PHARMACOLOGY AND CHEMISTRY

PHARMACOLOGICAL PROPERTIES
Dried aerial parts have produced an antifungal action against some species of fungi.[P31] Antihypertensive activity[P32] has been demonstrated but no significant antimalarial activity[P33] has been observed, despite traditional use of this herb for treating malaria. Additional pharmacological activities exhibited by this species include antioxidant,[P34] anti-inflammatory,[P34] antidiabetic,[P35] antidiarrhoeal[P36] and antimalarial[P36, P37] effects.

COMPOUNDS REPORTED
Diterpenes, such as ajugarin B, have been isolated from leaves,[P38] while some steroids, such as cyasteron, have been found in both leaves and roots.[P39] The steroidal lactone, ajugalactone,[P17] is also present. Investigation of the aerial parts yielded diterpenoids (ajugarin-I, ajugarin-II)[P40] and iridoid glycoside.[P40]

Ajugarin B

Cyasteron

a. *Albizia amara*   Indigenous

Common names Albizia, Bitter Albizia • **Local names** Boria (Bor.), Ruga (Luo), Kiundua / Kyundua (Kam.), Ruga (Luo), Orperelon'go (Maa.), Panan / Papan (Pok.), Gissrep / Gessreb (Som.), Mutinda (Tha.), Gotutwet / Kotutwo (Tug.), Muhogolo (Gogo), Mkengehovu (Lugu.), Mtanga (Mwe.), Mpogolo / Mtangala (Nyam.), Mufoghoo (Nyir.), Msisiviri (Ran.), Mpogolo (Suk.), Mkarasaritu (Zin.)

Description and ecology

Small to medium-sized, many-branched, deciduous acacia-like tree, often with rounded or spreading crown, 4(–13)m tall, frequently smaller. **Bark** thin, green at first, but scaly, dark brown and roughly cracked in older trees. **Leaves** paripinnately compound, 10–20cm long, with 15–30 pairs of bright pale green feathery leaflets, the leaves and branchlets with distinctive soft, golden hairs. **Flowers** small, creamy white or pinkish white, crowded at ends of branches, in showy globulous clusters 2.5cm in diameter. **Fruits** large, flat, straight pods, greyish brown, 10–22cm long, bulging over the seeds, indehiscent. **Seeds** 6–13, compressed, ovate, hard, brown. Widespread in Africa in wooded grassland, thickets and *Acacia–Commiphora* bushland and scrubland, at 400–1,900m.

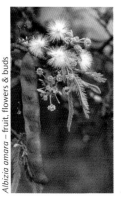

Albizia amara – fruit, flowers & buds

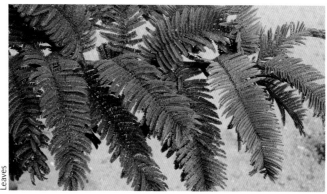

Leaves

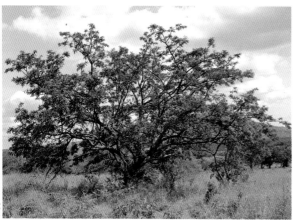

Tree

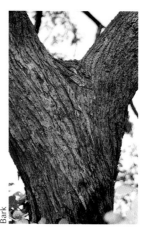

Bark

PARTS USED Roots, bark, leaves, seeds and flowers.
TRADITIONAL MEDICINAL USES Bark decoctions are taken as an emetic to induce vomiting and to treat malaria.[M4, M70, M71] Leaves are used to dress wounds.[M4, M70] A root infusion is drunk to treat pneumonia, tuberculosis, infertility in women and as an aphrodisiac.[M112, M115] Root or bark decoctions are used as a purgative, as an anthelmintic or to treat stomach ailments.[M4, M70] A paste of leaves and root bark is used to treat skin diseases, warts and poisonous insect bites.[M115, M126] The fruit pods are emetic and are also used in the treatment of malaria and coughs.[M111, M115] Flowers are used as a remedy for coughs, ulcers, dandruff and malaria;[M126] seeds are used for haemorrhoids, diarrhoea and gonorrhoea.[M126]

PREPARATION AND DOSAGE
WOUNDS Apply crushed fresh leaves directly to open bleeding wounds.
MALARIA AND EMETIC Boil a tablespoon of bark powder in a litre of water for 10 minutes. Drink a cup of the decoction 3 times a day.
ANTHELMINTIC AND PURGATIVE Boil a tablespoon of root or bark powder in a litre of water for 10 minutes. Drink a cup of the decoction 2 or 3 times a day before meals.

b. *Albizia anthelmintica*
Indigenous

Common names Albizia, Worm-cure Albizia • **Local names** Hobocho (Bon.), Howacho (Bor.), Mwowa / Kyowa (Kam.), Olmugutan (Maa.), Kitangwa (Mar.), Habacha (Orm.), Kamakitan / Mukotonwo (Pok.), Olmukutan (Sam.), Mporojo (Swa.), Habasho / Reidep / Reidup (Som.), Mwaawra / Muguta (Tha.)

Description and ecology
Deciduous shrub, bush or tree 3–9(–13)m tall. **Bark** smooth, pale grey but later brown, rough, deeply reticulate, branches often with sharp tips. **Leaves** bipinnately compound, with 2–4 pairs of pinnae, each with 1–4 pairs of hairless leaflets 1–4cm long. **Flowers** white or creamish yellow, in half-spherical fluffy heads up to 2.5cm across, usually on leafless twigs, stalk 0.5–5mm long. **Fruit** pods bright green when young but glossy pale brown or pale yellow when mature, 7–16cm long, usually hairless, tapering at both ends, containing 3–5 flat, round seeds. Most common in dry bushland on lava or along seasonal rivers, also in wooded grassland but less common in bushed grassland or woodland, and rarely occurs in evergreen coastal bushland, at 50–1,300m.

PARTS USED Bark, twigs and roots.
TRADITIONAL MEDICINAL USES Root decoctions are said to cure gonorrhoea[M111] and fever and to act as a sexual stimulant in women.[M70] Infusions of the bark are used as an emetic and for treating tapeworm and malaria.[M70, M112] Root or stem bark decoctions are taken as an anthelmintic and purgative.[M1, M70, M111, M112] The twigs can serve as toothbrushes for oral hygiene.[M111]

PREPARATION AND DOSAGE
MALARIA AND EMETIC As with *Albizia amara*, boil a tablespoon of bark powder in a litre of water for 10 minutes. Drink a cup 3 times a day.
ANTHELMINTIC AND PURGATIVE As with *A. amara*, boil a tablespoon of either root or bark powder in a litre of water for 10 minutes. Drink a cup of the decoction 2 or 3 times a day before meals.

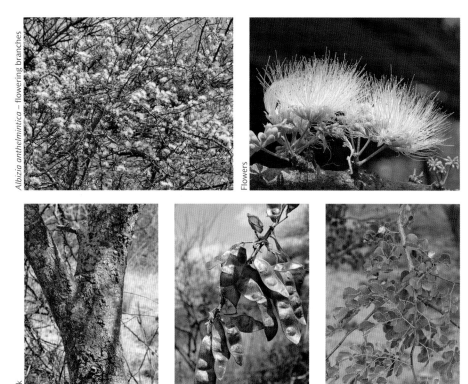

Albizia anthelmintica – flowering branches

Flowers

Old tree bark

Young fruit

Leaves

c. *Albizia coriaria*

Indigenous

Common name Giant Albizia • **Local names** Mukurue (Kik.), Mugavu (Swa.), Ober (Luo), Omubele / Kumupeli (Luh.), Etek / Etekwa (Ate.), Mugava (Lug.), Chesovio / Kumoluko (Lugi.), Mubere (Lugwe.), Latoligo / Ayekayek (Luo-A), Omogi, Ober (Luo-J), Itek / Bata (Luo-L), Musita (Luso.), Oyo (Madi), Muyenzayenze (Ruki.), Musisa / Murongo (Runyan.), Musisa (Runy., Ruto.)

Description and ecology
Deciduous tree 6–36m tall, heavily branched, with a spreading, dome-shaped crown and a straight, cylindrical bole. **Bark** grey-black, rough and flaking, young branches rather hairy. **Leaves** bipinnately compound, with 3–6 pairs of pinnae, each with 6–11 pairs of medium-sized to large leaflets, all of roughly equal size, up to 30mm long, narrowly oval-oblong, rounded and often wider at the bases, rounded at the tips. **Flowers** numerous, white, in half-spherical heads, fragrant, stamen filaments red above and not hanging out beyond the flower tube. **Fruits** oblong, flat, papery, purple-brown pods, often shiny, 10–14(–20) × 3–3.6cm, non-hairy, narrowing at tip and base. **Seeds** round and flattened, 9–12 × 8–9mm. Found from West Africa to Sudan and south to Angola. Grows in a variety of soils in Kenya and Uganda. Common in riverine forest edges, dry forest, particularly in wooded grassland, woodland and thickets, at 850–1,700m.

PARTS USED Bark, leaves and roots.

TRADITIONAL MEDICINAL USES The bark is often used in traditional medicine, being considered an astringent and vermifuge.[M112, M115] Root decoctions are used to treat venereal diseases. Decoctions of the leaves are used externally for headache and as a wash or steam inhalation against fever (including malaria) and toothache; also applied as a wash to kill head lice.[M112, M115] Dried, powdered roots, boiled in water and steam, are used to relieve sore eyes.[M1, M4, M70] A warm infusion of pounded fresh leaves is administered as an enema to induce abortion.[M112, M115] A decoction of bark taken internally is said to be helpful in treating menorrhagia and postpartum haemorrhage. A decoction of bark applied externally is said to soothe sores, pimples and other skin complaints.[M112, M115] Bark infusions are taken as a remedy for malaria.[M4, M70]

PREPARATION AND DOSAGE

GONORRHOEA Boil a handful of fresh roots or 5g of root powder in a litre of water for 10–15 minutes and filter the mixture. When cool, drink a cup 3 times a day.

MALARIA Soak a handful of pounded fresh bark in a litre of water and boil for 10 minutes. Drink a cup of the infusion 2 or 3 times a day.

SKIN PROBLEMS (PIMPLES, ACNE, SORES) Boil a heaped tablespoon of dried powdered bark in half a litre of water for 10 minutes. Sieve it and apply the warm mixture on affected areas.

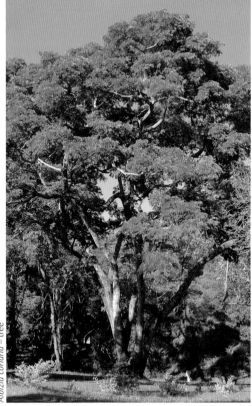

Albizia coriaria – tree

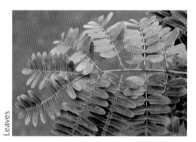

Leaves

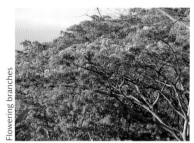

Flowering branches

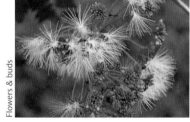

Flowers & buds

d. *Albizia gummifera*

Indigenous

Common name Peacock Flower • **Local names** Mukhonzuli / Kumulukhu (Luh.), Mwethia / Musya / Kisya (Kam.), Mkurwe / Mukurue (Kik.), Seet / Seyet (Kip., Nan.), Omugonjoro (Kis.), Kiririgiri / Kiririgiti (Tav.), Msarawachi (Tai.), Se / Set / Seot (Mar., Tug.), Mchani mbao (Swa. Ken.), Ol-osepakupes / Olsamakupe / Ormoso (Maa.Ken.), Mukuruwe (Mer.), Ses (Pok.), Sogore / Sogorogurri (Sam.), Ekakwait / Ekeweit (Tur.), Sangupesi / Olsanguuwezi (Aru.), Mboromo / Mduka / Mfuranje (Chag.), Ol-geturai / Osangupesi (Maa.Tan.), Msame / Msanga (Pare), Mkenge (Swa. Tan.), Mkengemaji (Ngu.), Mshai (Samb.), Chiruku / Kirongo (Lugi.), Mushebeya (Ruki.), Mulera / Mushebeya (Runyan.), Mulongo (Ruto.), Swessu (Sebei)

Description and ecology

Large, deciduous forest tree often about 15m tall but can reach 25–30m, with thick branches and a flattened, open canopy and straight, cylindrical bole 75–100cm in diameter. **Bark** smooth, grey. **Leaves** bipinnately compound, with 5–7 pairs of pinnae, each with up to 12 pairs of shiny, dark green leaflets 1–2cm long, almost rectangular, midribs diagonal, one outer corner rounded. **Flowers** in very attractive, pink-and-white clusters, stamens protruding, long, bright red. **Fruits** glossy reddish-brown pods, profuse, clustered in bundles, thin, flat, glabrous, with raised edges, 20 × 3cm, often shorter. Found mainly in East Africa, but also in Ethiopia, the DR Congo, Madagascar and West Africa, extending from dry or wet lowlands, through riverine forests to upland forest edges, at 0–2,300m.

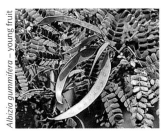

Albizia gummifera – young fruit

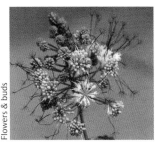

Flowers & buds

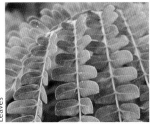

Leaves

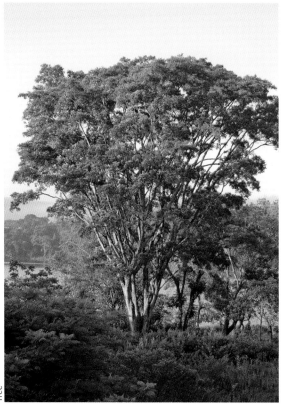

Tree

PARTS USED Bark, leaves, roots and pods.
TRADITIONAL MEDICINAL USES A bark decoction or infusion is used to treat malaria and as an emetic.[M4, M70, M71, M112, M115] The roots and leaves are purgative and are used to treat diarrhoea.[M115] An extract from crushed fresh pods is taken for stomach pain.[M1, M4, M71] Roots are used to treat skin conditions such as acne and eczema.[M70, M71] Pounded bark is used as a snuff to treat headache and is applied externally to treat scabies and psoriasis.[M112, M115] Freshly pounded leaf paste is applied to skin sores and fractures.[M112, M115]

PREPARATION AND DOSAGE
SKIN CONDITIONS (ACNE, ECZEMA, RASHES, ITCHING) Bath in warm water to which pounded fresh roots have been added.
MALARIA AND EMETIC As with *Albizia amara*, boil a tablespoon of bark powder in a litre of water for 10 minutes. Drink a cup 3 times a day.
STOMACH ACHE Steep a handful of pounded fresh pods in a litre of warm water for 15 minutes. Drink from the infusion at intervals until symptoms abate.

PHARMACOLOGICAL PROPERTIES
Seeds of *Albizia amara* have shown cytotoxic activity against some cancer cell lines,[P41] while a molluscicidal activity[P42] has also been observed. Dried roots of *A. gummifera* show antitrypanosomal[P43] and antimalarial[P23] activities, while bark from the species has acted as a strong uterine stimulant with abortifacient effects.[P44] Budmunchiamine K and other spermine alkaloids account for the antiplasmodial activity of *A. gummifera*.[P45] *A. anthelmintica* produced anthelmintic activity against gastrointestinal nematodes in naturally infected sheep.[P46]

COMPOUNDS REPORTED
Histamine, a potent vasodilator found in normal tissues and blood during hyposensitisation, is present in *A. anthelmintica*.[P46] Seeds of *A. amara* contain spermine alkaloids[P47] and lipids such as arachidic acid.[P48] Flavonoids (e.g. melacacidin) have also been extracted from the heartwood.[P49] Stem bark of *A. gummifera* contains spermine alkaloids such as budmunchiamine K, as well as triterpenes, of which the most common is lupenone.[P50] From the leaves of *A. anthelmintica* eight flavonol glycosides with antioxidant activities have been reported.[P51]

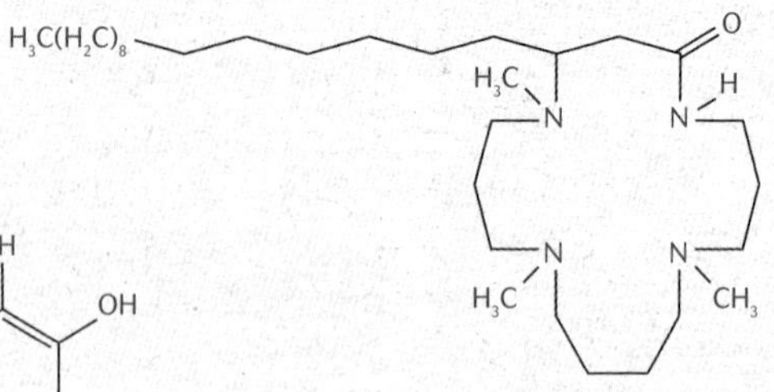

Budmunchiamine K

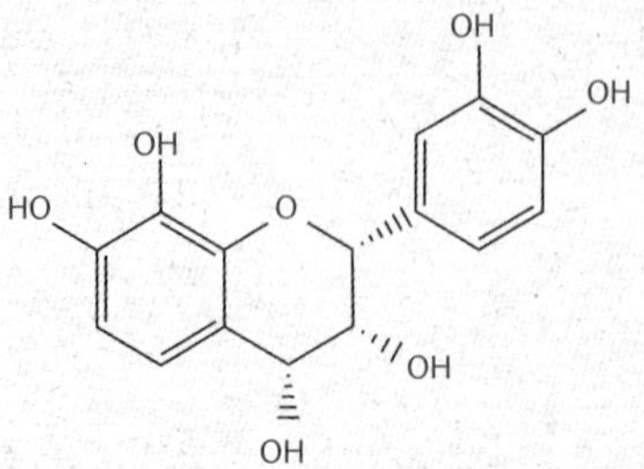

Melacacidin

a. *Allium cepa*

Native to southwestern Asia,
Iran and Middle East

Common names Onion, Bulb Onion • **Local names** Kitunguu / Vitunguu (Swa.), Dungari (Guj.),
Piyaz (Urd., Hind.), Piyaj (Punj.)

Description and ecology

Herbaceous, biennial bulbous plant of many types differing widely in colour, 20–50cm high. It is the most widely cultivated species of the genus *Allium*. Forms the bulb during the first year, the stem growing during the second year, whereupon the plant can bloom and bear fruit. Bulbs are shortened, compressed, underground stems surrounded by fleshy modified scales (fleshy, bluish-green leaves) that cover a central bud at the tip of the stem. **Flowers** white, borne in a globular umbel. **Seeds** glossy, black, triangular in cross section. Bulbs develop better in cooler climates in fertile, well-drained soils. Widely used medicinally in Africa and Asia, besides serving as a basic food ingredient in a variety of cooked meals, pickles and salads.

AS39

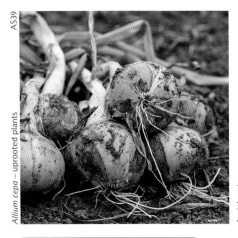

Allium cepa – uprooted plants

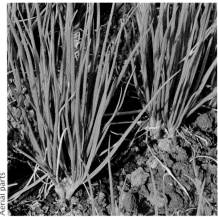

Aerial parts

USAGE AND TREATMENT

PARTS USED Aerial parts, bulb and seeds.
TRADITIONAL MEDICINAL USES *Allium cepa* is used to treat coughs, sore throat, bronchitis, fungal infections, abscesses, earache, high blood pressure and urinary tract infections.[M6, M8] It is used to protect against some epidemic diseases, notably cholera.[M7] Onion poultices are said to be an effective remedy for abscesses, pimples, acne, boils and furuncles.[M7] Applied externally, raw onion is said to act as an antibiotic to counter bacteria that infect the skin, helping to repair the damage caused by wounds, fungal infections, ringworm, insect bites, burns and acne.[M9] Eaten regularly, raw onions may help to improve the memory and soothe tonsillitis, laryngitis and bronchial asthma. Raw onions are also taken in the treatment of gastrointestinal infections, high blood pressure and diabetes. Known for its diuretic and hypotensive effects,[M6, M9] raw onion is strongly recommended in the diet of people with thrombosis as it helps to thin the blood and improve circulation.[M9] Raw onion is prescribed for hepatic disorders, especially chronic hepatitis. Fresh onion juice is used as a vermifuge.[M9]

PREPARATION AND DOSAGE

CHOLERA Mix a tablespoon of fresh onion juice with half a teaspoon of fresh lemon juice and drink at intervals of 3 to 4 hours for 3 days.

SKIN AILMENTS (ABSCESSES, PIMPLES, ACNE, BOILS AND FURUNCLES) Make a hot poultice from baked or boiled onion and apply directly to affected areas. This can help to ripen abscesses and to cleanse the skin of pimples, acne and other blemishes. Alternatively, crush raw onions and apply the fresh juice 2 or 3 times daily.

BOILS IN THE EAR Fresh onion juice administered in the form of eardrops may encourage the boil to burst.

WOUNDS, BURNS, FUNGAL INFECTIONS (ESPECIALLY RINGWORM) AND INSECT BITES (INCLUDING SCORPION AND WASP STINGS) Apply

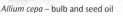

Allium cepa – bulb and seed oil

raw onion juice externally 2 or 3 times daily to aid the healing process. For ringworm and insect bites, add a little vinegar to crushed onion and apply 2 hours before taking a bath. For relief from fungal infections and painful insect bites, grind onion seeds in lime juice and rub gently onto the affected areas.

COUGHS, SORE THROAT, TONSILLITIS, LARYNGITIS, BRONCHITIS AND BRONCHIAL ASTHMA A drink combining fresh onion juice with honey is a widely used traditional cure. Mix half a cup of chopped onions in half a cup of water, add a little honey and stir thoroughly. Then sip at intervals during the day. Gargling with onion broth (onions boiled in water) will reduce inflammation in the throat and can be useful in treating tonsillitis.

GASTROINTESTINAL INFECTIONS, HIGH BLOOD PRESSURE, DIABETES, URINARY TRACT INFECTIONS, THROMBOSIS AND HYPERTENSION Half a cup of raw chopped onions, consumed daily in the diet, can be taken as an effective antidote.

CHRONIC HEPATITIS AND JAUNDICE Crush white onions. Add sugar or jaggery to taste and a quarter of a teaspoon of turmeric powder. Consume 2 or 3 times daily for 10 days.

VERMIFUGE (FOR INTESTINAL PARASITES) A tablespoon of fresh onion juice, fed to children twice daily for 3 or 4 days, can help to eliminate intestinal worms.

 WARNING! Raw onions are not recommended for people who suffer from hyperacidity or who have gastric, intestinal or abdominal ulcers.

b. *Allium sativum*   Native to Central Asia

Common names Garlic, Clove of Garlic • **Local names** Kitunguu aumu (Swa.), Lassan (Guj., Hind., Urd.)

Description and ecology

Erect, herbaceous bulbous plant 30–60cm high (sometimes as tall as 90cm in favourable conditions), with central bulbous roots comprising 5–15 bulblets or cloves. **Leaves** long, slightly folded, up to 30cm long, smooth, with prominent midrib. **Flowers** whitish or reddish. Grown in well-drained, fertile soils in many tropical countries, garlic is an essential ingredient in regional cuisine over much of the world, including Africa. On the Indian subcontinent, it is used as a spice, along with onions and ginger, in meat and vegetable curries and salads. It is also eaten raw as a medicine.

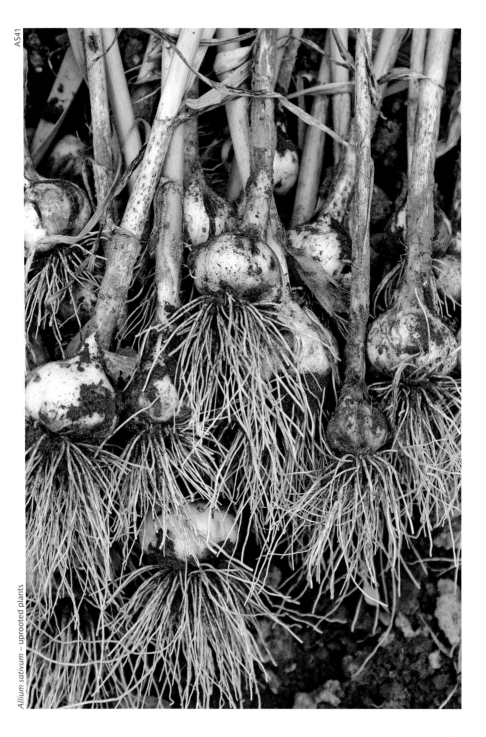

PARTS USED Aerial parts and cloves.

TRADITIONAL MEDICINAL USES Garlic has been used since ancient times to treat many diseases. Modern scientific research has vindicated most of its longstanding medicinal uses. Garlic helps to treat diabetes and reduces both high blood pressure and blood cholesterol levels.[M9, M10] It can be useful in treating tuberculosis, coughs, colds, a sore throat, sinusitis, asthma and whooping cough.[M6, M7] It acts as a powerful vermifuge in children.[M7, M8] Its use is recommended for treating typhoid, malaria, urinary tract infections, skin infections (fungal, viral and bacterial) and intestinal infections (diarrhoea, dysentery).[M9, M10] It helps to relieve gout, arthritis and rheumatic afflictions and is also a remedy for warts, corns, abscesses and boils.[M6] Infusions of the bulb are taken orally as an emmenagogue and anthelmintic.[M10]

PREPARATION AND DOSAGE

COUGHS, COLDS, SINUSITIS, SORE THROAT, WHOOPING COUGH, INFLUENZA AND ASTHMA Eat one or two garlic cloves 2 or 3 times a day with meals. One clove, crushed and mixed in honey, can be given to children twice a day. Alternatively, drink a teaspoon of garlic oil twice a day.

HYPERTENSION, THROMBOSIS, ARTERIOSCLEROSIS, HEART CONDITIONS AND DIABETES Garlic is strongly recommended for people suffering from high blood sugar levels, high blood cholesterol and high blood pressure. Chew one or two cloves of fresh raw garlic every day, preferably in the mornings. Alternatively, a paste made from fresh crushed garlic mixed with honey or 5–10 drops of garlic oil can be taken twice a day.

ABDOMINAL INFECTIONS, DYSENTERY, DIARRHOEA, COLITIS AND URINARY INFECTIONS Chop fresh garlic cloves into very small pieces and swallow a heaped teaspoonful with some tea, 3 times a day for 5 days (do not chew, as it might cause 'bad breath').

INTESTINAL WORMS Fresh garlic cloves are a potent vermifuge against intestinal parasites that cause anal itching in children. A teaspoon of fresh garlic clove paste mixed with honey, given twice daily for 3 days, can help eliminate cases of intestinal worms.

FUNGAL INFECTIONS (RINGWORM, ATHLETE'S FOOT), VIRAL INFECTIONS (HERPES) AND INFECTIONS OF THE SKIN (PIMPLES, WARTS, CORNS, ABSCESSES AND FURUNCLES) Apply either the fresh juice of crushed garlic or garlic oil to affected areas 2 or 3 times daily until symptoms abate. Mashed garlic applied to a wart or corn and covered with a plaster or bandage will soften the excrescence in 2 or 3 days, reducing inflammation.

TYPHOID, TUBERCULOSIS AND OTHER INFECTIONS Two or three fresh garlic cloves, taken with meals, can be of help in treating typhoid fever, bacillary dysentery, tuberculosis, cholera and sleeping sickness, while helping to prevent malignant intestinal cancers.

TEETHING IN BABIES Rubbing the gums of a teething baby with a garlic clove produces a soothing effect. Pressing a garlic clove against aching gums can also relieve toothache.

HIV/AIDS AND IMMUNE RESPONSE BOOSTER Garlic stimulates the body's immune response system and is being used with some success to complement HIV/AIDS management and treatment regimens. Inclusion of raw onions and garlic in the diets of AIDS sufferers can reduce the likelihood of acquiring other diseases such as tuberculosis, malaria and pneumonia.

SCORPION STINGS, INSECT BITES Apply fresh garlic cloves, ground into a paste, to the sting or bite area. One or two cloves of garlic can be eaten at the same time.

EAR PIMPLES Apply eardrops of pressed fresh garlic juice twice a day to relieve the pain. Continue treatment until the pimple ruptures, releasing the pus.

 WARNING! A continuous high intake of garlic is not recommended during pregnancy. Also, since garlic has a blood-thinning effect, its ingestion – raw or in extracts – is not recommended in cases involving excessive bleeding, such as heavy menstruation or haemorrhage as experienced after an accident (where coagulation of the blood may be inhibited).

PHARMACOLOGICAL PROPERTIES

All fresh aerial parts of *Allium cepa* have shown strong antioxidant,[P52] antihyperglycaemic[P53] and antimutagenic[P54] activities. From the bulbs, anti-asthmatic activity has been documented in people suffering from bronchial asthma.[P55] The antibiotic, mucolytic (easing the expulsion of mucus through making it more fluid) and anti-inflammatory properties of onion help to prevent respiratory infections. In addition, bulbs have shown antihypercholesterolemic and antihyperlipemic activities.[P56] Science has established that onion contains fibrinolytic substances that break up blood clots. By acting as a platelet anti-gatherer, onion prevents excessive build-up of blood platelets in thrombi or clots.[P56] Raw onion juice acts as an antibiotic against various bacteria that cause skin infections, including golden staphylococcus.

History attributes many properties to *A. sativum*. Most of these have been scientifically proven, including the antifungal[P57] and antibacterial[P58, P59] activities of both the aerial parts and bulbs. Antioxidant activity has been found only in fresh aerial parts.[P60] Bulbs have shown antihypercholesterolemic, cholesterol synthesis inhibition, fatty acid synthesis inhibition and antihypertriglyceridemic activities.[P61] From bulbs, antihyperlipemic,[P62] antihypertensive[P62] and antitumour[P63] activities have been observed in human adults. A gastroscopic screening survey showed bulbs have wound-healing acceleration properties.[P64] Immunostimulant,[P65] uterine stimulant,[P66] antioxidant[P67] and anti-ascariasis[P68] activities have also been reported in the case of bulbs. Ajoene, a component of this plant, has been found to produce antimalarial activity when used in combination with chloroquine.[P69]

COMPOUNDS REPORTED

A. cepa as a whole plant contains a volatile essence, rich in sulfured glycosides, of which the most important is allylpropyl disulfide. Other sulfur compounds present in the bulb include ajoene[P70] and certain flavonoids such as chrysanthemin, which has a diuretic action.[P71] Onions also contain many enzymes, which help in digestion, and some important trace elements (sulfur, iron, potassium, magnesium, calcium and phosphorus) and vitamins (A, B complex, C and E).

The numerous sulfur compounds isolated from *A. sativum* include ajoene from the bulb.[P72] The whole plant, especially the bulb, contains alliin as well as lipids (e.g. allium cerebroside AS-1-1)[P73] and carbohydrates (e.g. allium fructan K-1).[P74] Bulbs contain vitamins, including A, B1, B2, C and niacin. Alliin and diallyl disulfur are highly volatile substances that act on the whole body, particularly on those organs (the bronchi and lungs, kidneys and skin) through which they are eliminated.

Ajoene

Chrysanthemin

Alliin

a. *Aloe kilifiensis* Indigenous

Common name Aloe • **Local names** Kisimamleo (Swa.), Jolonji (Dig.), Kippa (Tai.)

Description and ecology

Evergreen, perennial, succulent plant with a rosette of leaves, often stemless but with age can develop a short, thick stem up to 30cm tall, often producing suckers to form small clumps. **Leaves** white-dotted, 18–20 × 6–9cm, exuding yellow latex when cut. **Flowers** regular, in racemes, orange-red, very decorative. **Fruit** a many-seeded capsule. **Seeds** winged, papery, released when fruit dries out. Occurs in dryland areas in open grassland and *Acacia* woodland. Can be grown as an ornamental in dry lowland areas. This species is one of the acaulescent, spotted aloes and is easily confused with the other spotted aloes of East Africa, especially *A. lateritia*.

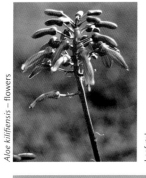

Aloe kilifiensis – flowers

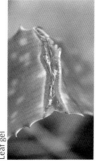

Leaf gel

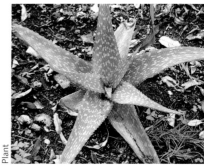

Plant

USAGE AND TREATMENT

PARTS USED Fresh leaves and roots.
TRADITIONAL MEDICINAL USES Juice from roasted leaves is used to treat burns, skin irritations and itching[M6, M70], body swellings[M1, M70, M112, M115] and also as a cure for malaria.[M11] Decoctions of leaves and roots are used for abdominal pain and to relieve constipation.[M70]

PREPARATION AND DOSAGE
BODY SWELLINGS AND SKIN RASHES Roast some leaves and apply the mucilage to the swollen area. Leaf sap can be applied externally to rashes, bruises and cuts.
ABDOMINAL PAIN AND CONSTIPATION Dissolve 1 or 2 spoons of squeezed juice in a cup of water, fruit juice or milk. Drink 3 times a day.

b. *Aloe lateritia* var. *graminicola* Indigenous

Common name Aloe • **Local names** Olkos (Pok.), Sukoroi (Sam.), Kiiruma (Kik.), Msubili (Swa.)

Description and ecology

Acaulescent, perennial, succulent aloe. **Leaves** in a sessile rosette, triangular, white-spotted or streaked, 18–20 × 5–6cm, with serrate edge, oozing gel-like yellow exudate when cut. **Flowers** red-orange, in rounded branching heads on long stems. **Fruits** dry oval capsules, many-seeded. **Seeds** ovoid, winged. Common on dry, sandy grassland or in scrub or lightly wooded areas, at up to 2,100m.

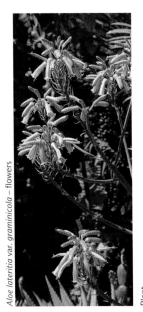

Aloe lateritia var. _graminicola_ – flowers

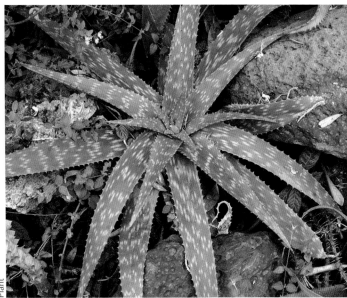

Plant

PARTS USED Fresh leaves.
TRADITIONAL MEDICINAL USES The leaf juice is used to cure stomach ailments, colds and malaria.[M70, M112] A decoction of boiled leaves in water induces vomiting and diarrhoea, providing relief from stomach upsets, malaria, liver problems and rheumatism.[M1, M70] Leaf sap is used to treat wounds, burns, skin rashes and itching.[M70]

PREPARATION AND DOSAGE
STOMACH AILMENTS AND LIVER PROBLEMS Boil 1 or 2 spoons of leaf sap in a cup of water and drink 3 times a day before meals.
SKIN BRUISES, BURNS AND CUTS Apply leaf sap directly to the affected areas.

c. _Aloe secundiflora_

Indigenous

Common name Bitter Aloe • **Local names** Harguessa (Bor.), Kitori (Gir.), Kiluma (Kam.), Ogara (Luo), Tangaratwet / Tangaratuet (Tug.), Olkos / Sikorowet (Pok.), Esuguroi (Maa.), Kigaka / Lineke (Mar.), Sukoroi (Sam.), Kisimamleo / Kisimando (Swa.), Echuchuka / Echichuviwa (Tur.), Magaka (Suk.)

Description and ecology

Succulent, evergreen, perennial herb, stemless or with a short stem up to 30cm high, usually growing solitarily but sometimes suckering at the base to form small groups, in dense rosettes of 15–20 leaves. **Leaves** long, ovate-lanceolate, thick, dull green, margin with sharp, dark brown teeth 3–6mm long. Inflorescence consisting of long racemes, 15–20cm long. **Flowers** dull red, arranged at one side of each raceme. **Fruit** an oblong-ovoid capsule, on maturity releasing many blackish-brown, speckled-winged seeds. This drought-resistant aloe is commonly found in open grassland, woodland and dry bushland in Kenya and Tanzania, at 600–2,000m.

PARTS USED Fresh leaves.
TRADITIONAL MEDICINAL USES Leaf sap is taken as an appetiser and also as a remedy for vomiting and nausea.M68 The leaf exudate is applied into the eyes to cure conjunctivitis.M68 Fresh leaf sap is used to treat chest pain, pneumonia, diarrhoea and oedema. Diluted leaf sap is drunk as a remedy for headache, malaria and typhoid fever.M68

PREPARATION AND DOSAGE
BODY SWELLINGS, WOUNDS AND BRUISES Roast some leaves and apply the sap to the swollen area. Leaf sap can also be applied directly, externally only, onto rashes, bruises and cuts.
MALARIA, TYPHOID FEVER, VOMITING AND NAUSEA Boil 1 or 2 spoons of leaf sap from the fresh leaves in a cup of water for 5 minutes. Drink 2 or 3 times a day.

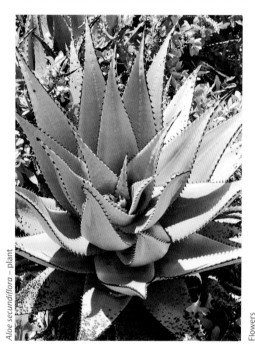

Aloe secundiflora – plant

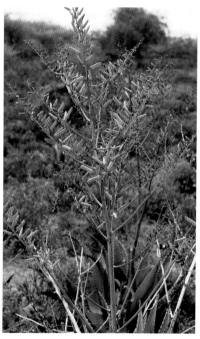

Flowers

d. *Aloe vera* — Native to southern Africa

Common name Bitter Aloe • **Local names** Msubili (Swa.), Kuvara (Guj.), Gheekuvar (Hind., Urd.)

Description and ecology

Evergreen, perennial, sessile or short-stemmed herb 60–100cm tall, with branches growing directly from the base. **Leaves** green to grey-green, thick, fleshy, lance-shaped, with toothed margin and streaky white spots from which a bitter, sticky yellow fluid oozes when cut. **Flowers** red or yellow (depending on the variety), protruding from the centre of the large stem or spike up to 90cm long. **Fruits** brownish-green, oval capsules, many-seeded. Widespread in hot desert areas of Central America, the West Indies and Asia, it is commonly grown in East Africa as an ornamental plant in gardens as well as for medicinal use.

PARTS USED The bitter yellow juice and transparent gel exuded by the leaves.

TRADITIONAL MEDICINAL USES The use of the gel and juice from this aloe has a long history in the external treatment of burns, wounds and skin conditions; drops for eye infections; and in formulations to soothe and enhance the appearance of the skin.[M7, M9, M70] Fresh leaf juice is also taken orally as an emmenagogue, a laxative, purgative, appetiser, blood purifier and for relief from stomach pain,[M9, M10, M70] asthma and a chronic cough. Whole leaves are used to relieve swellings of the glands between the thighs and in the armpits.[M7] A decoction of leaves is used as eyedrops to treat inflammation and redness of the eyes.[M6, M7, M70] A decoction of dry leaves is taken orally to induce abortion and to treat hepatitis.[M10]

PREPARATION AND DOSAGE

HEALING WOUNDS, SKIN ULCERS AND DIABETIC ULCERS Wash a leaf thoroughly in warm water. Cut away the flesh. A transparent, sticky, flavourless gel will ooze out with the juice. Rub the gel and juice over the wound. The remaining flesh can be applied as a poultice over the affected area. After each such treatment, clean the wound with cool paw-paw latex water (drops of paw-paw latex from the fresh unripe fruits, boiled in water). This aids the regenerative process and prevents scarring. Repeat this treatment 3 or 4 times a day. Leave the wound open to dry, out of reach of flies.

BURNS For minor (first-degree) burns, apply aloe gel and juice 3 or 4 times daily for 2 or 3 days, using the aloe flesh to make a poultice as well, if necessary. This will have a soothing effect, boosting the healing process and reducing scarring. For more severe burns, consult a doctor.

SKIN INFECTIONS The colourless gel from the inner leaf parts has anti-allergic and anti-inflammatory properties, highly efficacious in the treatment of eczema, acne, fungal infections (e.g. athlete's foot) and herpes. Apply the fresh gel to inflamed areas on the skin. Drinking 1 or 2 spoons of juice or gel dissolved in a cup of water 2 or 3 times a day will further aid the healing process. For infants, a few drops of fresh juice or gel mixed with baby lotion can be used to treat eczema and diaper rashes and will also relieve the itching. This mixture is helpful too in healing the skin after diseases such as chicken pox and measles.

SKIN CARE AND BEAUTY THERAPY A few drops of fresh aloe juice or gel, added to a moisturising lotion, will help to remove scars and prevent dryness and cracking of the skin. It leaves skin clear, fresh and smooth. Mixed with honey, a few dops of the juice or gel in water can also be taken orally as a tonic.

LAXATIVE AND PURGATIVE Wash a leaf in hot water and cut off the surface layer. Put the stripped leaf into a container, allowing the viscous yellow, bitter juice to drain. After 20–25 minutes, weigh the sap and mix with sugar of 2–3 times its mass. Leave this mixture, known as 'aloe sugar', in the sun to dry, under a net to keep flies away. The dry aloe sugar can be given to children as a laxative in doses of 0.5g. Adults can take 1–2g, either as a laxative or – for women – as an emmenagogue. The same procedure can be followed without adding sugar. This will produce a dark, shapeless mass of what is known as 'bitter aloe', which in doses of 0.1–0.2g can be used by adults as either a laxative or an emmenagogue. In doses of 0.4–0.5g, bitter aloe acts as a purgative.

GASTRITIS Boil half a cup of finely cut leaves in a litre of water and drink as a tea.

HAIR LOSS Mix the leaf gel with egg yolk and massage into the hair. Allow this mixture to soak in overnight before washing it out the following day.

GLANDULAR SWELLINGS Scrape one side of an aloe leaf with a stainless steel knife, removing the sharp tip and edges of the leaf. Sprinkle turmeric powder on the scraped leaf surface. Warm the leaf and press against the swollen glands, particularly under the armpits. The pain caused by such swellings will quickly dissipate.

 WARNING! Bitter aloe should not be taken during pregnancy or under circumstances of excessive menstruation. Aloe gel and juice can trigger allergic reactions (characterised by redness or itching) on the skin of some people.

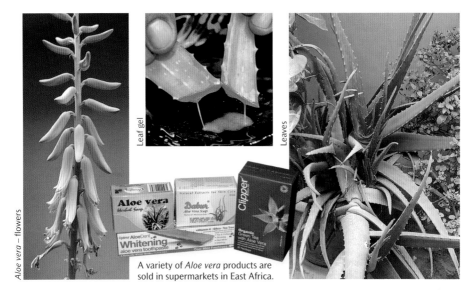

Leaf gel

Leaves

Aloe vera – flowers

A variety of *Aloe vera* products are sold in supermarkets in East Africa.

PHARMACOLOGY AND CHEMISTRY

PHARMACOLOGICAL PROPERTIES

The pharmacological activities that are documented for the leaf gel of species of *Aloe* include wound healing,[P75, P76] immunostimulation,[P77] antitumour, antiburn, antibacterial,[P78] analgesic, antifungal,[P79] anti-asthmatic,[P79] anti-inflammatory[P79] and antipyretic[P79, P81] effects. Roots of *Aloe lateritia* have shown antibacterial[P80] activity. Studies of fresh leaf juice of *A. vera* have revealed an anti-ulcer[P82] activity. In vitro studies on the efficacy of crude extracts of *A. secundiflora* on *Candida albicans* showed the inhibition of the growth of *C. albicans*.[P83]

COMPOUNDS REPORTED

Leaves of bitter aloe contain 20% aloin and 40–80% resin, plus carbohydrates (acemannan) and an anthraquinonic glycoside considered to be the active compound.[P84] Aloe leaves also contain quinoids such as aloin A[P85] and homonataloin A,[P86] while the roots of *A. lateritia* contain aloesaponarin I.[P87] The main chemical components of the leaf exudate of *A. secundiflora* include the anthrones aloenin, aloenin B, aloin A (barbaloin) and other aloin derivatives.[P88] The leaf exudate also contains chromones and phenylpyrones, and the phenyl-ethylamine alkaloid N-methyltyramine.[P88] The presence of naphthoquinones from the roots of this plant has also been reported.[P89]

Aloin A

Aloesaponarin I

Southwestern Asia or southeastern Europe

Common names Dill, Indian Dill • **Local names** Suwa / Suwa dhana (Guj., Hind., Punj., Urd.)

Description and ecology

Erect, herbaceous, blue-green annual plant 0.5–1.5m tall. Stems slender, hollow, 12mm in diameter, much-branched, softer and weaker in very young plants. All parts with strong smell when crushed. **Leaves** alternate, green, softly delicate, 10–20cm long, strongly aromatic, finely divided into needle-shaped leaflets. **Flowers** yellow, in compound umbel 4–16cm in diameter and on long hollow stalk up to 30cm long. **Fruit** a small, flattened, lens-shaped schizocarp 2.5–6 × 2.4mm, dark brown with whitish to pale brown margins, dehiscent, splitting at maturity into two 1-seeded mericarps. **Seeds** 1mm thick, straight to slightly curved. A very common garden herb, dill is widely used in Indian and Mediterranean cuisine. It is among the earliest herbal ingredients used in Indian homeopathic and Ayurvedic medicines. Even the ancient Egyptians, Greeks and Romans knew this plant and used it medicinally and for seasoning and spicing food. Dill can become a weed. It thrives in full sun, in moist, well-drained soils, at 0–2,200m.

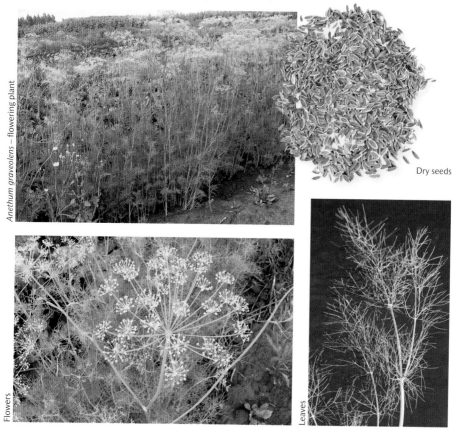

Anethum graveolens – flowering plant

Dry seeds

Flowers

Leaves

USAGE AND TREATMENT

PARTS USED Leaves, dry seeds.

TRADITIONAL MEDICINAL USES Most of East Africa's indigenous communities have been slow to appreciate the medicinal importance of dill. By contrast, the Indian community, domiciled in East Africa for more than 100 years, has long used dill as both a medicine and an aromatic spice in cooking. Dill seeds have strong appetising, carminative and diuretic properties.[M7, M9, M25, M70] They are used as a mild sedative and as an emmenagogue.[M9, M70] The seeds stimulate lactation in breast-feeding mothers, serve as a remedy for hiccups in children and provide relief from excessive stomach gas, intestinal flatulence and indigestion in adults.[M70] Dill is also very useful for improving the eyesight and fortifying the stomach. It is used to treat fever, diarrhoea and stomach disorders and may induce a pleasant mild burning sensation in the hands and feet.[M7, M70]

PREPARATION AND DOSAGE

STOMACH GAS, INTESTINAL FLATULENCE AND INDIGESTION Boil a tablespoon of dry dill seeds in a cup of water for 10 minutes. Give the warm mixture to children at intervals during the day for 2 or 3 days. For adults, roast a tablespoon of dill seeds, add a pinch of table salt, and eat 3 times daily after meals.

STRENGTHENING THE STOMACH, IMPROVING EYESIGHT AND INDUCING A MILD BURNING SENSATION IN THE HANDS AND FEET Mix half a teaspoon of dill seed powder and an equal quantity of coriander powder with half a teaspoon of brown sugar. Eat 3 times daily after meals or take a tablespoon of powdered dill seeds in the mornings.

DIURETIC, A GALACTOGOGUE AND FOR DIARRHOEA Fry a tablespoon of dill seed powder in half a teaspoon of ghee with a little brown sugar added. Take in the morning and evening.

MENSTRUATION Add a pinch of table salt and a pinch of turmeric powder to a tablespoon of dill seeds and roast in a frying pan for 5 minutes. Eat 3 times daily after meals to restore normal menstruation after childbirth or to regulate the menstrual cycle thereafter.

PHARMACOLOGY AND CHEMISTRY

PHARMACOLOGICAL PROPERTIES

The essential oil of *Anethum graveolens* is thought to possess carminative, emmenagogue, diuretic, galactogenic, mild sedative and mild diuretic properties.[P90] Aqueous extracts of *A. graveolens* showed a broad-spectrum antibacterial activity against *Staphylococcus aureus*, *Escherichia coli*, *Pseudomonas aeruginosa*, *Salmonella typhimurium*, *S. typhi* and *Shigella flexneri*.[P91, P92] Two flavonoids have been isolated from seeds reported with antioxidant activity.[P92]

COMPOUNDS REPORTED

Phytochemical screening of plants showed that leaves, stems and roots were rich in tannins, terpenoids, cardiac glycosides and flavonoids.[P92] Two flavonoids have been isolated from *A. graveolens* seed: quercetin and isoharmentin. Essential oil obtained from seeds contains a relatively high percentage of carvone (75.21%) and limonene (21.56%).[P93]

Carvone   Limonene

a. *Artemisia afra* — Indigenous

Common names African Wormwood, Wild Wormwood • **Local names** Mutasia / Muhato (Kik.), Sisimwet (Kip.), Nyumba (Luo), Ol-tikambu (Maa.), Sesimwa (Mar.), Ushemeli (Suk.)

Description and ecology

Multi-stemmed, woody perennial herb or shrub 0.5–2m high and with ridged, woody stems, growing in clumps, strongly aromatic and exuding a pungent, sweet smell when any part is cut or bruised. **Leaves** grey-green above, grey-silver below, finely divided, fern-shaped and softly feathery. **Flowers** pale yellow, in pendulous heads, along branch ends, inconspicuous, 3–5mm across. Usually confined to grassland, upland bush and forest edges, occasionally forming pure stands, also grows in damp areas such as along streams, at 1,500–3,700m. Very common in South Africa, extending northwards through tropical eastern Africa to Ethiopia.

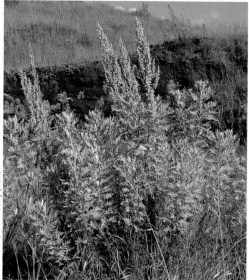

Artemisia afra – woody plant

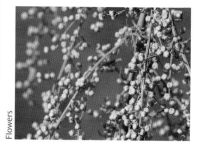

Flowers

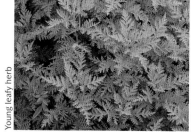

Young leafy herb

USAGE AND TREATMENT

PARTS USED Mainly the leaves, but occasionally the roots as well.

TRADITIONAL MEDICINAL USES Roots, stems and leaves are used in many different ways and taken as enemas, poultices, infusions, body washes and lotions, and are also smoked, snuffed or drunk as a tea.M116 Leaves are used to treat a sore throat and fever and for treating indigestion.M1, M4 A root decoction is taken for relief from abdominal pain, M4 and as a remedy for intestinal worms. Fresh leaves serve as an emetic and are also used as a purgative.M69 They furthermore help to ease and regulate menstruation. In South Africa, aerial parts (mainly leaves) are widely used to treat coughs, colds, influenza, asthma, fever, headache, malaria, earache, loss of appetite, colic, intestinal worms (vermifuge), diabetes, rheumatism and inflammation of the heart. Roots are used to treat colds and fever.M2, M69, M116

PREPARATION AND DOSAGE

VERMIFUGE AND EMETIC Boil a tablespoon of pounded fresh roots or dry ground roots in half a litre of water. Drink the decoction 2 or 3 times a day. This can help to expel intestinal parasites, while also serving as an emetic.

EMMENAGOGUE (IN REGULATING MENSTRUATION) Add 6–8g of dry leaf powder to a cup of cold or warm water, leave for 30 minutes and drink at least twice a day. This infusion should be taken in the week prior to the expected onset of menstruation. It can help to normalise the menstrual cycles of women who experience painful or irregular menstruation.

DIGESTIVE DISORDERS, COLITIS, APPETITE LOSS AND DYSPEPSIA (BLOATED STOMACH) Wash some fresh leaves and dry them in the sun. Grind them into a powder and add 5–10g of the dry leaf powder to a litre of boiled water. Leave for 15–20 minutes. Sieve the solution and drink small quantities of the decoction 3 or 4 times daily for 2 days.

COLDS AND BLOCKED NOSE Insert fresh leaves in the nostrils or inhale the fumes of fresh leaves boiled in water.

MALARIA, HEADACHE, FEVER, SORE THROAT AND EARACHE Add 5g of dried leaf powder to half a litre of boiled water. Leave for 15 minutes. Drink the infusion 3 or 4 times daily for 5 days. Alternatively, add 5g of dried leaf powder to half a litre of cold water. Leave for 30 minutes and drink 3 times daily for 5–7 days.

b. *Artemisia annua*   Native to China and Vietnam

Common names Sweet Wormwood, Sweet Annie, Annual Wormwood

Description and ecology

Erect, woody, many-stemmed perennial herb or shrub, reaching 0.7–2.5m. **Leaves** soft, dark green, 3–5cm long, finely divided, sweetly aromatic. **Flowers** inconspicuous, 2–2.5mm in diameter, greenish yellow turning brown with age, arranged in loose panicles. **Seeds** 0.6–0.8mm in diameter, brown achenes. Grows in well-drained soils, at 1,000–1,500m. Traditionally cultivated by herbalists in its native China for more than 2,000 years for use in treating fever and malaria. More recently, its cultivation as a medicinal plant has spread to many countries in East, southern and West Africa, North America, Europe and elsewhere.

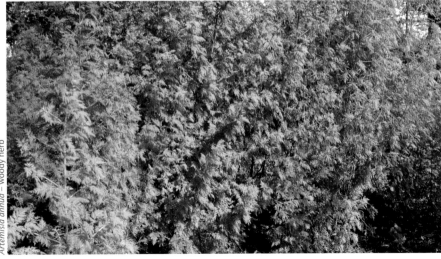

Artemisia annua – woody herb

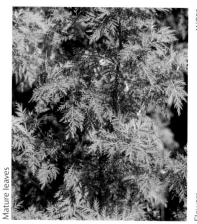
Mature leaves

WC53

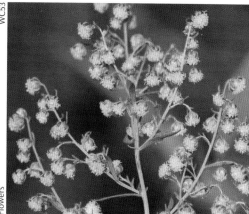
Flowers

PARTS USED Leaves.

TRADITIONAL MEDICINAL USES This antimalarial herb is widely used in East Africa. A tea made from *Artemisia* leaves (fresh or dry) is used to treat even the problematic cerebral malaria,[M12, M13, M70, M71, M112] still East Africa's number one killer disease. Leaf decoctions are taken for gastrointestinal problems, indigestion and appetite loss, and can also be used as a vermifuge, as an emetic [M6, M12, M70, M71] and as an emmenagogue for regulating menstrual cycles in women. Infusions are taken as an aphrodisiac and for treating of haemorrhoids.[M6] *Artemisia* tea is recommended for HIV/AIDS sufferers because it boosts the body's immune system. It is also used to treat schistosomiasis.[M6] An infusion of leaves is used internally to treat fever, colds and diarrhoea, and externally the leaves are poulticed onto a nose bleed, boils and abscesses.[M112]

PREPARATION AND DOSAGE

MALARIA AND SCHISTOSOMIASIS (BILHARZIA) For adults, add 5g of dried leaf powder or 25g of fresh leaves to a litre of boiled water. Leave to brew for 15–20 minutes and drink 3 or 4 times daily for 7 days. For children aged 11–13 years, use 4g of dried leaf powder or 18g of fresh leaves in a litre of boiled water and serve 2 or 3 times daily for 5–7 days. For children under the age of 10, use 3g of dried leaf powder or 10g of fresh leaves in a litre of boiled water.

COUGHS, COLDS AND SINUSITIS Boil fresh *Artemisia* leaves in water. Keep the tea boiling on low heat. Inhale the hot steam vapour for 10 minutes 3 times a day.

HAEMORRHOIDS Boil 1.5g (about a teaspoon) of dried leaf powder in a litre of water for 10 minutes. Sieve and drink at intervals during the day for a week.

ABSCESSES Wash a few fresh leaves, then boil in a little water for 10 minutes. Pound them into a paste and apply this to open abscesses. On closed boils, use a bandage to cover the application.

VERMIFUGE OR EMETIC Boil a tablespoon of pounded fresh roots or ground dry roots in a cup of water. Drink the decoction 2 or 3 times a day. Alternatively, add a tablespoon of powdered dry roots to a cup of cold water and leave to brew for 30 minutes. Drink the infusion 2 or 3 times a day.

REGULATING MENSTRUATION Add 6–8g of dry leaf powder to a cup of cold or warm water and leave for 30 minutes. Drink at least twice a day in the week prior to the expected onset of menstruation. This can help normalise the menstrual cycles of women who are prone to painful and irregular menstruation.

COLITIS, GASTROINTESTINAL PROBLEMS AND APPETITE LOSS Add 5g of dried leaves to a litre of water. Boil for 10–15 minutes and sieve. Drink small quantities at intervals through the day for 2 or 3 days.

NOTE *Artemisia* tea can be sweetened with honey or sugar to overcome the bitter taste. There are no known side effects, provided correct dosages are adhered to. External use may cause skin irritation, however.

 WARNING! Do not exceed the recommended doses. Taken in high doses, thujone has convulsive, neurotoxic and hallucinogenic effects that may trigger convulsions, vertigo, shaking and other harmful effects. *Artemisia* is not recommended for pregnant women (since it can have abortifacient effects), breast-feeding mothers and people suffering from abdominal ulcers or gastritis.

PHARMACOLOGY AND CHEMISTRY

PHARMACOLOGICAL PROPERTIES

In addition to the well-established antimalarial properties of *Artemisia annua*, some species of the genus have shown antifungal, antioxidant and antibacterial activities.[P94, P95] The antiviral, antibacterial, anti-inflammatory and antidepressant activities of *A. afra* have been reported.[P95] The volatile oils in the leaves have shown decongestant,[P94] vermifuge and emetic[P96] effects. Some studies report antihistamine, narcotic and analgesic activities.[P97] Dyspeptic effects have been demonstrated, and most species of *Artemisia* are also powerful emmenagogues.

COMPOUNDS REPORTED

Sesquiterpenes such as artemisinin (the active antimalarial ingredient of *A. annua*) have been isolated,[P98] along with flavonoids, including quecetagetin-4'-methyl ether. Some flavonoids markedly enhance the antimalarial activity of artemisinin.[P98] The essential oil of *A. afra* contains monoterpenoids (α-thujone, ß-thujone, 1,8-cineole, camphor and borneol) that are responsible for the antioxidant and antimicrobial activity of this plant.[P94] In addition to sesquiterpenes, monoterpenes and flavonoids, the presence of phenylpropanoids (e.g. ferulic acid), benzoic acid derivatives (e.g. gallic acid) and coumarins (e.g. scopoletin) has been reported from various species of *Artemisia*.[P99]

Artemisinin

Quecetagetin-4'-methyl ether

a. *Asparagus africanus* Indigenous

Common names Bush Asparagus, African Asparagus, Wild Asparagus • **Local names** Embare baba (Maa.), Lwafumbo (Tai.), Murikano (Gir.), Kapalangánga (Hehe)

Description and ecology

Perennial, scrambling shrub up to 1m tall or a climber with woody, prickly, scrambling stems up to 3m long, with rhizomatous roots, producing many slender stems from a fibrous rootstock, older stems smooth, hairless and with brown spines. '**Leaves**' (cladodes) small, clustered, needle-like, 10mm long, hanging downwards in bunches. **Flowers** small, white, in clusters amid the leaves. **Fruits** red, 1-seeded berries, green at first, turning orange-red when ripe. Common along forest edges, in bushy wooded areas and grassland, often on rocky terrain, at 100–2,700m.

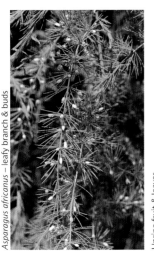

Asparagus africanus – leafy branch & buds

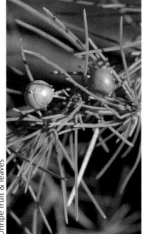

Unripe fruit & leaves

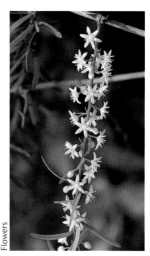

Flowers

USAGE AND TREATMENT

PARTS USED Leaves, shoots, stem and root tubers.
TRADITIONAL MEDICINAL USES The shoots, roots and the underground stems of *A. africanus* are used to make medicines for treating ailments such as rheumatism, arthritis, eye problems, nausea, colic, pulmonary tuberculosis, and bladder and kidney infections.[M112, M116] Dry leaves are used to treat wounds. Fresh root juice is taken as a remedy for a sore throat and cough.[M1, M70] Infusions of roots are used to treat venereal diseases, notably gonorrhoea and syphilis.[M70, M112] Infusions of branches, leaves and roots are used in treatments for depression and mental illnesses.[M112, M115] The shoots, roots and underground stems are also used in traditional South African medicine.[M72]

PREPARATION AND DOSAGE

HEALING WOUNDS Dry some leaves, crush into a powder and apply directly to the wound.
COUGHS AND SORE THROAT Chew some fresh roots.
DEPRESSION Soak 2–3g of pounded fresh stems, leaves or roots in a cup of boiled water and drink the resulting infusion 2 or 3 times a day.

b. *Asparagus flagellaris* Indigenous

Common name Wild Asparagus • **Local names** Mwimbana Muthumbi (Mer.), Lukalanganjoro (Nyam.)

Description and ecology
Erect to straggly, climbing, woody, spiny perennial, with twisted, grooved, greenish cylindrical stems, sometimes scrambling over rocks, branches mostly solitary. 'Leaves' (cladodes) numerous, small, needle-like, stiff, erect, tapering at the end; flowering shoots with cladodes few or absent, but fruiting branches with many cladodes. **Flowers** small, white, usually in axillary pairs, on stalks joined near base. **Fruits** fleshy orange berries, 1-seeded. Widespread in tropical Africa, mostly confused with *A. africanus*, which occurs in dry areas throughout East Africa. Common in dry bushland, sometimes scrambling over rocks, at 800–2,200m.

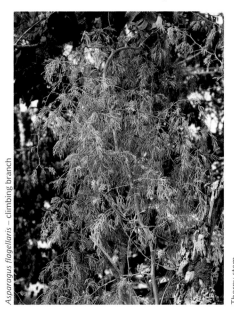

Asparagus flagellaris – climbing branch

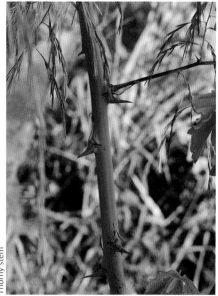

Thorny stem

USAGE AND TREATMENT

PARTS USED Leaves and roots.
TRADITIONAL MEDICINAL USES The plant is used as a diuretic and laxative.[M112] Dry leaf or root powder is used to treat wounds.[M1, M70] The root is chewed or macerated and gargled for throat troubles.[M115] Fresh roots are chewed as a remedy for a sore throat and cough.[M70] Young branches, stems or roots are used for the treatment of depression and mental disturbances. A root decoction is gargled against a sore throat.[M73] A root infusion or decoction is a treatment against syphilis, gonorrhoea and other sexually transmitted diseases.[M112, M115]

PREPARATION AND DOSAGE
HEALING WOUNDS As with *Asparagus africanus*, apply dry leaf powder directly to the wound.
COUGHS AND SORE THROAT Chew some fresh roots.
DEPRESSION Soak 2–3g of pounded fresh stems, leaves or roots in a cup of boiled water and drink the resulting infusion 2 or 3 times a day.

c. *Asparagus officinalis*

Native to Europe, Western Asia and northwestern Africa

Common names Asparagus, Garden Asparagus

Description and ecology
Upright, herbaceous plant reaching 1.5–2m, with a rhizome. Stems smooth, green, with protruding soft needles. 'Leaves' (cladodes) tiny, fine needles, flattened and produced in a cluster. Flowers small, bell-shaped, yellow or greenish yellow, male and female flowers borne on separate plants. Fruits red berries containing up to 6 black seeds. Cultivated on commercial farms in East Africa for consumption in soups and other dishes, especially as part of Chinese cuisine.

USAGE AND TREATMENT

PARTS USED Young stems and roots.
TRADITIONAL MEDICINAL USES Young *Asparagus officinalis* stems are eaten for relief from chronic constipation.[M9, M70] Infusions of young stems and roots have a very pronounced diuretic effect on the kidneys, stimulating a huge increase in urine production.[M70] Stems are also useful in stimulating renal function, especially in cases of oedema.[M9, M70] The stems, raw or cooked, are often included in diets for countering obesity as they are low in calories. Fresh root or stem paste helps to treat chronic eczema.[M9, M70]

PREPARATION AND DOSAGE
DIURETIC Add 50g of dry young stem or root powder to a litre of water. Drink 3 cups of this infusion daily.
ECZEMA Rub pounded fresh roots or stem paste onto affected areas of the skin.

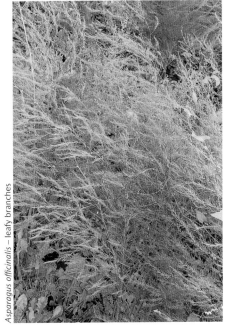

Asparagus officinalis – leafy branches

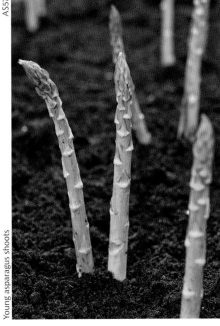

A57

Young asparagus shoots

PHARMACOLOGY AND CHEMISTRY

PHARMACOLOGICAL PROPERTIES

Asparagus officinalis has diuretic, depurative and also laxative properties.[P17] Extract of the roots of *A. africanus* has shown both antimalarial and antileishmanial activity.[P100]

COMPOUNDS REPORTED

A. officinalis contains steroidal glycosides, asparagosides A and B, saponins, asparagine glycosides, coniferine, vanillin, rhutine and tannins.[P17, P84] Roots have produced saponins and sugars. A sapogenin (muzanzagenin) and a norlignan (nyasol) have been isolated from roots of *A. africanus*[P100]. Nyasol has shown potent antileishmanial and moderate antiplasmodial activities.[P100] From *A. racemosus* (not described here), a plant traditionally used as a female reproductive tonic, steroidal saponins (shatavarins I–IV), flavonoids, alkaloids, proteins, starch, tannin, glycosides of quercetin, rutin and hyperosides have been reported.[P101]

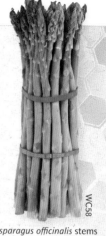

Asparagus officinalis stems

Muzanzagenin

Nyasol

a. *Aspilia mossambicensis* Indigenous

Common names Wild Sunflower, Aspilia • **Local names** Muti (Kam.), Mutanzi / Muhepe (Dig.), Raywetigo (Luo), Lilelie (Luny.), Ihwula (Suk.), Eraji (Nyan.)

Description and ecology

Woody, much-branched herb or shrub, growing to 0.5–1m, or straggling bush up to 2.5m high, with rough, hairy branches. **Leaves** elliptic-lanceolate to ovate, 2–10 × 1–3cm, opposite, sessile or with short stalk up to 1cm long, margin smooth or serrate, apex pointed, base rounded, rough on both surfaces, 3-veined from the base. **Flower** heads bright yellow, roughly 2cm across, solitary or in loose terminal groups. **Fruits** brown, obovoid achenes, 4–5mm long, hairy. Very common throughout East Africa except in the driest areas. Where not controlled by burning, it can become extensive and may scramble over neighbouring bushes. Grows in almost any habitat from woodland, wooded grassland, bushland and grassland to forest margins, rivers, lakes and seasonal swamps, at 50–2,300m.

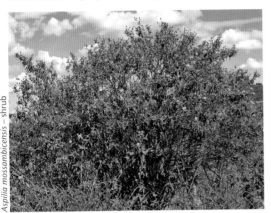

Aspilia mossambicensis – shrub

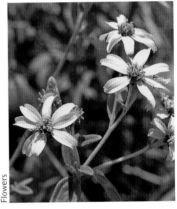

Flowers

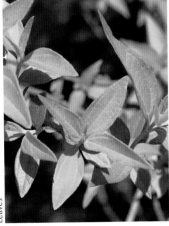

Leaves

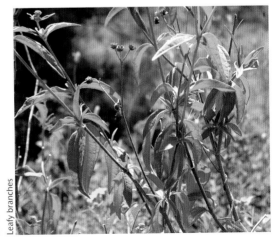

Leafy branches

PARTS USED Roots, leaves, stems and bark.

TRADITIONAL MEDICINAL USES Leaves are used to treat hepatic (liver), skin and abdominal diseases as well as to heal fresh wounds and cuts[M75] and to treat conjunctivitis. Bark is used to treat backache and abdominal problems, notably those arising from intestinal worms (hookworm). Roots are used as a remedy for cystitis and venereal diseases, mainly gonorrhoea.[M1, M75] A leaf decoction is taken as a remedy for intestinal worms, respiratory diseases and malaria.[M75]

PREPARATION AND DOSAGE

WOUNDS, CUTS AND FUNGAL INFECTIONS (RINGWORM) Pound fresh *A. mossambicensis* leaves and apply directly to affected areas of the skin. Repeat 2 or 3 times daily for at least 2 days.

ABDOMINAL PAIN AND USE AS A VERMIFUGE (TO EXPEL INTESTINAL WORMS) Pound a handful of fresh leaves or take a tablespoon of dry leaf powder and heat in half a litre of water. Take this leaf decoction in small quantities 2 or 3 times a day.

LIVER PROBLEMS (HEPATITIS) Add a tablespoon of pounded leaves to 2 cups of cold boiled water. Steep for 15 minutes, stir and strain. Take this infusion 2 or 3 times a day.

b. *Aspilia pluriseta*

Indigenous

Common names Aspilia, Dwarf Aspilia • **Local names** Muti / Wuti (Kam.), Shilambila (Luh.), Ololyabase (Maa.)

Description and ecology

Perennial, suberect, woody herb with branches 0.5–0.7m tall, or sometimes a small scrambling shrub up to 1.5m high, usually much branched. Leaves ovate to narrowly ovate, 2–5(–8) × 0.8–2(–3.5)cm, opposite, margin toothed, base rounded, apex pointed, rough on both surfaces, 3-veined from the base, with or without a very short stalk 0–3(–5)mm long. Flower heads yellow or orange-yellow, 1.6–1.8cm in diameter, solitary or in loose terminal groups, on stalks 0.5–0.6cm long. Fruits small, obovoid, dry, 1-seeded achenes, 2.5–4.5mm long, hairy. This variable plant can reach a large size as a scrambler. It grows abundantly in black cotton soils in dry bush, woodland and grassland, at 1,050–2,250m.

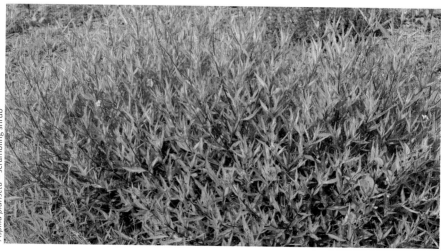

Aspilia pluriseta – scrambling shrub

PARTS USED Leaves, stems and bark.

TRADITIONAL MEDICINAL USES Pounded fresh leaves are used to treat skin afflictions such as ringworm and to heal bruises, burns, fresh cuts or wounds.[M1, M70, M74] Infusions of pounded fresh leaves soaked in cold water are taken as a remedy for liver problems.[M70]

PREPARATION AND DOSAGE

FRESH CUTS, BRUISES OR WOUNDS, FUNGAL INFECTIONS Pound some fresh leaves. Apply directly to the skin.

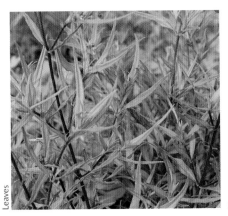

Leaves

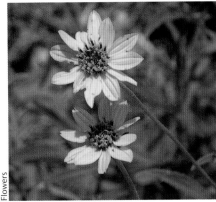

Flowers

PHARMACOLOGY AND CHEMISTRY

PHARMACOLOGICAL PROPERTIES

Dried leaves of *Aspilia pluriseta* have shown antitrichomonal[P102] and antiviral (HIV-1)[P103] activities. From dried leaves and stems, immunomodulator activities[P104] have also been recorded.

COMPOUNDS REPORTED

Sulfur compounds (e.g. thiarubrine) have been found in the leaves[P105] of some species of *Aspilia*. Diterpenes (e.g. ent-kaur-16-en-19-al) have been isolated from roots,[P106] and sesquiterpenes (e.g. germacrene D) from aerial parts.[P106] From roots and aerial parts of *A. pluriseta* and *A. mossambicensis*, ent-kaurane-type diterpenoids and other phytochemicals, which include steroids, triterpenes and a phenylpropanoid, have been reported.[P107]

Germacrene D

Ent-kaur-16-en-19-al

Native to India, Sri Lanka, Bangladesh and Southeast Asia

Common names Neem Tree, Indian Lilac • **Local names** Mwarubaini / Mkilifi / Mwarubaini kamili (Swa.), Neem (Urd., Hind., Punj.), Karwu limbru (Guj.)

Description and ecology
Hardy, fast-growing, deciduous tree 15–20m tall, rarely reaching 25–30m, with wide and spreading branches and dense rounded crown 20–25m in diameter. **Bark** rough, grooved, grey-brown. **Leaves** pinnately compound, alternate, crowded near end of branches, 20–40cm long, stalk short, leaflets 20–30, medium to dark green, 3–8cm long, with long, sharply pointed apices, asymmetrical at the bases, with coarsely serrate margins. **Flowers** small, creamy white, sweetly scented, hanging in long axillary sprays. **Fruit** a 1-seeded drupe, oval or round, green turning yellow when ripe, 1–2cm long. Celebrated in its native India, neem is now one of Africa's most widely planted trees. Long cultivated on the East African coast, it is common in arid and semi-arid regions, being drought resistant and flourishing in poor soils, at 0–1,500m.

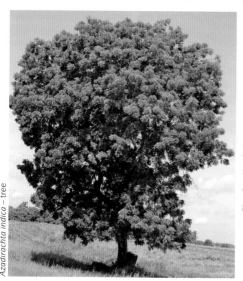

Azadirachta indica – tree

PB60

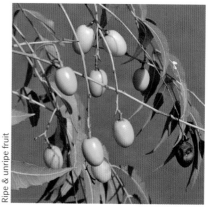

Ripe & unripe fruit

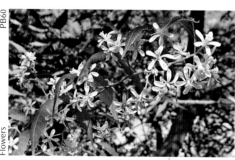

Flowers

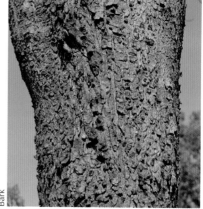

Bark

USAGE AND TREATMENT

PARTS USED Bark, leaves, twigs, fruits and seed oil.

TRADITIONAL MEDICINAL USES Neem oil can be used to treat skin diseases (including leprosy), fungal infections and eczema.M4, M70, M111 The twigs contain antiseptic ingredients that are used to maintain healthy teeth and gums.M4, M70 The bark is bitter and astringent; a decoction thereof can be applied externally to haemorrhoids. M112 Leaves are used in the treatment of malaria,M14, M15, M70 intestinal worms, diarrhoea and dysentery.M6, M112 Bark,

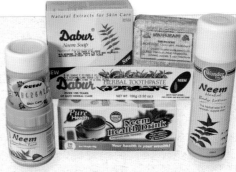

A variety of neem health care products is available in health shops and supermarkets in East Africa.

leaves and ripe fruits can help in blood purification and are used as a remedy for intestinal worms.M6, M15, M70 The leaf juice is applied externally to skin ulcers, cuts, wounds, boils and eczema.M111, M112

PREPARATION AND DOSAGE

BOILS, ULCERS AND ECZEMA Boil a few crushed leaves in a small volume of water and apply as a poultice over open ulcers and boils. For blind boils, apply a poultice of unboiled fresh leaves.

INFECTED BURNS Boil a handful of fresh leaves in a litre of water for 15–20 minutes. Filter, cool and use immediately to wash infected burns. Wash the burns at least 3 times a day, and keep affected areas away from flies and other vectors of infection, using a net if necessary.

MALARIA AND SLEEPING SICKNESS Add 5g of dried leaf powder or 20–30 fresh leaves to a litre of boiling water. Drink at intervals for 3 days to treat malaria. Drink every day for sleeping sickness.

PROTECTIVE CLEANING OF THE MOUTH AND TEETH Use the twigs as toothbrushes for cleaning the mouth and teeth. Neem bark contains substances that have an antibiotic effect against germs and infection.

CANDIDA (THRUSH) Mix 2 drops of neem oil with 20 drops of castor or vegetable oil. Apply locally to treat candida of the skin or the vagina. For candida in the mouth, add 2 drops of neem oil to 20 drops of honey.

SKIN INFECTIONS Immerse fresh neem leaves in boiling water for 10 minutes. Use this decoction to wash affected areas of the skin. Alternatively, mix 5g of neem oil with 50g of any locally applied ointment or cream. To treat athlete's foot, rub a paste or ointment of crushed leaves onto the affected areas. For warts, apply the oil directly to the skin.

GASTROINTESTINAL UPSETS (DIARRHOEA, DYSENTERY) Immerse about 30 leaves in half a litre of boiling water for 5–10 minutes. Sip the resulting tea in small quantities at intervals during the day for 3 days, along with plenty of other rehydration liquids and water.

HEAD LICE AND SCALP DANDRUFF Apply the oil to the hair twice a day for 4 days to kill head lice, or rub onto the scalp to get rid of dandruff. Alternatively, make a paste from neem seeds (after removing their hard outer skins), then every evening after washing the hair, rub 2 teaspoons of the paste into the hair and scalp. Continue this treatment for 4 or 5 days.

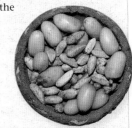

Ripe fruit and dry seeds

 WARNING! Internal use of neem is not recommended for pregnant women. Prolonged internal use may cause irritation of the liver or the kidneys.

PHARMACOLOGICAL PROPERTIES

Studies have reported a wide range of biological activities for both bark and leaves. These include antimalarial,[P108] anti-ulcer[P109] and cytotoxic[P110] effects. Fresh bark and leaves have shown anti-inflammatory effects,[P111] but no antibacterial activity is reported for dried bark and leaves.[P112] The seeds have shown antimalarial[P113] and antifungal[P114] activities. Insecticide activity against a variety of insects[P115] has been ascribed to the seed oil.

COMPOUNDS REPORTED

Numerous compounds have been isolated from neem, including triterpenoids (e.g. azadiradione) and limonoids (e.g. azadirachtin) from the

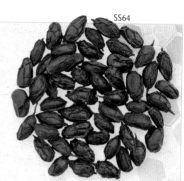

Azadirachta indica – dry fruit

seeds.[P116] Azadirachtin is the most active insecticidal and antimalarial constituent of neem,[P108] which also produces phenolics such as gallic acid and epicatechin that inhibit inflammation.[P108] Several bioactive phytochemicals, including nimocinol (anti-breast cancer), azadiradione (treatment of neurodegenerative diseases) and nimbidin (anti-inflammatory, antifungal, hypoglycaemic, antibacterial), have been reported.[P117]

Azadirachtin

Gallic acid

13 *Balanites aegyptiaca* ZYGOPHYLLACEAE

Indigenous

Common name Desert Date • **Local names** Baddan (Bor.), Mwambangoma (Dig.), Baddana (Gab.), Mkongo / Konga (Gir.), Mulului / Ndului (Kam.), Othoo (Luo), Olng'oswa / Olokwai (Maa.), Ngoswa (Mar.), Baddan (Orm.), Tuyunwo / Tuyun (Pok.), Lowai (Sam.), Kullan / Kullung (Som.), Mjunju / Mchunju (Swa.), Kiwowa (Tai.), Lungoswa (Tav.), Ng'eswo / Ngosyek (Tug.), Eroronyit (Tur.), Mohoromo (Chag.), Mduguyu (Gogo), Mkongo (Lugu.), Mduguyu / Myuguyu (Nyam.), Mfughuyu (Nyat.), Iteru / Mkisingo / Mkonga (Pare), Myuguyugu / Nyuguyu (Suk.), Muwambangoma (Zig.), Mruguhu (Zin.), Echoma / Ekorete (Ate.), Musongole (Lug.), Loba / Logba (Lugb., Madi), Zomai (Lugi.), Kinachoma (Lugw.), To (Luo-A), Loba / Logba (Madi), Mutete (Runy.), Chomiandet (Sebei)

Description and ecology

Multi-branched, slow-growing, spiny shrub or tree 6–10m high and with a rounded crown, the arching branches with long, straight, green spines up to 8cm long. **Bark** smooth, green in young trees but dark and deeply fissured when old. **Leaves** 2-foliolate, the pair of bright green leaflets leathery, obovate-elliptic and with entire margins. **Flowers** in greenish or yellow-green clusters at the leaf bases, fragrant. **Fruit** an oblong or narrowly ellipsoid drupe, 4–5cm long, rounded at both ends, green at first, turning brownish yellow when ripe, with brown or brown-green sticky edible pulp and a hard stone seed. Common tree of arid and semi-arid regions to subhumid savanna of East Africa, found in dry bushland, bushed grassland, wooded grassland and woodland, but also grows along rivers, at 0–2,000m.

AS65

Balanites aegyptiaca – tree

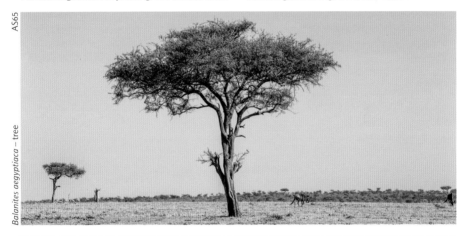

Branch, thorns & flowers

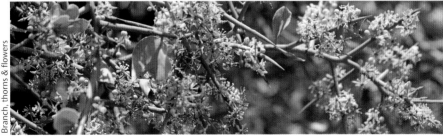

PARTS USED Stem bark, leaves, root bark, fruits and seeds.
TRADITIONAL MEDICINAL USES An infusion of stem bark can be used as an anthelmintic and to treat syphilis.[M17, M70] A root and/or bark infusion may help malaria.[M3, M71, M76, M111] Dried stem bark is taken as a cough remedy. Leaf decoctions are used to treat sleeping sickness. Infusions of roots are used as anthelmintics,[M1, M70, M76] purgatives, vermifuge[M111, M112] and to treat abdominal pain.[M18] The fruit and seeds are poisonous to freshwater snails and have been used as a purgative in treatments for schistosomiasis (bilharzia).[M4, M19] (The parasites that cause schistosomiasis live in certain freshwater snails.) The fruits are used to treat a cough and sore throat. Dry root bark may be used in the treatment of asthma, snakebite and impotence.[M20, M70] Roots boiled in a soup can be used for the treatment of oedema and stomach pain.[M111, M112]

PREPARATION AND DOSAGE

MALARIA Add 4g of dry bark or root powder to half a litre of hot (or cold) water. Leave for 20 minutes, stir and strain. Drink the infusion twice daily for 2 days.
ANTHELMINTIC, PURGATIVE AND ABDOMINAL PAIN Add 4g of pounded fresh roots to half a litre of boiled water. Leave for 10–15 minutes, stir and strain. Drink before breakfast.
COUGHS AND ASTHMA Add a pinch of table salt to half a teaspoon of dried stem bark powder. Place this dose on the tongue twice a day. It will dissolve and be absorbed.

PHARMACOLOGICAL PROPERTIES

Some antibacterial and antifungal activities have been reported for *Balanites* bark.[P118, P119] Bark extracts have shown spermicidal and molluscicidal effects[P119, P120, P121] coupled with both antiviral activity against HIV5 and antihepatotoxic activities.[P122]

COMPOUNDS REPORTED

Several sapogenins and saponins, such as diosgenin[P119, P123] and cryptogenin,[P119, P124] have been isolated from *Balanites* species. The presence of flavonoids (e.g. astragalin[P125]) has also been reported. Leaves contain saponin, furanocoumarin and glucosides.[P119] Fruits contain steroidal saponins, while oil from the kernel contains fatty acids, mainly palmitic, stearic, oleic and linoleic acids.[P119]

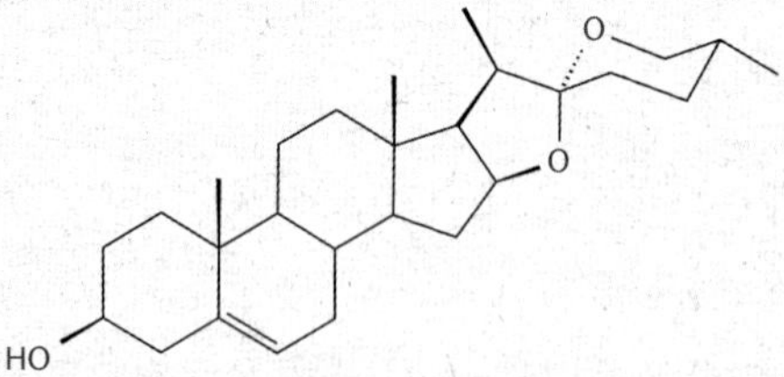

Diosgenin

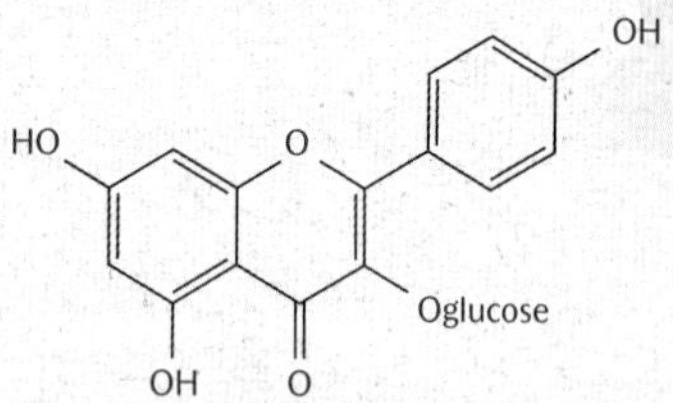

Astragalin

Indigenous

Common name Winged Bersama • **Local names** Muthandi / Murumia andu (Kik.), Cheptoroguet / Ororuewet / Toroguet (Kip.), Omubamba (Kis.), Shirikamabinga / Kumusikiria (Luh.), Olobayie-tiang'ata (Maa.Ken.), Kipset / Kasagas (Mar.), Muthandathande (Mer.), Kibuimetiet (Nan.), Kipumetiet (Tug.), Iranguwe (Aru.), Moosa / Manguwe (Chag.), Muyungula (Haya), Alasoki / Engoisiki (Maa.Tan.), Mpeme / Mnyatoma / Mbasamono (Hehe), Mwangwakwao (Swa.), Gishombe / Shigishombe (Lugi.), Mukaka (Ruki.), Muhungura (Ruto.), Sigirwo (Sebei)

Description and ecology

Evergreen shrub or well-foliaged tree 7–12(–15)m tall. **Bark** light brown, smooth at first, becoming rough with age. **Leaves** compound, clustered at ends of branches, leaflets 7–10cm long, in 5–10 opposite pairs plus a terminal one. **Flowers** whitish pink to cream, aromatic, on thick upright spikes up to 30cm, candle-like and hairy. **Fruits** thick, woody capsules, rounded, up to 2.5cm across, with golden hairs at first, opening into 3–5 sections to reveal bright orange-red seeds, each with a yellowish-green, fleshy aril. Found on banks in wooded river valleys, on upland grassland along montane and riparian forest edges and in open woodland, at 1,300–2,400m.

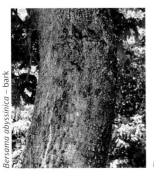
Bersama abyssinica – bark

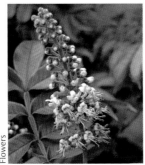
Flowers

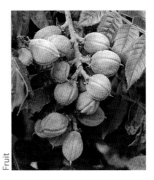
Fruit

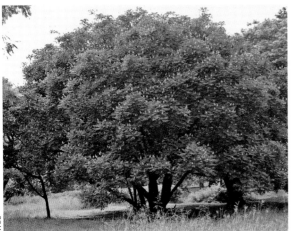
Tree

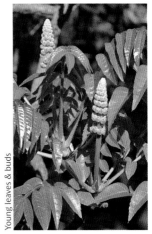
Young leaves & buds

PARTS USED Leaves, twigs, bark and roots.
TRADITIONAL MEDICINAL USES Snuff made from powdered leaves or bark can be used to treat colds and headache.[M4] Fresh leaves are chewed as an aphrodisiac.[M1, M70] A bark poultice is applied to the back for treating muscle and lower back pain, and a leaf decoction is drunk for back pain.[M112, M115] Decoctions of dried bark powder are fed to young children as an anthelmintic and emetic.[M70] Juice from fresh bark is used as a purgative. Infusions of young twigs are used in the treatment of dysentery and intestinal worms.[M4, M70] Root decoctions are taken to treat epilepsy and haemorrhoids, and are also used to wash wounds.[M1, M4, M70] Bark or root decoctions are taken to relieve menstrual pain and to treat infertility. Bark, leaf and root decoctions are widely taken as a purgative to treat a range of stomach disorders such as abdominal pain, colic, diarrhoea, cholera, intestinal worms, amoebiasis and dysentery.[M112, M115]

PREPARATION AND DOSAGE
COLDS AND HEADACHE Grind some sun-dried leaves or bark into a fine powder. Either use as snuff or mix with water and apply as nasal drops.
PAIN IN THE MUSCLES AND JOINTS OF THE LOWER BACK Apply a few pieces of fresh bark or 5g of dried powdered bark as a poultice on the painful areas.

 WARNING! All species of *Bersama* contain highly toxic compounds that can affect the heart, so internal use of any part of these plants should be undertaken with extreme caution.

PHARMACOLOGICAL PROPERTIES
Fruits of *Bersama abyssinica* have shown cytotoxic activity,[P126] but the leaves have proved inactive against bacteria, fungi, yeast[P127] and viruses.[P128] Dried roots produce strong activity against some organisms such as *Escherichia coli* but are inactive towards other bacteria.[P13] Cytotoxic effects of the bufadienolides in *B. abyssinica* are well documented.[P129] The presence of poisonous heart glycosides in species of *Bersama* is well known but research has not shown conclusively whether these compounds have any pain-relieving or curative function.

COMPOUNDS REPORTED
Species of *Bersama* are known to contain bufadienolides, such as bersaldegenin-1,3,5-orthoacetate in the case of *B. abyssinica*.[P129] Cardenolides (e.g. abyssinin), benzenoids (e.g. gallic acid) and triterpenes (e.g. oleanolic acid) have been isolated from *B. abyssinica* root bark.[P130] Recently, three new bufadienolides (paulliniogenin A, B and C) that suppress the proliferation of the human epidermoid carcinoma KB-3-1 cell line have been isolated from stem bark of *B. abyssinica*.[P131]

Abyssinin

Paulliniogenin A

15 *Boscia* species CAPPARACEAE

a. *Boscia angustifolia* Indigenous

Common names Narrow-leaved Boscia, Rough-leaved Shepherd's Tree • **Local names** Kalkaj (Bor.), Mlalambuzi / Musambweke (Gir.), Mulule (Kam.), Bware / Ayiergweng (Luo), Oloireroi (Maa.), Chieh (Som.), Lito (Kip., Tug.), Likwon (Pok.), Lororoi (Sam.), Emejen (Tur.)

Description and ecology

Evergreen shrub or tree 6–14m high. Bole often short but massive, twisted and grooved, crown rounded, with ascending branches. **Bark** silver-grey, smooth. **Leaves** simple, alternate, entire, leathery, non-hairy, grey-green, elliptical to obovate, 1.5–5(–7)cm long, tip sharply pointed, base rounded. **Flowers** cream or greenish yellow, stalk 0.5–1.5cm long, in short, many-flowered axillary or terminal spikes or umbel-like racemes up to 6cm long, glabrous to shortly hairy. **Fruit** a globose to slightly ellipsoid berry, 0.5–1.5cm across, orange-yellow to reddish grey, up to 7-seeded. **Seeds** globose, compressed. Commonly seen in dry bushland, woodland and wooded grassland, on termite mounds and sometimes in dry riverbeds, at 0–2,100m.

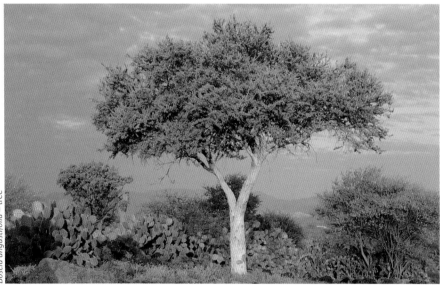

Boscia angustifolia – tree

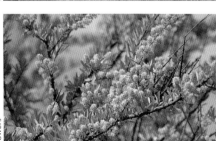

Flowers

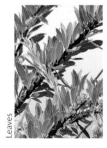

Leaves

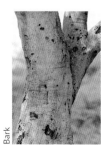

Bark

PARTS USED Bark, leaves and fruits.
TRADITIONAL MEDICINAL USES Fresh bark is used as a treatment for malaria.[M1, M4, M70] Fresh leaves are chewed as an anthelmintic and as a remedy for stomach ache.[M4, M70] Bark decoctions are used to treat backache.[M70] The fruit can work as a laxative.[M111, M112]

PREPARATION AND DOSAGE
ANTHELMINTIC AND STOMACH ACHE Wash a few fresh leaves before chewing them, swallowing the juice.
MALARIA Chop 5g of fresh bark into fine pieces. Then boil in half a litre of water for 5–10 minutes. Drink the decoction in small quantities at least 3 times daily.

b. *Boscia coriacea* Indigenous

Common name Boscia • **Local names** Galgacha-Hareh (Bor.), K'alk'acha (Gab.), Muthiu (Emb., Mbe.), Isivu (Kam.), Engamuluki (Maa.), Sorichon (Pok.), Ghalangai (Som.), Mnafisi (Swa.), Chariso (Tai.), Muthiuthiu (Tha.), Eedung (Tur.), Kalkalch (Orm.), Nyaror / Lyoror / Yoror (Ren.), Siriko / Sirkwa (Tug.)

Description and ecology
Twiggy, usually multi-stemmed, evergreen shrub or small tree usually 2–7m tall. **Leaves** simple, alternate, grey-olive-green, oval 6 × 1.8cm, with sharp tip, hard and leathery, stalk 4–8mm long. **Flowers** white or yellowish, in dense axillary or terminal clusters or many-flowered racemes, fragrant. **Fruits** rounded, 1–2cm across, densely and softly hairy, olive-green when young becoming orange-yellow when ripe. **Seeds** enclosed in a tough white skin. Grows in arid coastal lowlands but is most commonly found in *Acacia–Commiphora* bushland and semi-desert scrub, often in rocky areas, at 1–1,200m.

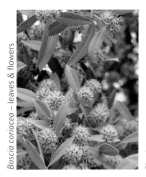

Boscia coriacea – leaves & flowers

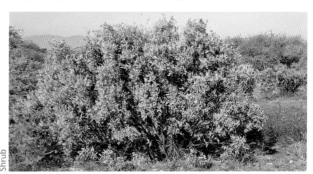

Shrub

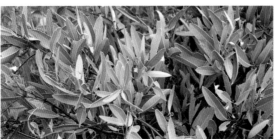

Leaves

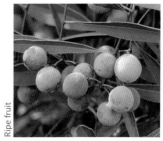

Ripe fruit

PARTS USED Leaves and roots.
TRADITIONAL MEDICINAL USES Fresh leaves are used to treat stomach ache or as an anthelmintic.[M115] Root decoctions are taken as a remedy for venereal diseases, notably gonorrhoea,[M1, M3, M70, M115] as well as for headaches.[M3, M70]
NOTE Another *Boscia* species, *B. salicifolia*, common in both Kenya and Tanzania, is also very widely used in traditional medicine.

PREPARATION AND DOSAGE
ANTHELMINTIC AND FOR TREATING STOMACH ACHE As with *B. angustifolia*, wash a few fresh leaves and then chew them, swallowing the juice.
GONORRHOEA Chop 5g of fresh roots into fine pieces. Boil in half a litre of water for 10 minutes, cool and filter. Drink in small quantities through the day for 3 days.

PHARMACOLOGY AND CHEMISTRY

PHARMACOLOGICAL PROPERTIES
Roots of *B. angustifolia* have shown antibacterial activity against various organisms.[P132] A leaf extract of *B. coriacea* showed antifungal activity against *Aspergillus flavus*, which is the leading aflatoxin-producing fungus.[P133]

COMPOUNDS REPORTED
Phytochemical screening on the leaf extract of *B. coriacea* indicated the presence of flavonoids, alkaloids and cardiac glycosides.[P133] From *B. senegalensis* a flavonol glycoside named bosenegaloside A has been found, along with known glycosides of flavonoids, phenylpropanoids and terpenes.[P134]

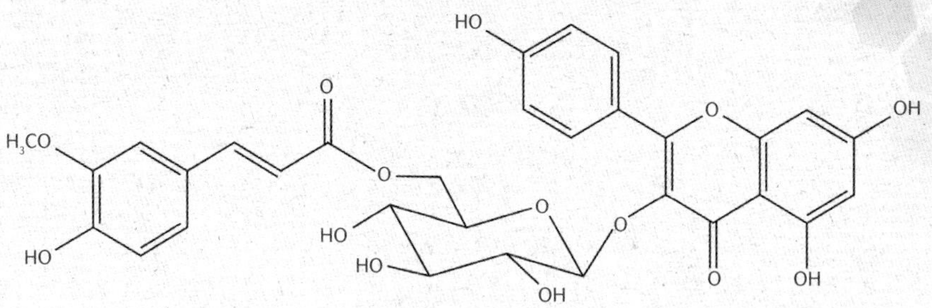

Bosenegaloside A

16 *Bulbine abyssinica*   ASPHODELACEAE

Indigenous

Common name Bushy Bulbine

Description and ecology
Erect, succulent, perennial herb growing in small clusters from a vertical rhizome with fleshy roots. **Leaves** soft, erect, fleshy, up to 35cm long, narrow and grass-like, thornless. **Flowers** star-shaped, bright yellow, in dense clusters on ascending stalks up to 35mm long. **Fruit** a black capsule, spherical, 4–5mm in diameter. It frequently forms small colonies and is commonly found in dry bushland or grassland, often on shallow soil over rock, at 600–2,250m.

WC72

Bulbine abyssinica – plant with flowering shoots

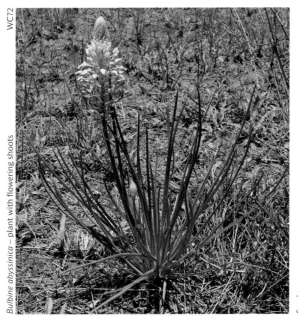

Seeds

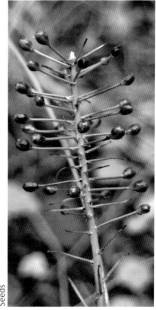

USAGE AND TREATMENT

PARTS USED Roots, leaves and fruits.
TRADITIONAL MEDICINAL USES Infusions of roots or fruits of *Bulbine* species are used for treating malaria.[M11, M70] Leaves are used to heal wounds, burns, rashes, itching, herpes and fungal diseases, notably ringworm.[M2, M77] Crushed leaves serve as a dressing for burns, while leaf sap can be applied to cracked lips.[M77] Another species, *B. frutescens* (with yellow-and-orange flowers), is widely grown as an ornamental garden plant in East Africa.

PREPARATION AND DOSAGE
SKIN AILMENTS Apply sap from crushed fresh leaves to affected areas 2 or 3 times a day.
MALARIA Steep a handful of crushed roots in a litre of cold boiled water for 15 minutes. Strain and drink 2 or 3 cups daily.

PHARMACOLOGY AND CHEMISTRY

PHARMACOLOGICAL PROPERTIES

The leaf gel of *Bulbine* species has wound-healing effects. Glycoproteins such as aloctin A and B may account for this.[P135] Phenylanthraquinones (e.g. isoknipholone and jozknipholone A) produce potent antiplasmodial activities.[P80, P136]

COMPOUNDS REPORTED

The roots of *Bulbine* contain phenylanthraquinones, including gaboroquinone B,[P137] knipholone[P138, P139] and simple anthraquinones such as chrysophanol. Some anthraquinone dimers such as abyquinone A have been reported from the fruits of *B. abyssinica*.[P140] The leaf gel contains glycoproteins such as aloctin A and aloctin B.[P135] In addition to anthraquinones, species of *Bulbine* also elaborate isofuranonaphthoquinones and naphthalene derivatives, flavonoids, phenolics and triterpenes.[P141]

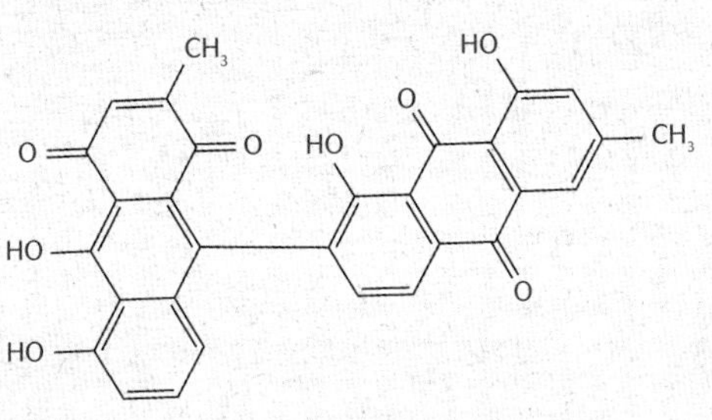

Abyquinone A

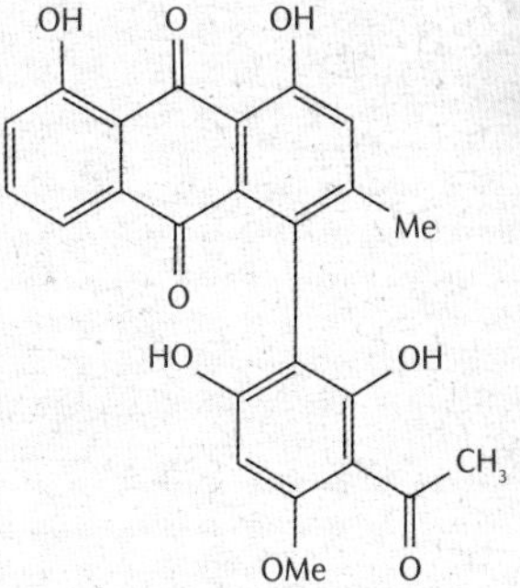

Knipholone

Indigenous

Common names Cadaba Bush, Herd-boy's Fruit • **Local names** Dekoku (Bor.), Deekuku (Gab.), Kalaqacha (Ilw.), Porowet Ap Teta (Kip.), Akado marateng (Luo), Olamalogi (Maa.Ken.), Kalkalch-hare (Orm.), Arerenyon (Pok.), Geikuku (Ren.), Larasoro (Sam.), Dumei / Galgnal / Tukh (Som.), Kibilazi-Mwitu / Mvunja-vumo (Swa.), Msimaguare / Msimakwari (Tai.), Birirwet (Tug.), Eireng (Tur.), Mvumvu (Gogo), Mkubange (Haya), Luharamira (Lugu.), Ngamalog (Maa.Tan.), Mtundusuvuya (Nyam.), Mnyukapala (Zig.), Kaninigwa Msagwasagwa (Suk.)

Description and ecology

Evergreen, twiggy, much-branched shrub 2–3m high, rarely a small tree reaching 5m. **Bark** yellowish grey, strongly grooved, branches stiff and sharp. **Leaves** simple, alternate, oblong or elliptic, greyish green, apex rounded, margin smooth. **Flowers** creamy yellow to pale pink, solitary or in small, terminal, few-flowered, flattish-topped racemes, with pedicel 5–15mm long. **Fruits** cylindrical greyish pods, 4–5cm long, with many rounded or kidney-shaped seeds embedded in an orange-red pulp. A shrub of arid and semi-arid areas, of dry *Acacia* scrubland and bushed or wooded deciduous grassland, but also grows in riverine and coastal thickets and bushland, at 0–1,900m.

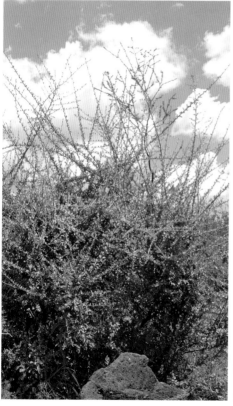

Cadaba farinosa – shrub

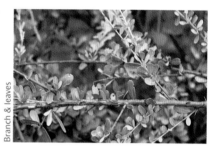

Branch & leaves

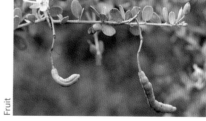

Fruit

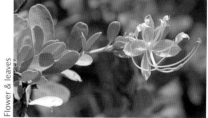

Flower & leaves

PARTS USED Leaves and roots.

TRADITIONAL MEDICINAL USES Plant parts of *Cadaba farinosa* are widely used as an anti-inflammatory agent and for the treatment of colic, conjunctivitis, stomach ache and snakebite.[M115] Ash of the burned plant is rubbed into the skin to relieve general body pain. Roots are burned and the ash can be used to neutralise venom from snakebite.[M115] Roots are also used in treatments for chest colds.[M4, M33] Infusions of roots may be taken for protection against sexually transmitted diseases.[M33, M70] A leaf decoction can be used in treatments for gonorrhoea[M1, M4, M70] and syphilis.[M78] Ground leaf powder is used to treat skin ulcers.[M1, M70] Leaves are used as a purgative and as a remedy for coughs, rheumatism, fever, colds, dysentery and as a poultice for sores on the skin.[M78, M115] Leaves can also be used as an anthelmintic.[M115]

PREPARATION AND DOSAGE

COLDS AND HEADACHE Dig out some fresh roots. Wash them thoroughly and chew them raw, swallowing the juice.

GONORRHOEA Add a handful of fresh leaves to half a litre of hot water. Leave for 15 minutes, until cool. Drink the decoction at intervals during the day.

SKIN ULCERS AND SORES Apply dry, ground leaf powder directly to affected areas of the skin.

PHARMACOLOGICAL PROPERTIES

A leaf extract of *Cadaba farinosa* has showed hepatoprotective, antioxidant, antiprotozoal, schistosomicidal and antifungal activities.[P142]

COMPOUNDS REPORTED

C. farinosa contains spermidine alkaloids, phenylpropanoids and benzoic acid derivatives.[P142] Sesquiterpenes, including cadabicilone, have been isolated from stem bark.[P143] The entire plant contains alkaloids such as cadabicine.[P144] The presence of flavonol triglycosides in the aerial parts[P145] and a novel macrocyclic dibenzo-diazacyclododecanedione along with five known compounds from the roots[P146] of *C. farinosa* have been reported.

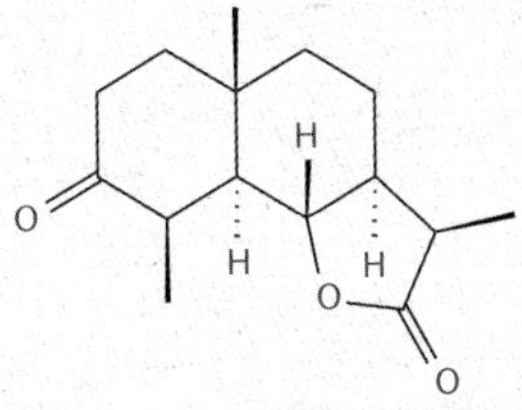

Cadabicilone

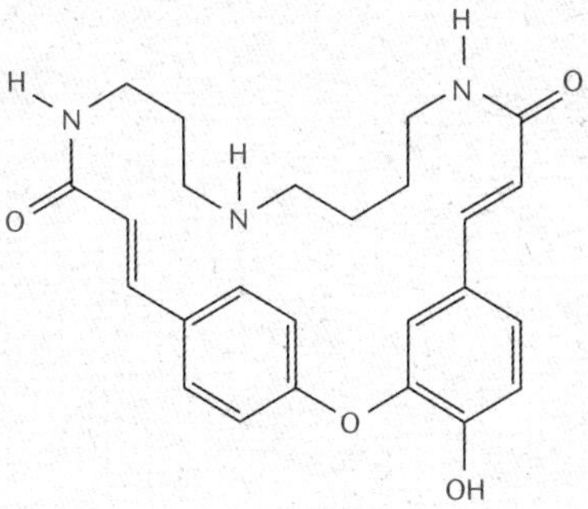

Cadabicine

18 *Calotropis procera* APOCYNACEAE

Indigenous

Common names Giant Milkweed, Apple of Sodom, Dead Sea Fruit • **Local names** K'obbo (Gab.), Ilumbu / Muvuthu (Kam.), Okwot-pu (Luo), Ararat (Mar.), Muk-rugha (Orm.), Labechi / Laibeleh (Sam.), Etetheru / Etithuru (Tur.), Boah (Som.), Mpamba-mwitu (Swa.), Akado / Akh (Guj.), Madar / Karnataki (Hind., Urd.)

Description and ecology

Large, erect, spreading shrub or small to medium-sized tree 2–6m tall, with a soft, woody stem when young, exuding copious latex when broken. Older trees with rough, fissured, corky bark. **Leaves** opposite, simple, rounded or oval, 15–30 × 2.5–10cm, thick, waxy, hairy below, prominently veined, stalkless, tip pointed. **Flowers** cup-shaped, creamish white to pink with dark purplish tips, clustered. **Fruits** large, grey-green, turning brown at maturity, oblong, inflated like a small balloon, 10cm or more in diameter. **Seeds** numerous, covered by tuft of long, silky white hairs. Common in dry areas, often along seasonal watercourses and roadsides, at 300–1,200m.

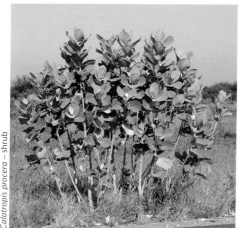
Calotropis procera – shrub

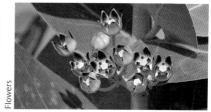
Flowers

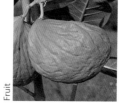
Fruit

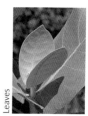
Leaves

USAGE AND TREATMENT

PARTS USED Root bark, stem bark, leaves, flowers and latex.
TRADITIONAL MEDICINAL USES Root infusions are taken as a remedy for coughs and are also used to treat snakebite.[M4, M70] Decoctions of roots can help for hookworm and are also taken as an emetic.[M1, M4, M111, M112] Dried leaves or roots are used as snuff for bronchial catarrh, acute and chronic bronchitis, pneumonia, headache, colds and nasal congestion. The latex is a remedy for ringworm, scorpion stings and venereal sores[M7, M70, M111, M112] and is also used as a laxative and purgative.[M111, M112] An infusion of bark powder is used as a treatment for leprosy and elephantiasis.[M111, M112] Leaf poultices can relieve pain and swelling of the joints caused by rheumatic afflictions. The flowers are used for fortifying the stomach, increasing the appetite and expelling rheumatic phlegm.[M7, M70] Root bark is administered in cases of cholera. Ash from the whole plant can treat asthma, coughs and rheumatism.[M70] The leaf sap may help to relieve earache.[M7]

PREPARATION AND DOSAGE

RHEUMATISM, LUMBAGO AND SCIATICA Boil a handful of crushed dry leaves in half a cup of sesame oil. Rub the warm oil onto the painful swellings. Massage and then cover with a bandage. Apply at least 3 times daily until the painful swelling has abated.

ASTHMA, BRONCHITIS, PNEUMONIA, MIGRAINE AND HEADACHE, COLDS AND COUGHS Grind the dry leaves or roots into a fine powder. Use this as snuff 3 times a day. Sneezing will follow and the nose will start running as congestion clears, bringing relief from the associated headache. For bronchitis and in the early stages of pneumonia, boil a teaspoon of ground dry roots in a cup of water for 10 minutes. Drink 1 or 2 cups daily.

RINGWORM Cases of ringworm that stubbornly resist more conventional treatments have been known to be eliminated quickly by applying latex from this plant directly to affected areas of the skin. Application can be painful, however. A second treatment may be necessary a few days after the first.

EARACHE Heat a ripe yellow leaf over a fire for a few minutes to warm it. Once warm, squeeze the leaf between the fingers, inserting 1 or 2 drops of the warm leaf juice into the ear. Do this twice a day.

EMETIC AND ANTHELMINTIC Boil a teaspoon of dried root powder in half a litre of water for 10–15 minutes. Drink this decoction before breakfast for 2 days.

> ⚠ **WARNING!** The whole plant contains some toxic glycosides and may cause poisoning if consumed fresh. Although these substances disappear with drying, all internal treatments should be administered with caution.

PHARMACOLOGY AND CHEMISTRY

PHARMACOLOGICAL PROPERTIES

Aerial parts of *Calotropis procera* have shown antimalarial,[P147, P148] anti-inflammatory[P149] and antipyretic[P149] activities. These parts have also produced a neuromuscular blocking activity.[P149, P150] The entire plant has a uterine stimulant effect[P26] as well as smooth-muscle stimulant activity.[P151] The latex shows strong fibrinolytic activity in human plasma.[P152] *C. procera* appears to also have hepatoprotective activity.[P153]

COMPOUNDS REPORTED

Unusual pentacyclic triterpenes such as calotropis triterpene 1 have been isolated from root bark.[P154] Cardenolides such as ascleposide[P26] and flavonoids such as rutin occur in the entire plant.[P155]

Ascleposide

Rutin

19 *Cannabis sativa* CANNABACEAE

Native to Central Asia

Common names Hemp, Marijuana • **Local names** Mbangi (Swa.), Ganja / Hashish (Guj., Hind.), Bhang / Ganja / Hashish (Urd.)

Description and ecology

Erect, predominantly dioecious, annual herb with male and female flowers on separate plants, 1–5m high, with stems smooth and hollow. **Leaves** soft, palmately compound, divided into 5–7 leaflets with toothed edges. **Flowers** both male and female flowers are greenish yellow, inconspicuous, in terminal clusters. **Fruit** a black-brown achene, oval, 1.5–4mm long. This is a well-known narcotic plant (one that alters normal mental function and induces sleepiness) whose cultivation and trade is illegal in many countries and strictly regulated in others. *C. sativa* grows as a weed along roadsides and also in abandoned fields and gardens.

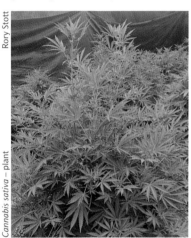

Rory Stott

Cannabis sativa – plant

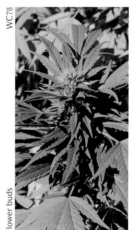

WC78

Flower buds

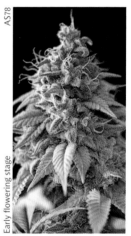

AS78

Early flowering stage

USAGE AND TREATMENT

PARTS USED Leaves, flowers and seeds.

TRADITIONAL MEDICINAL USES Marijuana can be used to treat vomiting and nausea in cancer patients after chemotherapy and to boost appetite and energy in AIDS patients.[M2, M6, M127] It can reduce chronic pain and muscle spasms.[M127] It can also help to ease neuralgic and rheumatic pain[M6, M9, M25] and may help to treat asthma, depression, psychotic crying,[M6, M70] glaucoma and spasmodic cough.[M25] A tea made from the seeds may decrease levels of cholesterol in the blood.[M7, M9] Leaves may help to relieve pain or swelling of the testicles and soothe earache; use of the plant may inhibit malarial fever.[M7] This plant produces a peculiar intoxication that enhances appetite, sleep and relaxation, while reducing stress.[M7, M70] As with other intoxicants, its prolonged use is harmful, resulting in appetite loss, insomnia and a deterioration of mental function, sometimes leading to insanity.[M7, M70]

NOTE In East Africa, marijuana is not widely used medicinally. The smoking of hashish, though illegal, is a common practice and the plant is also widely used as an ingredient in many of the region's illegal alcoholic brews.

PREPARATION AND DOSAGE

DEPRESSION, APPETITE LOSS, NAUSEA AND EXTREME PAIN IN CANCER AND AIDS SUFFERERS Dry some flowering heads of a female plant (easy to identify by the stigmas in the flowers). Roll the flowerheads into a cigarette. Depending on the pain, smoke one or two of the cigarettes daily; the effect can be immediate and will last for 3 or 4 hours. **(Before embarking on this course, be sure to obtain the health authorities' official permission. It will require a doctor's prescription as proof that the treatment is strictly for medicinal purposes.)** Alternatively, *Cannabis* tea can be prepared by adding a tablespoon of dry seed powder to a cup of warm boiled water and then steeping it for 10–15 minutes. Drink 2 or 3 cups of this infusion daily. It may take about an hour for this preparation to take effect but once it does, the results will last for 7–8 hours.

NEURALGIC AND RHEUMATIC PAIN Add a tablespoon of dried flower and leaf powder to half a litre of 50% alcohol in a sealed glass bottle. Leave for 4 or 5 days, shaking the bottle periodically. Rub 15–20 drops of the mixture as a massage lotion on the affected areas of the body.

 WARNING! The prolonged, habitual smoking of hashish can cause memory loss and atrophy of the genital organs, resulting in sterility and impotence. Its regular intake in high doses, while inducing a state of euphoria, can cause hallucinations, senselessness and, ultimately, insanity. The extent of the mental suffering resulting from prolonged misuse is well documented.

PHARMACOLOGY AND CHEMISTRY

PHARMACOLOGICAL PROPERTIES

Antispasmodic, analgesic, narcotic and cerebral sedative effects are reported for this plant,[P156] whose tetrahydrocannabinols (THC) act as a bronchodilator, increasing hypotension and decreasing intra-ocular pressure.[P96] THCs strongly affect the central nervous system[P84] (despite having a low toxicity), causing slowed speech, co-ordination problems, euphoria, relaxation, laziness, sleepiness, low motivation or the complete loss of motivation if used to excess.[P84, P156] One of the main uses of *Cannabis* is relief from chronic pain. Other uses include the antitumour effect of cannabinoids, which also have a potentially therapeutic effect in patients with irritable bowel syndrome (IBS).[P157]

COMPOUNDS REPORTED

Chemical compounds found in *Cannabis* include phenolic terpenoids, notably cannabinoids[P156] (e.g. cannabinol), which are the major active components in leaves and flowers.[P96] The fruits, seeds and stems do not contain cannabinol.[P84, P96] The principal psychotropic compounds are the 'tetrahydrocannabinols' found mainly in the bracts and in resin produced by the glands of the female flowers.[P84, P156]

Tetrahydrocannabinol (THC)

Cannabinol

20 *Capsicum frutescens* SOLANACEAE

Native to South and Central America

Common names Chilli Pepper, Hot Red Pepper, Hot Green Pepper • **Local names** Pili-pili (Swa.), Lal-mirch / Hari-mirch (Hind., Urd.), Lal-mirchi / Hari-mirchi (Punj.)

Description and ecology

Small, much-branched perennial plant 1–2m tall. Stems erect, usually zigzagging, angular, becoming woody near the base. **Leaves** dark green, linear or oblong,1.3–5(–12)cm long, veins prominent, tip pointed, margin entire. **Flowers** star-shaped, white or pale green, 2–4 flowers per branch or leaf axil. **Fruits** smooth, ovoid to narrowly conical, elongated berries, 8–20 × 3–6mm, variable in shape, green when young, turning bright red or occasionally orange when fully ripe. **Seeds** yellow to orange-yellow, ovoid, 3–3.5 × 2–3mm, with thickened margin. Cultivated as a vegetable or spice in almost all tropical and warm countries. Hot red pepper, also known as chilli pepper, is historically one of the most widely used spices on the Indian subcontinent, in China and the Far East. Today its popularity is universal. Grows in rich, well-drained soils from very low to very high altitudes.

USAGE AND TREATMENT

PARTS USED Fruits and leaves.
TRADITIONAL MEDICINAL USES The fruit is taken with food as a remedy for nausea, bloated stomach, lack of appetite and indigestion.[M70, M79] Hot peppers boost production of gastric and intestinal juices, thus enhancing the digestive functions.[M9, M70, M79] They are also used in treatments for toothache, stomach ache, rheumatism, lumbago, arthritis, muscular pain, numbness, leg pain, sciatica, sprains and a stiff neck.[M6, M9] The bell or sweet pepper or paprika (*C. annuum*) has laxative and antiflatulent properties and can be used in the treatment of diabetes and obesity.[M9, M70] Hot peppers are used locally to treat skin diseases. Decoctions of leaves and hot green fruits can be an effective treatment for schistosomiasis.[M9, M70] According to Indian herbalists, consumption of peppers in the daily diet prevents heart attacks. Applied to wounds, hot peppers are thought to boost the healing process, even to the extent of neutralising poisons in the bites of infected dogs and other animals.[M7] Hot peppers are also used to relieve earache and migraine.[M70]

PREPARATION AND DOSAGE
RHEUMATISM, LUMBAGO, ARTHRITIS, MUSCULAR PAIN, NUMBNESS, LEG PAIN, SCIATICA, SPRAINS AND A STIFF NECK Prepare either a chilli ointment or chilli oil. Add a teaspoon of finely ground dry chilli powder or pounded fresh green chilli to 50g of clear butter or ghee (to make the ointment) or to a teaspoon of vegetable oil (to make the oil). Mix thoroughly. Rub vigorously on affected areas 2 or 3 times a day. Keep the affected areas warm between massages.
SKIN AILMENTS, HERPES ZOSTER (SHINGLES) Apply chilli oil or chilli ointment (prepared as in the treatment above) directly to the affected areas.
FLATULENCE, OBESITY, DIABETES AND AS A LAXATIVE Eat sweet pepper (paprika) either raw or roasted (but do not fry).

 WARNING! People with abdominal ulcers, gastritis, colitis and haemorrhoids should avoid eating hot pepper, as should women suffering from cystitis and men with prostate problems, as it can cause inflammation of the urinary bladder. After handling hot chillies, always wash hands thoroughly. Prevent hot chillies from coming into contact with the eyes, nose, anus or with open wounds. Eat hot pepper sparingly in meals; excessive intake can cause anal inflammation and irritation during bowel movement.

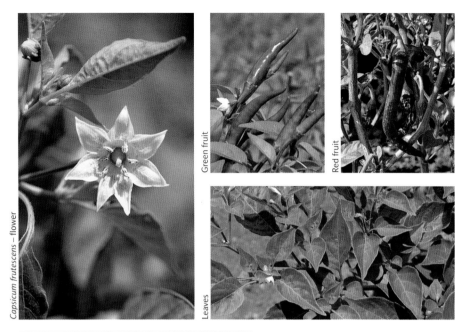

Capsicum frutescens – flower

Green fruit

Red fruit

Leaves

PHARMACOLOGY AND CHEMISTRY

PHARMACOLOGICAL PROPERTIES

As sweet peppers contain carotene (provitamin A) and are low in carbohydrates and fats, they are recommended for diabetic and obese patients.[P156] Hot chilli peppers have rubefacient (irritation of the skin and mucous membranes) and revulsive properties, which help reduce congestion among internal organs and tissues, providing relief from muscular aches, sprains, arthritis, lumbago and rheumatism.[P156] People who consumed fresh chilli peppers were indicated to be less likely to die of cancer or diabetes.[P158]

COMPOUNDS REPORTED

The pungency of *Capsicum* fruits is due to alkaloid capsaicinoids of which capsaicin is the most prevalent. The other members of this group are dihydrocapsaicin, norcapsaicin, nordihydrocapsaicin, nornordihydrocapsaicin, homocapsaicin and homodihydrocapsaicin;[P156, P158, P159] capsaicin is present in higher concentrations in hot peppers.[P159] Capsaicin was suggested to play a potential role in management of cardiometabolic diseases such as obesity, hypertension, dyslipidemia, diabetes and atherosclerosis.[P158] It also provides pain relief, gastrointestinal protection and antioxidant properties such as antitumour, anticancer and anti-inflammatory effects.[P160] Carotene and vitamins, especially vitamin C and palmitic acid,[P159] also occur in species of *Capsicum*.

Capsaicin

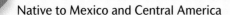

21 *Carica papaya*   CARICACEAE

Native to Mexico and Central America

Common names Paw-paw Tree, Papaya • **Local names** Mpapai (Swa.), Papaali (Lug.), Mupapaali (Luso.), Papai (Guj.), Papita (Urd., Hind.)

Description and ecology

Fast-growing evergreen tree reaching 3–10m, usually with only one trunk. Trunk or stem hollow, cylindrical, 10–30cm in diameter, with soft fibrous wood, narrowing to a crown of leaves. **Bark** pale grey, smooth, well marked with leaf scars. **Leaves** simple, spirally arranged, clustered towards the top of the trunk, deeply 7-lobed, blade large, 50–80cm in diameter, prominently veined, lobes deeply and broadly toothed. The species is dioecious, the male and female flowers typically on separate trees, but cultivars are bisexual. **Flowers** small, creamy white, about 2cm long, tubular or funnel-shaped, sweetly scented, solitary or clustered, borne in the leaf axils. **Fruit** a large, fleshy, hollow berry, green at first, turning yellow or orange when ripe, round to oval, containing sweet edible flesh, bearing several black seeds. Cultivated in all wetter areas of the tropics. Naturalised and well established throughout East Africa, growing best at altitudes below 1,500m.

USAGE AND TREATMENT

PARTS USED Leaves, roots, flowers, seeds, ripe and unripe fruits.
TRADITIONAL MEDICINAL USES A veritable pharmacy unto itself, the paw-paw is widely used medicinally in Africa, as it is throughout the world. It has been used to treat worms and amoebic dysentery.[M6, M70] Leaves and especially unripe fruit have been used to treat coughs, constipation, indigestion, malaria, high blood pressure, diarrhoea, yellow fever, asthma, bronchitis, hepatitis, gonorrhoea and urinary tract infections.[M6, M80] The juice or latex of unripe fruit may help infected wounds, boils, ulcers, cancerous tumours, burns and fungal infections.[M10, M112] Juice of the fruit has been used to dissolve warts.[M80] A hot-water extract of young green fruit latex may have a strong laxative effect [M9, M70] and has been used as an anthelmintic[M24] and a children's vermifuge.[M80] The seeds can act as a gentle purgative to rid the body of worms.[M112] Immature seeds are swallowed to treat diarrhoea.[M80] Ripe fruits, rich in vitamins A, B and C,[M9, M6] are recommended for colitis and chronic constipation.[M9, M10] Decoctions of roots and/or seeds may be taken orally as an anthelmintic,[M10] while a hot-water extract of unripe fruit juice or leaves has been taken as an abortifacient.[M10] Leaves and seeds are used as a vermifuge for tapeworms and roundworms.[M80] Juice of the fruit has been used to treat diabetes and hypertension.[M112] The ripe fruit is said to be a mild laxative, and a decoction of ripe fruit has been used to treat persistent diarrhoea and dysentery in children.[M112]

PREPARATION AND DOSAGE
ANTHELMINTIC AND VERMIFUGE (AGAINST INTESTINAL PARASITES) Latex (sap) can be harvested from unripe fruits by making incisions in the fruits while still hanging on the tree. Latex can also be taken from the tree trunks. Add a teaspoon of latex, half a teaspoon of juice from freshly ground leaf tissue and a tablespoon of pure honey to half a cup of hot water. Leave to cool and then drink this mixture at breakfast in the morning or on an empty stomach. After 2 hours, swallow a tablespoon of castor oil to complete the treatment – and eliminate intestinal parasites, including both tapeworm and hookworm. Alternatively, add 30g of powder made by grinding some fresh leaves to a litre of water, and drink 2 or 3 cups of this infusion daily for 2 days.
INDIGESTION, CHRONIC CONSTIPATION AND ULCEROUS COLITIS After meals, swallow a few drops of paw-paw sap or chew on pieces of a leaf or 3 or 4 seeds. Eating the fresh ripe fruits can normalise the digestive process, restoring regular intestinal function in cases of chronic constipation.

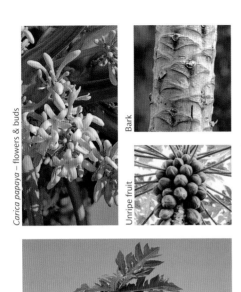

Carica papaya – flowers & buds

Bark

Unripe fruit

Leaves

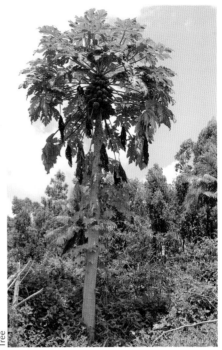

Tree

AMOEBIC DYSENTERY Chew on a piece of paw-paw leaf (5 × 5cm) once a day or on a tablespoon of dried seed powder until symptoms abate. For severe dysentery, boil a handful of paw-paw leaves together with a handful each of young green mango leaves and guava leaves in a litre of water for 15 minutes. Filter and sip portions of the mixture at intervals through the day. For mild dysentery, immerse a handful of paw-paw leaves or roots in a litre of water and boil for 5–10 minutes. Leave to cool, then filter and drink in small quantities through the day. An alternative for mild cases is to chew a teaspoon of fresh paw-paw seeds 3 times a day for 5 or 6 days. Quantities should be halved in doses administered to children.

INFECTED WOUNDS, OPEN BOILS AND SUPPURATING BURNS Add a tablespoon of paw-paw sap or latex, harvested from fresh, unripe, hanging fruits, to half a litre of cool, boiled water. Use this several times a day to wash burns or to clean wounds and open sores. Make sure that all cutting, measuring and stirring instruments are clean, sterile and rust free. To treat infected wounds, add 100ml of 70% denatured alcohol (or tincture) to 10g of dried leaf powder in a sterilised glass bottle sealed with a cork. After a week, press and filter the mixture. Apply to the wound at intervals during the day.

MALARIA Add a handful of fresh paw-paw leaves to a litre of hot, boiled water. Leave for 15 minutes to cool, then filter. Drink at intervals during the day. Children should consume only half of the adult dose.

COUGHS, BRONCHITIS AND ASTHMA To soothe persistent coughs, boil a handful of fresh paw-paw roots for 15 minutes in a litre of water. Filter. Adults should drink a cup of this decoction 3 times daily. For children aged 1–4 years, the dose is a quarter of a cup, and for children aged over 5, half a cup. To treat asthmatic attacks, the young dried leaves can be smoked in a pipe or rolled into a cigarette and either smoked or left to burn beside the sufferer's bed so that the smoke can be inhaled.

LIVER DISEASES, HEPATITIS, JAUNDICE AND YELLOW FEVER Add a handful of male flowers or bark to a litre of boiled water and steep for 15–20 minutes. Drink this decoction for 3 or 4 days. Alternatively, boil a handful of paw-paw roots in a litre of water for 10–15 minutes, leave to cool, then drink the decoction at intervals during the day. Eaten regularly as a vegetable, the cooked unripe fruits will help to normalise liver function. Ripe fruit, eaten regularly, can also help to rectify cases of enlarged liver or spleen. A daily intake of one or two slices of unripe fruit, left to stand in vinegar for 8–10 days, can also be effective.

FUNGAL INFECTIONS (RINGWORM) Add half a teaspoon of latex or sap to a tablespoon of vegetable or olive oil. Mix thoroughly. Rub the mixture onto affected areas of the skin 3 times daily. Prepare a fresh mixture every time. Alternatively, add 10 drops of fresh paw-paw latex and a tablespoon of olive or vegetable oil to a handful of freshly ground *Senna alata* leaves. Mix thoroughly, and apply 3 times daily for 3 or 4 days.

GONORRHOEA AND URINARY INFECTIONS Dry some paw-paw seeds either out in the sun or in an oven at low heat. Crush the dry seeds into a fine powder. Then take a tablespoon of this powder 3 times daily for 6–12 days.

 WARNING! Pregnant women should avoid using paw-paw in oral or internal treatments. Papain may cause stomach ache. Care should be taken to ensure that raw paw-paw latex does not come into contact with the eyes. Only small doses should be given to children, in accordance with their age.

PHARMACOLOGY AND CHEMISTRY

PHARMACOLOGICAL PROPERTIES

All parts of the papaya, including leaves, latex, seeds of ripe fruits and the pulp of unripe fruits, contain papain, a protein-splitting enzyme known primarily as a worm killer.[P84] All contain several active compounds of proven medicinal value, such as flavonoids, antibiotics, fungicides and enzymes.[P161] The juice or latex has shown antioxidant and antimicrobial activities.[P162] In fresh unripe fruits, anti-ulcer effects are documented.[P162] Rich in vitamins A and C, ripe paw-paw helps digestion and normalises intestinal function.[P84]

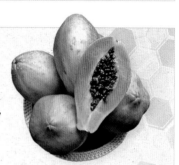

Ripe fruit and seeds

COMPOUNDS REPORTED

Papaya seed oil contains lipids, including arachidic acid and eicosatetraenoic acid.[P163] Ascorbic acid (vitamin C) has been isolated from the fruits.[P164] Steroids such as 5-dehydroavenasterol[P165] have also been identified in the fruits. The latex of the fruit and leaves contains the enzyme papain.[P84] Oleic acid was identified as the antipathogenic drug against *Klebsiella* PKBSG14.[P166]

Ascorbic acid

Oleic acid

Indigenous

Common names Bush Plum, Simple-spined Carissa • **Local names** Mulimuli (Bon.), Dagams (Bor.), Mtambuu (Dig.), Mukawa (Emb., Mbe.), Mtandambo (Gir.), Mukawa (Kam., Kik.), Ochuoga (Luo), Legetiet (Kip.), Omonyangateti (Kis.), Shikata / Kumurwa / Sirwa (Luh.), Olamuriaki (Maa.), Kamuria / Nkawa mwimbi (Mer.), Legetetuet (Nan.), Lakatetwa / Lokotetwo (Pok.), Godhoom boor (Ren.), Lamuriai (Sam.), Mtandamboo (Swa.), Kirumba / Kirimba (Tai.), Legetetwa / Legetetik (Tug.), Ekamuria (Tur.), Manka (Chag.), Muyanza / Muyonza (Haya), Mfubeli (Nyam.), Mchofwe (Pare), Mkabaku (Ran.), Mfumba / Mkumbaku (Samb.), Emuriai (Ate.), Muyonza / Nyonza (Lug.), Achuga (Luo-A, Luo-L), Muyonza (Ruki.), Muyonza (Runy.)

Description and ecology

Spiny, much-branched, multi-stemmed, evergreen shrub or small tree 1–6m tall, adopting a scrambling habit, young branches green, smooth, covered with hairs. **Bark** dark grey, smooth, with paired, straight, woody spines that are up to 5cm long and sometimes forked. **Leaves** simple, opposite, leathery, dark glossy green above, pale green below, with or without hairs, base rounded, apex pointed, margin smooth, the short leaf stalk up to 5mm long. **Flowers** reddish pink outside, white inside when open, highly scented, in terminal clusters. **Fruits** fleshy berries, round or ellipsoid, 0.6–1.5cm in diameter, green often tinged red or purple, but turning dark purple (almost black) and glossy when ripe, then sweet and edible, 2–4-seeded. Widespread in bushland and thickets, often in riverine vegetation or on termite mounds and in dry forest edges, at 0–2,500m. In common use as a medicinal plant throughout East Africa.

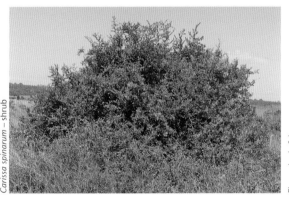

Carissa spinarum – shrub

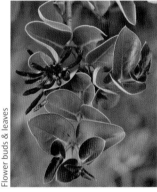

Flower buds & leaves

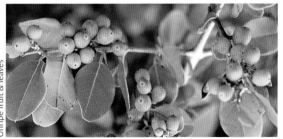

Unripe fruit & leaves

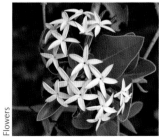

Flowers

PARTS USED Roots, bark, leaves, twigs and fruits.

TRADITIONAL MEDICINAL USES Decoctions of roots are taken as a painkiller and to treat malaria,[M4, M70, M81, M82] headache, indigestion[M81] and fever in children.[M3] Ripe fruits are used to treat both dysentery and gastrointestinal complaints.[M28, M81] Root decoctions are taken orally for chronic chest pain and as a remedy for coughs,[M1, M3, M81, M112] lower abdominal pain, back pain, indigestion, swollen glands and diarrhoea, as well as for strengthening the bones, as an astringent[M29, M70, M82] and health drink for general fitness, as a snake repellent and as a treatment for both malaria and dysentery. Infusions of dried leaves are taken orally to control diabetes.[M70] Decoctions of dried roots are sometimes mixed with paw-paw and taken orally to treat venereal diseases, especially gonorrhoea, and also for stomach ailments.[M26, M27, M70, M82] A root infusion is drunk to ease stomach ache and as a cough remedy, and also used as eyedrops for cataract problems.[M81] This plant has been used successfully in treating herpes simplex virus.[M81]

PREPARATION AND DOSAGE

MALARIA, FEVER, STOMACH ACHE, HEADACHE, BACK AND OTHER BODY PAINS Dig out and wash a handful of fresh roots. Boil in a litre of water for 15 minutes. Drink small quantities of this decoction while it is still warm at intervals during the day and before going to bed.

INDIGESTION, DYSENTERY AND GASTROINTESTINAL AILMENTS Wash some ripe fruits in water and eat fresh, 5 or 6 fruits at a time, 3 times a day.

PHARMACOLOGICAL PROPERTIES

Dried leaf extracts have shown antihyperglycaemic activity.[P167] Studies of dried roots have recorded weak antibacterial activity.[P168] Stem extracts have produced antischistosomal activity.[P169] Stems of *Carissa spinarum* have shown activity against herpes simplex viruses (HSV I and II).[P172, P173]

COMPOUNDS REPORTED

Several compounds are reported, particularly from the roots. These include lignans (e.g. carissanol),[P170, P173] benzenoids (e.g. 2-hydroxyacetophenone)[P171] and sesquiterpenes (e.g. carissone).[P171, P173] Phytochemical investigation[P172] of the stems of *C. spinarum* led to the isolation of 12 compounds: a coumarin, two cardiac glycosides and nine lignans. These compounds were tested[P172] for bioactivities, and the cardiac glycoside evomonoside showed moderate activity against herpes simplex virus types I and II, while cytotoxicity was observed for the lignans (-)-carinol, (-)-carissanol and (-)-nortrachelogenin against breast (MCF7) and lung (A549) cancer cells.

Carissanol

Carissone

a. *Cassia abbreviata*
Indigenous

Common names Long-pod Cassia, Long-tail Cassia • **Local names** Kang (Bon.), Rabiya (Bor.), Muhumba mkulu (Dig., Gir.), Mualandathe / Kyathandathe / Malandesi (Kam.), Domader / Domaderi / Rabuya (Som.), Mbaraka (Swa.), Msoko / Mkangu (Tai.), Mulimuli (Gogo, Hehe), Mulundalunda / Munzoka (Nyam.), Mzangazi (Samb.), Nundalunda (Suk.)

Description and ecology
Deciduous shrub or small, much-branched tree 4–6(–8)m tall, with a rounded, open crown. **Bark** reddish when young, becoming brown or blackish and cracked with age. **Leaves** compound, with 7–12 pairs of oblong leaflets, each 4–6cm long, tips rounded, young leaflets hairy on undersurface. **Flowers** yellow, in heads of up to 9cm, usually on bare tree. **Fruits** brown-black cylindrical pods, 30–90cm long, thick, cylindrical, hairy or non-hairy, indehiscent. **Seeds** numerous, 9–12 × 8–9mm, brown to blackish. Common in coastal areas and dry thorn bush, especially *Acacia–Commiphora* bushland, but also grows in woodland and wooded grasslands, at 50–1,500m.

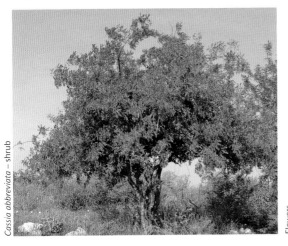
Cassia abbreviata – shrub

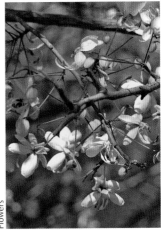
Flowers

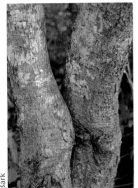
Bark

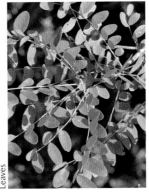
Leaves

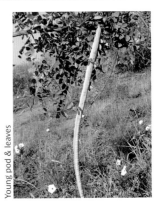
Young pod & leaves

PARTS USED Leaves, roots and stem bark.

TRADITIONAL MEDICINAL USES Decoctions of leaves, roots and bark are used to treat stomach disorders.[M33, M70] A decoction of stem bark can be used as a purgative and a treatment for malaria and diarrhoea.[M112, M115] Powdered stem bark is applied to abscesses.[M83] A root infusion may be used as an eyewash to soothe eye inflammation (ophthalmia).[M83] Root decoctions are taken for relief from pneumonia and other chest complaints and for treating malaria[M112, M115] as well as for afflictions of the uterus and fungal ailments. Roots are chewed, producing a juice said to be a remedy for gonorrhoea and syphilis.[M1, M4, M70] Fresh roots are chewed and swallowed to relieve toothache. Root decoctions or dried powdered roots in water are taken as a purgative, stomachic, aphrodisiac, abortifacient and vermifuge[M112, M115] and are also taken to treat pneumonia, schistosomiasis and heavy menstruation.[M83, M112, M115]

PREPARATION AND DOSAGE

STOMACH PROBLEMS AND CONSTIPATION Add a teaspoon of dried leaf powder or root bark to a cup of boiling water. Leave for 15 minutes and filter. Drink just before going to bed; the mixture will take effect after 8–10 hours. Drink plenty of water at the same time so as to avoid becoming dehydrated.

FUNGAL INFECTIONS AND OTHER SKIN DISEASES Crush a handful of fresh leaves and apply the pounded leaves to affected areas 2 or 3 times daily. Pound new leaves for the treatments on each successive day.

INFLAMMATION IN THE EYE (OPHTHALMIA) Wash, then pound and mix fresh roots in a glass of water. Let it stand for 30 minutes. Stir the mixture, sieve it and wash the infected eye.

b. *Cassia alata* (*Senna alata*)

Native to South America

Common names Candle Bush, Candlestick Cassia, Ringworm Shrub, Ringworm Bush

Description and ecology

Attractive multi-stemmed, deciduous shrub 3–4m tall. **Bark** dark brown, woody, branches greenish brown, finely ribbed. **Leaves** paripinnately compound, large, up to 75cm long, leaflets about 12 pairs, 6–11cm long, oblong or obovate, bases and apices rounded, hairless above, with few hairs below. **Flowers** golden yellow with darker veins, in erect, axillary, candle-like spikes up to 25cm long. **Fruits** long, boat-shaped pods, 6–16cm long, green when young but dark brown to black when dry, splitting open on the plant releasing numerous brown, pointed seeds. Commonly found on lakeshores, near riverine areas and as a weed on cultivated land, at 0–1,200m.

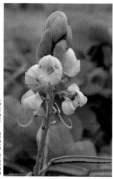
Cassia alata – flower

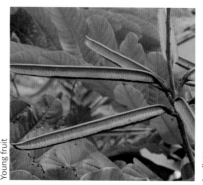
Young fruit

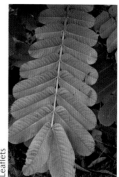
Leaflets

PARTS USED Leaves and roots.
TRADITIONAL MEDICINAL USES Leaves and roots are used to treat various fungal infections (notably ringworm),[M4, M6, M70, M115] impetigo, scabies,[M6] leprosy and eczema.[M10] Decoctions of leaves are used as an anthelmintic and as a laxative for relief from constipation.[M10, M70, M115] The disinfectant function of leaf decoctions in the treatment of infected wounds is well documented.[M6] Skin problems treated with *Cassia alata* include ringworm, impetigo, syphilis sores, psoriasis, herpes, scabies, rash and itching. Skin problems are most often treated by applying leaf sap or by rubbing fresh leaves on the skin.[M115]

PREPARATION AND DOSAGE
FUNGAL INFECTIONS, RINGWORM, IMPETIGO, SCABIES AND PSORIASIS Grind a handful of fresh leaves. Apply directly to the skin or mix with castor, palm or vegetable oil and rub on the affected areas 2 or 3 times daily. Use newly picked leaves every time. Add 8–10 drops of fresh latex from an unripe paw-paw when treating fungal infections or impetigo.
STOMACH PROBLEMS, CONSTIPATION, LAXATIVE AND ANTHELMINTIC USE Add a teaspoon of mixed dry leaf and root bark powder to a cup of boiling water. Leave for 15 minutes, then filter. Drink before going to bed; the mixture will take effect after 8–10 hours.
INFECTED WOUNDS Dry some fresh leaves and pound them into a fine powder. Add a cup of this powder to a 50% alcohol solution in a sterilised glass bottle. Leave for a week. Sieve and apply as a wound disinfectant. For larger, more severe wounds, seek treatment at a hospital.

c. *Cassia didymobotrya (Senna didymobotrya)* — Indigenous

Common names African Senna, Candle Bush, Peanut-butter Cassia, Wild Senna • **Local names** Ithaa / Inyumganai (Kam.), Mwino / Mwinu (Kik.), Senetwet (Kip., Nan., Mar.), Luvino / Lubino (Luh.), Ovino / Owinu (Luo), Osenetoi (Maa.), Kirao / Murao (Mer.), Mbinu / Mshua (Tai.), Senetiet (Tug.), Lakera (Ach.), Mukyula (Lug.), Mubenobeno / Kebenobeno (Lugi.), Mugabagaba (Runyan.), Senetwa (Sebei)

Description and ecology

Hardy, deciduous, multi-stemmed, bushy shrub 1–6m tall, young stems hairy. **Leaves** spirally arranged, compound, with 8–16 pairs of leaflets, each 6.5cm long, elongated oval in shape, apices rounded or obtuse. **Flowers** bright yellow or orange, on candle-like axillary raceme 10–30cm long, open flowers on the lower part and unopened buds at the tip of the raceme. **Fruit** a flat brown legume pod, oblong, linear or slightly curved, 8–12 × 2cm, splitting open on the plant to release numerous oblong, blackish-brown seeds. Confined to lowland scrub, woodlands, evergreen thickets, often to riparian edges along lakeshore and riverine areas and to forest edges in wetter areas of East Africa, at 700–2,100m.

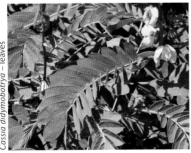

Cassia didymobotrya – leaves

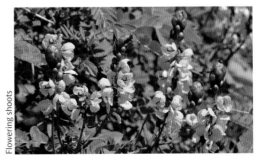

Flowering shoots

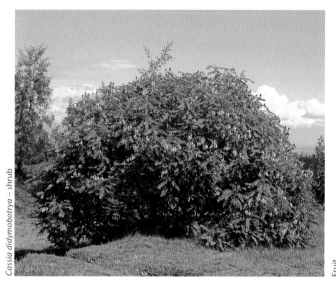

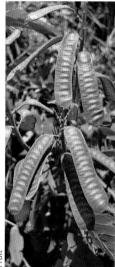

Cassia didymobotrya – shrub

Fruit

USAGE AND TREATMENT

PARTS USED Leaves, stems and roots.

TRADITIONAL MEDICINAL USES Leaf infusions or decoctions are used as an emetic in treating malaria; the stems and roots are also used in malaria treatments.[M4, M70] Decoctions of leaves, stems and roots are taken as a laxative or purgative for the treatment of abdominal pain, while large quantities are taken as an emetic.[M84, M115] Such decoctions are also used as a remedy for gonorrhoea and can relieve backache in women.[M1, M70] An infusion of roots is drunk to treat diarrhoea.[M84] Roots are used as an antidote to general poisoning. A warm leaf mixture is applied to the skin of people suffering from measles and is also taken orally for stomach disorders.[M70] Decoctions of roots and leaves are given to people suffering from headache, fever and excessive bile,[M4, M70] **but these remedies are always administered with caution**. A root decoction is drunk for the treatment of malaria, other fevers and jaundice.[M84, M115] A decoction of leaves, either on its own or in mixtures, can be used to treat external parasites such as ticks. Leaves and young stems are pounded to a pulp and applied to the skin to treat skin diseases, ringworm, itching, abscesses, sores and venereal diseases.[M115]

PREPARATION AND DOSAGE

FEVER AND MALARIA Add some crushed fresh leaves to a pot of boiling water. The inhaled steam acts as a vapour bath for relieving the symptoms of high fever.

STOMACH DISORDERS, LAXATIVE AND PURGATIVE USE Add a teaspoon of mixed dry leaf, stem and root powder to a cup of boiling water. Leave for 15 minutes and then filter. Drink before going to bed; the mixture will take effect in 8–10 hours. Drink plenty of water at the same time to avoid becoming dehydrated.

NOTE Other treatments are similar to those outlined for *C. abbreviata* (page 87), *C. alata* (page 88) and *C. occidentalis* (page 91).

> ⚠ **WARNING!** *Cassia didymobotrya*, like other species of *Cassia* (*Senna*), is poisonous. Decoctions from all plant parts can cause violent vomiting and diarrhoea and may be fatal. It is recommended that pregnant women and children take only a small dose.

d. *Cassia occidentalis* *(Senna occidentalis)* Indigenous

Common names Stinkingweed, Coffeeweed, Coffee Senna • **Local names** Mwengajini (Swa.), Inglatiang' (Luo), Segusse (Suk.), Imindi (Luny.)

Description and ecology
Erect, unarmed annual herb up to 0.5m high, sometimes a slightly woody undershrub reaching 2m, but usually smaller. Stem angled, branched, greyish black, slightly hairy. **Leaves** alternate, compound, with 3–7 pairs of leaflets that are ovate-oblong, sometimes lanceolate, 2–10cm long, non-hairy. **Flowers** yellow, in short racemes from upper axils. **Fruit** pods narrow, semi-flattened, woody, straight or slightly recurved, green at first, turning dark brown with pale margins, subcompressed, dehiscent, subglabrous, 20–40-seeded. **Seeds** flattened, 3–5mm in diameter, olive-brown. A common weed of cultivation, roadsides, pastures and waste ground near villages and buildings, this plant is also found in grassland and on lakeshores, at 0–1,200m.

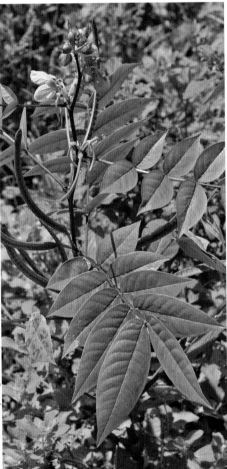

Cassia occidentalis – young flowering plant

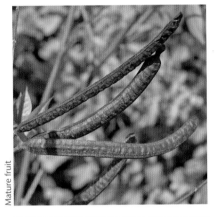

Mature fruit

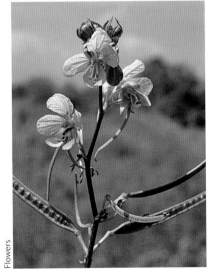

Flowers

PARTS USED Leaves, roots and seeds.

TRADITIONAL MEDICINAL USES Leaf decoctions are used in the treatment of constipation, haemorrhoids[M6, M70] and fever, including malaria. Leaf and root decoctions are taken for oedema. Fresh leaves are used in treatments for fungal diseases,[M6, M112] inflammation and swellings, bruises, furuncles and sprains. Root decoctions are taken as a remedy for convulsions, palpitations and ophthalmia, while also serving as a purgative, an anthelmintic and abortifacient, a remedy for postpartum problems, a treatment for oedema, colds and abdominal pain,[M34] and for a hernia, dysmenorrhoea and sterility in women.[M35, M70] Infusions of roots are used for malaria, kidney disease, fatigue, indigestion, colic and stomach ache.[M23, M70] The seed is a febrifuge and sedative. An infusion is drunk to calm the nerves and as a treatment for kidney problems, haemorrhage, worms, and for cleaning the womb and Fallopian tubes.[M112] A decoction of boiled roots can be used to treat swollen testicles. Leaves are used in treatments for snakebite and kidney ailments. Seeds are consumed as a purgative and as a substitute for coffee. The entire dried plant may be used as a diuretic and for expelling intestinal parasites.

PREPARATION AND DOSAGE

PURGATIVE FOR CONSTIPATION AND OTHER STOMACH AILMENTS Add 3g of pounded fresh roots to half a litre of cold water. Stir the mixture and allow it to settle. The clear solution has a strong and very bitter taste and should be taken in doses of a tablespoon 3 times daily for relief from constipation-related stomach ache. Alternatively, boil a teaspoon of dried leaf powder in a cup of hot water. Leave for 15 minutes and filter. Drink before going to bed, also drinking plenty of water to avoid becoming dehydrated. For use as a purgative, crush a teaspoon of dry seeds and use it to prepare a coffee-like beverage, which can be drunk 2 or 3 times daily.

HAEMORRHOIDS Add a teaspoon of ground dry leaves to half a litre of boiling water. Filter after 15–20 minutes. Drink at intervals during the day.

FEVER AND MALARIA Add some crushed fresh leaves to a pot of boiling water. The inhaled steam acts as a vapour bath, relieving the symptoms of high fever.

INFLAMMATION, SWELLINGS, BRUISES, FURUNCLES, SPRAINS, FUNGAL INFECTIONS, RINGWORM, SCABIES AND PSORIASIS Apply a poultice of ground fresh leaves mixed with castor, palm or vegetable oil, or simply rub this mixture on affected areas of the skin 2 or 3 times daily. A handful of seeds, ground and mixed with vinegar, should be rubbed into the scalp for relief from head itching.

OEDEMA AND PALPITATIONS Add a tablespoon of dried leaf or root powder to a litre of water. Boil for 15 minutes. Filter and drink in small portions during the day. Add honey as a sweetener.

ANTHELMINTIC AND FOR DYSMENORRHOEA Boil 30–50g of ground roots in a litre of water until the liquid level is reduced to a third. Strain and sweeten with honey. Take 2 tablespoons 3 times a day with meals. Women suffering from painful menstruation should add a tablespoon of dried root powder to a litre of water, stir and leave for 20 minutes, then take the mixture twice a day starting 3 or 4 days before the anticipated onset of menstruation.

 WARNING! Women should avoid all internal use of *Cassia* (*Senna*) during lactation or pregnancy. Prolonged oral or internal use and excessive doses should be avoided as they may cause stomach pain, vomiting and diarrhoea.

PHARMACOLOGICAL PROPERTIES

Leaves and dried roots of *Cassia abbreviata* have shown antimalarial activity against multi-drug-resistant *Plasmodium falciparum*.[P174] Dried *C. abbreviata* roots show antibacterial activity against *Staphylococcus aureus* but show no activity against *Escherichia coli*.[P175] Extracts of dried aerial parts of *C. occidentalis* have shown weak antimalarial activity against *Plasmodium falciparum*.[P5] The best indication for an antispasmodic activity in roots of *C. occidentalis* is for dysmenorrhoea, which is usually caused by uterine spasms.[P84] Antifungal, antibacterial, anti-inflammatory, antihistamine, antispasmodic, analgesic and diuretic activities are all reported for *C. alata*.[P79]

COMPOUNDS REPORTED

C. abbreviata contains quinoids such as aloe-emodin[P176] in the flowers, and flavonoids, including (2R,3S)-guibourtinidiol, in the bark.[P177] Some parts of *C. alata* contain anthraquinones such as 5-hydroxy-2-methylanthraquinone, 1,5-dihydroxy-2-methylanthraquinone, chrysophanol, chrysophanol glucoside, sitosterol and tannin.[P79] Three new compounds along with 25 known compounds were isolated from roots and stems of *C. abbreviata*.[P178] Among these, the new compound cassiabrevone, which is a rare heterodimer, exhibited the most potent anti-HIV-1 activity with IC50 values of 11.89μM.[P178]

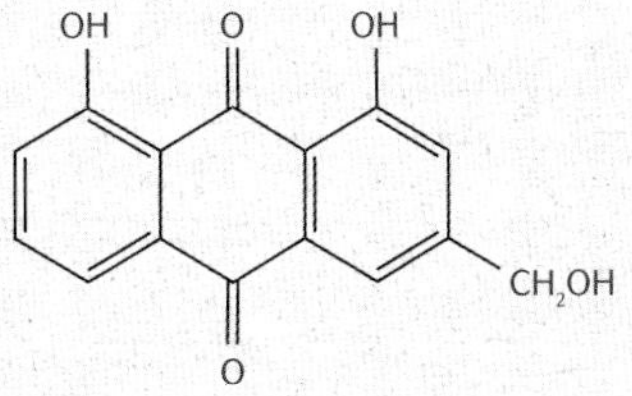

Aloe-emodin 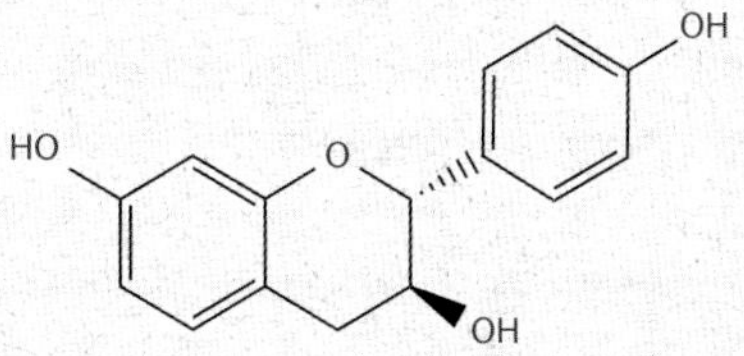   (2R,3S)-guibourtinidiol

Indigenous

Common names Miraa, Khat, Chat, Qat, Somali Tea, Abyssinian Tea • **Local names** Chai / Cati (Bor.), Miraa (Emb., Gir., Mer., Swa.Ken.), Mailyungi / Miungi (Kam.), Muirungi / Miirungi (Kik.), Tomoiyot (Kip.), Mairungi (Kis.), Ol-meraa (Maa.), Tumayot (Mar.), Mamiraa (Sam.), Quat / Chat / Jat (Som.), Wahawi (Goro.), Muhulo (Hehe), Morungi (Ran.), Mwandama (Samb.), Mrungi (Swa. Tan.), Muirungi (Ate.), Munyaga (Ruki.), Kitandwe / Lutandwe (Lugi.), Mutabungwa (Runyan.), Mutabungura (Runyar.), Tume-yondet (Sebei)

Description and ecology

Evergreen, multi-stemmed shrub 1–5m high or a tree growing to 10–12(–18)m, with dimorphic branching and a dense crown. **Bark** grey-green and smooth when young but becoming dark brown and flaking when old, young shoots green to red. **Leaves** simple, opposite, oblong to narrowly elliptic or obovate, 5–11cm long, with pointed apex and wavy margin, crimson-brown and glossy when young, becoming yellow-green and leathery with age. **Flowers** small, white to creamy yellow, borne in small axillary clusters (cymes). **Fruit** an oblong or ellipsoid, 3-lobed, woody capsule, 6–16 × 3–4mm, reddish brown when mature, with 1–3 seeds. Grows in moist upland forests, evergreen forests and their margins, in dry *Olea* and *Juniperus* forests, riverine forests and thickets in *Combretum* wooded grassland, at 1,200–2,400m.

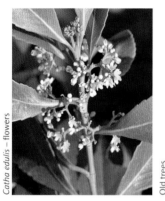

Catha edulis – flowers

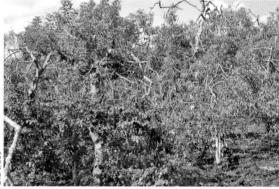

Old trees

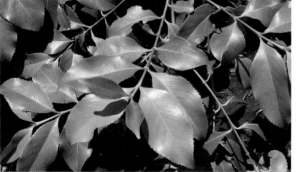

Mature & young leaves

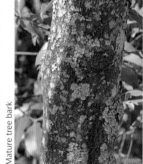

Mature tree bark

USAGE AND TREATMENT

PARTS USED Root, stem bark, young shoots and leaves.

TRADITIONAL MEDICINAL USES Decoctions of roots and stem bark are used in treatments for gonorrhoea.[M3, M70] Young leaves and shoots, and green bark are chewed as a stimulant and to allay hunger and prevent sleepiness[M1, M3, M70] as well as to treat malaria and coughs.[M1, M70] Both leaves and roots are used for influenza; the roots are used to soothe stomach ache as well. In South Africa, fresh leaves are used to relieve tiredness and to increase powers of mental concentration as well as to treat coughs, asthma and chest ailments.[M2, M70]

NOTE Chewing miraa or khat is an old tradition in African and Arab culture and probably originated in the Harar area of Ethiopia. Cultivation, sale, marketing and use of this plant is generally either prohibited or strictly regulated by law. Consumption induces mild euphoria and excitement, similar to the effects of strong coffee. Fresh young shoots with leaves are chewed daily as a stimulant in many communities, especially in Somalia and Meru and in some Swahili coastal areas and towns. It is particularly popular among drivers of long-haul trucks and lorries, who rely on its effects to stay awake and alert at the wheel. Chewing gum and miraa are normally masticated together, with large quantities of fluids (often soft drinks or spiced black tea) consumed during the chewing process. The leaves are used to make a strong beverage known as Somali or Abyssinian tea.

PREPARATION AND DOSAGE

GONORRHOEA Boil a handful of fresh stem bark in half a litre of water for 5–10 minutes. Drink a cup of the decoction as a tea twice a day.

MALARIA, CHEST AILMENTS (COUGHS, ASTHMA) AND FATIGUE Chew some fresh young shoots and leaves at intervals during the day for 2 days.

 WARNING! *Catha edulis* (miraa) should be used strictly for medicinal purposes only. Its prolonged use can trigger attitude and personality problems, often characterised by aggressive behaviour.

PHARMACOLOGY AND CHEMISTRY

PHARMACOLOGICAL PROPERTIES

The main effect of cathinone – the active principle in the plant – is the reduction of fatigue and tiredness in the body. Besides acting as a stimulant, cathinone has potentially harmful effects such as hypertension, anorexia, hyperthermia, arrhythmia and respiratory stimulation.[P179]

COMPOUNDS REPORTED

The stimulating properties of the plant may be a result of the many phenethylamines of which perhaps the main one is cathinone found in fresh leaves.[P180] In addition, alkaloids (dihydromyricetin), triterpenoids, monoterpenes and other compounds have also been reported.[P181] The flavonoids may possibly play a role in the antioxidant properties of miraa.[P181]

Cathinone

Dihydromyricetin

25 *Catharanthus roseus* APOCYNACEAE

Native to Madagascar

Common names Madagascar Periwinkle, Pink Periwinkle, Rose Periwinkle, Vinca •
Local names Maua (Luo), Vinka (Swa.)

Description and ecology

Erect, evergreen, much-branched undershrub or herbaceous plant up to 1m tall. Stems cylindrical, longitudinally ridged, green or dark red, hairy when young. **Leaves** opposite, dark green, glossy, with prominent midrib, elliptic-oblong, 2.5–9cm long, with short stalk 1–1.6cm long. **Flowers** pink with dark pink centre or white, axillary, borne in leaf axils, solitary or paired. **Fruits** two cylindrical follicles, 2–4cm long, green at first but turning brown when mature, dehiscent, 10–20-seeded. **Seeds** oblong, 2–3mm long, grooved at one side, black. This plant is salt tolerant and drought resistant but does not do well in severe heat. Widely grown as a garden plant in lowland, coastal and lake areas, but has become a weed along roadsides and on disturbed land in drier parts of East Africa, at 0–1,800m.

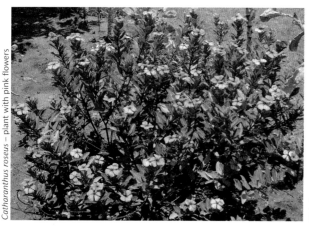

Catharanthus roseus – plant with pink flowers

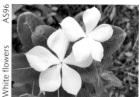

AS96

White flowers

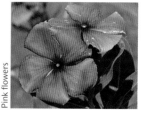

Pink flowers

USAGE AND TREATMENT

PARTS USED Whole plant (leaves, roots, branches and twigs).
TRADITIONAL MEDICINAL USES The leaves, dried or fresh, are used to treat diabetes, dysentery and leukaemia in children.[M6, M14, M70] Root and bark decoctions are used for treating high blood pressure. A root decoction is taken to treat dysmenorrhoea. A decoction of all parts of *Catharanthus roseus* is taken as treatment for malaria, dengue fever, diarrhoea, diabetes, cancer and skin diseases.[M85] Dried or fresh roots are a remedy for diabetes.[M10, M70] Extracts prepared from the leaves have been applied as antiseptic agents for the healing of wounds, against haemorrhage and skin rash, and as a mouthwash to treat toothache.[M85] The plant is used in different parts of Africa to treat gonorrhoea, diarrhoea and hepatitis. Leaves are used to heal wounds. In the *British Pharmacopoeia*, a tea made from leaves is registered as a diabetic medicine, and in France roots are used in an official drug for diabetes. In South Africa, the plant is used for treating diabetes and rheumatism.[M2, M70] Aerial parts are used to treat various forms of cancer, including breast and uterine cancer.[M2] Decoctions of aerial parts and roots are used as a menstrual regulator, and a decoction of dried roots is taken for fever and malaria.[M10, M70, M85] An infusion of leaves is taken to treat stomach ulcers.[M85]

PREPARATION AND DOSAGE

DIABETES, MALARIA AND DENGUE FEVER Steep a handful of fresh leaves, or 5g of dried leaf powder or 5g of fresh roots or dry root powder, in a litre of boiling water for 10–15 minutes. Filter and then drink in small quantities at intervals during the day. Alternatively, add 5g of dry leaf powder to a litre of cold boiled water, leave for 15 minutes, stirring intermittently, then filter and drink at intervals during the day. For children, maximum daily intake should be reduced to 500ml (for ages 10–12) and to only 200ml for children aged 2–4 years.

HIGH BLOOD PRESSURE Boil a teaspoon of pounded dry root bark in 2 cups of water for 10 minutes. Filter and drink before breakfast in the morning.

DYSENTERY (BACILLARY AND AMOEBIC) Make a tea from leaves or from dried leaf powder, following the same procedure and using the same dosages as for diabetes (above). In cases of severe amoebic dysentery, mix 4g of washed fresh leaves with 4g of fresh paw-paw leaves, 4g of fresh young mango leaves and 4g of fresh guava leaves. Boil in a litre of water for 15 minutes, then filter and sip at intervals during the day.

CANCER (LEUKAEMIA) Make a tea from leaves or from dried leaf powder, following the same procedure as for diabetes, malaria and dengue fever (above). Fresh leaves, boiled in water for a few minutes only and then pounded into a paste, can be applied externally to cancer-related wounds, along with the juice or latex of either unripe paw-paw or aloe leaves.

 WARNING! *Catharanthus roseus* should never be used during pregnancy. It is a poisonous plant, and overdosing and/or prolonged use can be harmful and may lower blood pressure and cause stomach ache.

PHARMACOLOGY AND CHEMISTRY

PHARMACOLOGICAL PROPERTIES

Catharanthus roseus is an important source of anti-leukaemic drugs.[P182] It contains alkaloids that produce antitumour activity,[P156, P159, P183] as well as hypotensive, vasodilator, hypoglycaemic, hyperglycaemic, astringent, vulnerary and sedative effects.[P156] Antifungal, antidiuretic, anti-inflammatory and antiviral activities are also reported for this plant.[P79]

COMPOUNDS REPORTED

More than 70 alkaloids,[P79, P159, P183] including leurosine, vindolinine, catharanthine,[P182] pubescine, vinine and vincamine,[P156] have been isolated from *C. roseus*. Two binary indole alkaloids, vincristine and vinblastine,[P156] have proved to be especially effective in cancer chemotherapy because of their antitumour activity.[P96, P159, P183] The plant also contains some flavonoids, pectin, organic acids, several mineral salts, ursolic acid, and robinoside. From the leaf extract of *C. roseus* a new indole alkaloid (vindogentianine), along with six known alkaloids, were isolated. The new compound showed hypoglycaemic activity, indicating potential against type 2 diabetes.[P184]

Vincristine

26 *Centella asiatica*

Native to Indian subcontinent and Southeast Asia

Common names Indian Pennywort, Asiatic Pennywort • **Local names** Nyonyo (Luo), Brahmi (Hind.)

Description and ecology

Creeping, herbaceous perennial plant about 20cm high with slender green to reddish-green stems, the creeping stolons connecting the plants to each other. Rootstock consists of rhizomes, growing vertically down, creamish and covered with root hairs. **Leaves** kidney-shaped or near circular, blade 2–7cm across, margin toothed, often with apical points on the teeth, leaf stalk 1–10cm long. **Flowers** white or crimson, small and inconspicuous, in groups of three. Grows as a weed in moist and swampy areas.

USAGE AND TREATMENT

PARTS USED Aerial parts, mainly leaves.

TRADITIONAL MEDICINAL USES A decoction of fresh or dry aerial parts is used to treat leprosy,M17 albinism, anaemia, asthma, skin ulcers and burns and also to dress wounds.M21 It is also used as a brain tonic, sedative, diuretic, purgative, antipyretic and analgesic.M22, M70 Fresh leaves are taken orally for stomach ulcers.M23 This plant has furthermore been used to treat fever and sexually transmitted diseases, especially syphilis.M2, M70 *Centella* is considered an essential herb in dermatological formulations for the treatment of skin allergies and acneM2 and is also an important herbal constituent of many homoeopathic remedies.

PREPARATION AND DOSAGE

ASTHMA AND AS A SEDATIVE Soak a few fresh or sun-dried leaves or other aerial parts in hot water for 5–10 minutes. Strain the resulting decoction and drink at intervals through the day.

WOUNDS, SKIN ALLERGIES AND ACNE Crush some fresh leaves and rub onto affected areas of the skin.

LEPROSY Bath twice a day in warm water to which a hot decoction of aerial parts has been added.

AS98

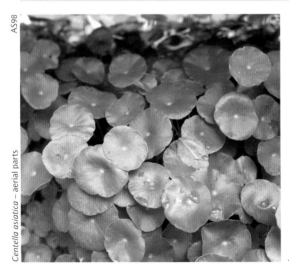

Centella asiatica – aerial parts

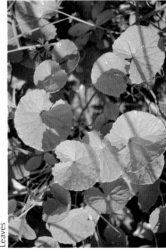

Leaves

PHARMACOLOGY AND CHEMISTRY

PHARMACOLOGICAL PROPERTIES

In clinical trials, aerial parts have shown accelerated wound-healing effects,[P185] along with other pharmacological activities that produce anticonvulsant,[P186] anti-allergic,[P187] antifungal,[P188] antibacterial,[P189] anti-inflammatory,[P185] peptic ulcer-healing, antipyretic, hypotensive and anti-tranquillising[P190] effects. In vitro and in vivo antitumour activities have also been reported.[P185]

COMPOUNDS REPORTED

The essential volatile oil contains many monoterpenoids and some sesquiterpenoids,[P191] such as β-acoradiene.[P192] The wound-healing properties are linked to triterpenoid saponins, principally

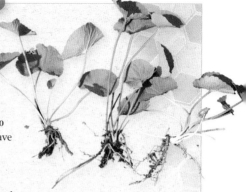

Centalla asiatica – uprooted herbs

asiaticoside,[P193, P194, P195] and to sapogenins (e.g. asiatic acid).[P193, P195] Benzenoids isolated from aerial parts of the plant include 1-methyl-4-(1,2,2,trimethylcyclopentyl)benzene.[P192] Triterpenoids, such as madecassic acid,[P193] may be responsible for the plant's antitumour properties.[P193, P196] Flavonoids, including luteolin, were reported to be responsible for anti-allergic, antibacterial and antifungal properties of the plant.[P197]

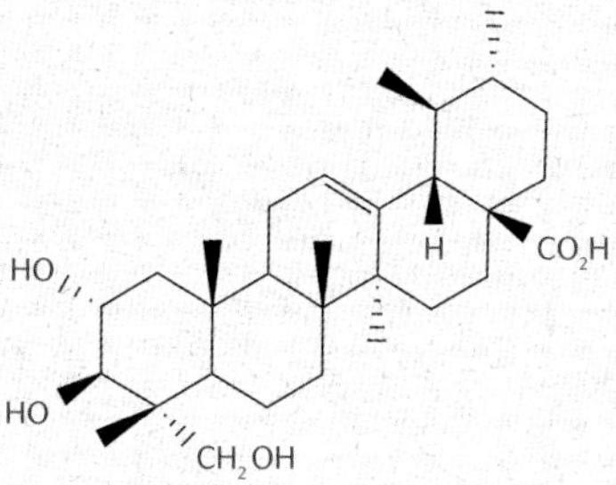

Asiatic acid

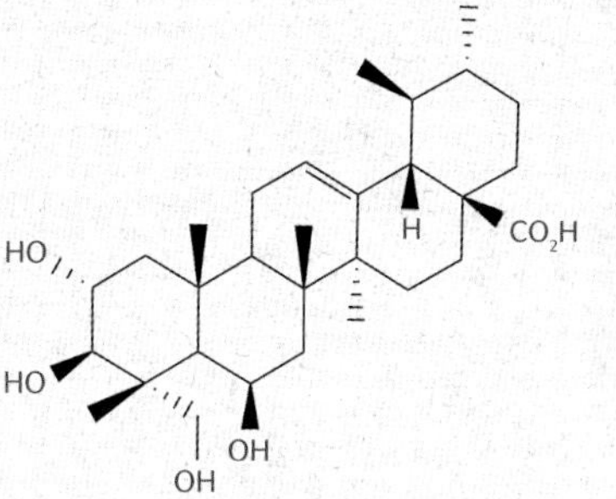

Madecassic acid

Common names True Cinnamon Tree, Ceylon Cinnamon Tree • **Local names** Taaj (Guj.), Dar Chini (Hind., Urd., Punj.)

Description and ecology

Small to medium-sized, evergreen tree 6–15m tall, with dense bushy canopy. **Bark** thick, smooth, pale brown, strongly aromatic. **Leaves** opposite, shiny dark green above, paler below, ovate to elliptic, 5–20cm long, strongly aromatic when crushed, stalk 1–2cm long. **Flowers** small, 3mm in diameter, numerous, yellowish green or creamy white, arranged in axillary or terminal panicles up to 10cm long. **Fruit** a 1-seeded drupe, green to black when ripe, ellipsoidal to ovoid, 1–2cm long. Grows both wild and cultivated in Southeast Asia (Sri Lanka in particular), India, East Africa and South America. Highly valued in Indian cuisine as a spice (either sticks or ground to a powder) but has also been used medicinally for centuries. Grows well at low altitudes and without shade.

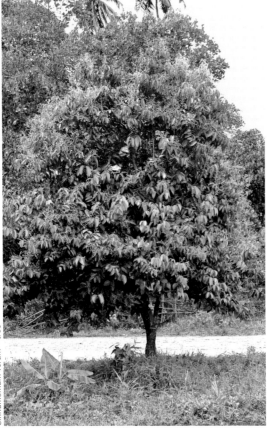

Cinnamomum verum – tree

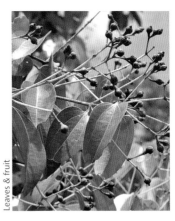

Leaves & fruit

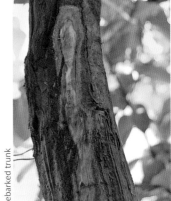

Debarked trunk

USAGE AND TREATMENT

PARTS USED Dried bark and leaves.
TRADITIONAL MEDICINAL USES Dried bark is an intestinal stimulant and an astringent and carminative.[M25, M70] It eases digestion and is used for treating vomiting and nausea.[M25] It is a remedy for appetite loss, flatulence, bloated stomach and other gastric ailments.[M7, M70] As a mild astringent, it helps to stop bleeding from cuts, wounds and other injuries.[M9, M70] Cinnamon oils extracted from the bark and leaves are widely used in the treatment of oral diseases and toothache.[M86] Oils are also used to treat rheumatism, wounds and fungal infections.[M86]

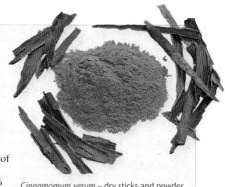
Cinnamomum verum – dry sticks and powder

PREPARATION AND DOSAGE
BLEEDING CUTS AND WOUNDS Sprinkle some fresh cinnamon and turmeric powder on a wound to help stop the bleeding.
INDIGESTION, BLOATED STOMACH, VOMITING AND NAUSEA Soak one or two sticks of cinnamon 8–10cm long in a cup of hot water. Add 1g of ginger powder and 1g of dry lemon powder or 2 slices of fresh lemon. Leave for 10 minutes and drink 3 times daily after meals.
TOOTHACHE AND WOUNDS Soak a cotton bud in cinnamon oil and apply directly on a painful tooth or wound.

PHARMACOLOGY AND CHEMISTRY

PHARMACOLOGICAL PROPERTIES
The anti-allergic, anti-ulcerogenic, antipyretic, anaesthetic and analgesic activities of cinnamon have all been verified.[P198] Cinnamon also mimics the function of insulin, stimulating insulin action in isolated adipocytes.[P198] Cinnamon inhibits various cancer cell lines.[P199] It could help in treatments for type 2 diabetes by reducing levels of glucose, triglyceride, total cholesterol and LDL cholesterol in plasma.[P200] It has a potent antioxidant activity and is a more effective radical scavenger than many of the common antioxidant food additives.[P201] It also has antioxidant, antimicrobial, anti-inflammatory, anticancer, antidiabetic, anti-HIV, anti-anxiety, antidepressant and wound-healing properties.[P202]

COMPOUNDS REPORTED
Chemical analysis of cinnamon extracts has revealed the presence of tannins, phenolic acids, cinnamaldehyde, eugenol, cinnamophilin, hydroxychalcone and coumarin.[P199, P202] The essential oil contains cinnamaldehyde, eugenol, caryophyllene, cinnamyl acetate and cinnamic acid as the major compounds.[P202]

Cinnamaldehyde

Cinnamophilin

a. *Citrus aurantium*

Native to Southeast Asia

Common names Sour Orange, Bitter Orange • **Local names** Mchungwa (Swa.), Muchungwa (Lug.), Narangi (Punj., Urd., Hind.)

Description and ecology

Evergreen shrub or small, much-branched tree 3–8(–10)m tall, with dense, rounded crown, young twigs angled and bearing short slender spines, but older branches with stout spines up to 8cm long. **Leaves** simple, alternate, dark green, ovate to elliptical, 7–10cm long, stalk 2–3cm long and narrowly to broadly winged.

Flowers white, in axillary clusters of 1–6, with sweet smell, petals 5, thick, 2–3cm across. **Fruit** a green to orange-yellow hesperidium, round, 4–8(–10)cm across, skin smooth or rough, strongly aromatic, pulp very sour, acidic and slightly bitter. **Seeds** numerous. Grown widely in both tropical and subtropical latitudes but not doing well in wetter high-altitude areas.

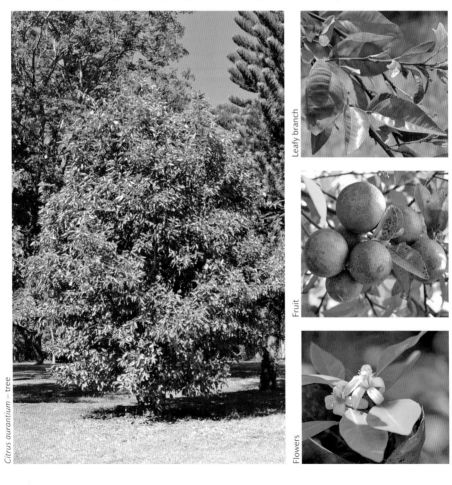

Citrus aurantium – tree

Leafy branch

Fruit

Flowers

PARTS USED Leaves, flowers, fruits, fruit peel and seeds.
TRADITIONAL MEDICINAL USES The peel is widely recommended for people suffering from oedema, varicose veins, haemorrhoids (bleeding) and blood-clotting dysfunction.[M9, M70] Leaf juice squeezed into the ears may help with earache.[M7] Flowers and leaves are taken in the treatment of insomnia, nervousness, migraine, digestive disorders (stomach spasms and gastric pains), palpitations

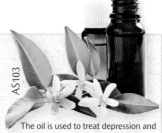

The oil is used to treat depression and is also an ingredient in perfumery.

and menstrual pain.[M25] The juice could help prevent scurvy, body weakness, malnutrition,[M25] anaemia, rickets, thrombosis, arteriosclerosis and problems related to blood circulation.[M9, M70] It also enhances the appetite and promotes fast emptying of the gall bladder. Leaf decoctions help to relieve asthma, coughs, fever and migraine, and in children act as a tranquilliser ensuring calm and peaceful sleep.[M25] The essential oil from the skin of the fruit is used to treat depression, tension and skin problems.[M87] Both the leaves and the flowers are antispasmodic, digestive and sedative. An infusion of leaves and flowers is used in the treatment of stomach problems and helps with digestion. The bitter fruit peel acts as an appetiser and digestive. The seed and the skin are used in the treatment of anorexia, chest pain, colds and coughs.[M87]

PREPARATION AND DOSAGE
ASTHMA, COUGHS AND MIGRAINE Boil a handful of fresh leaves in a litre of water for 2–3 minutes. Drink the decoction at intervals during the day.
MALNUTRITION, APPETISER, FATIGUE AND ANAEMIA Juice of the sweet orange (*C. aurantium* var. *sinensis*), contains vitamins A, B, C and P. Drink 2 or 3 glasses of freshly squeezed juice a day. All orange juice must be consumed fresh as vitamin C is quickly destroyed on coming into contact with oxygen, making the juice bitter.
INSOMNIA, NERVOUSNESS, DIGESTIVE DISORDERS, PALPITATIONS AND MENSTRUAL PAIN Add 3 or 4 crushed fresh leaves and 5 or 6 crushed flowers to a litre of water and leave for 15 minutes. Drink 3 or 4 cups of this infusion daily, including a cup just before going to bed to ward off sleeplessness. Children should be given a quarter of this dose as a tranquilliser.
OEDEMA, VARICOSE VEINS, HAEMORRHOIDS AND THROMBOSIS Cut the peel of some bitter oranges into small pieces and dry them in the sun or in an oven at low temperature. Add 30g of dry peel to half a litre of water and boil for 15–20 minutes. Add some honey to sweeten the mixture and drink a cup of this decoction after every meal.
HERPES LABIALIS LESIONS Apply the peel of a squeezed bitter orange directly to the herpes lesion or – if this is found to be painful – add a drop of soothing vegetable oil.

b. *Citrus limon*   Native to South Asia, northeastern India

Common name Lemon • **Local names** Ndimu / Mlimao (Swa.), Nimawa / Nnimu (Lug.), Limbu (Guj., Punj.), Nimbu (Urd., Hind.)

Description and ecology
Evergreen shrub or small tree 3–6m tall, open and with stout, stiff thorns. **Bark** grey-brown, branches greenish brown, armed with spines. **Leaves** shiny, pale green, 5–10cm long, tooth-edged, with sharp tip, emitting a spicy aroma when crushed, with short leaf stalk. **Flowers** small, solitary or clustered, white with purple streaks on the outside of the thick petals, sweetly scented. **Fruit** a hesperidium (as for all citrus), round or oval, 7–8cm long, green to yellow when ripe, flesh pale yellow, juicy, strongly acidic. Seeds few. Lemon trees grow at both low and higher altitudes, 0–1,800m, and require high temperatures to fruit well. One of the most widely grown fruit trees.

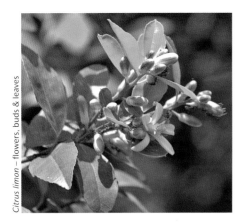

Citrus limon – flowers, buds & leaves

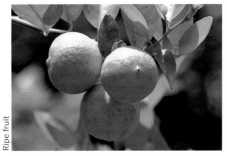

Ripe fruit

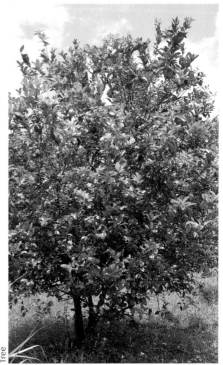

Tree

PARTS USED Leaves, fruits (ripe and unripe) and fruit rinds.

TRADITIONAL MEDICINAL USES Lemon juice in hot water is a popular remedy for fever, colds and influenza.[M7] Lemon juice stirred into cold boiled water is taken as a treatment for gout, arthritis and kidney stones. Leaf decoctions are taken for coughs. Decoctions of lemon peel in hot water are taken to ease bronchitis. By stimulating activity of the digestive organs, lemon juice is helpful in cases of dyspepsia and stomach upsets. It is also said to be useful for its sedative properties.[M7] Use of lemon is recommended for people suffering from obesity, nervousness, insomnia, palpitations, migraine and asthma.[M6, M7, M70] It has a vermifuge effect (on intestinal parasites) and also helps in the treatment of scurvy and scorbutus (both caused by a vitamin C deficiency).[M9, M25] Lemon juice also helps in cases of severe nausea and vomiting, especially during pregnancy.[M7] It may be used to treat jaundice and enlargement of the spleen. It helps to remove scars, acne, dry skin and other skin blemishes.[M70] It relieves pain and burning when applied to the stings of scorpions, wasps and bees. It is recommended for those suffering from high blood pressure, swollen legs, oedema, varicose veins, haemorrhoids and thrombosis.[M7, M9] It is a good antiseptic for use on skin ulcers, abrasions and wounds and also helps to remove scalp dandruff and to make the hair look shiny.[M7]

PREPARATION AND DOSAGE

FEVER, COLDS AND INFLUENZA Squeeze the juice of a lemon into 500ml of hot water (do not boil the mixture). Drink 2 or 3 times a day. Alternatively, chop 2 juicy lemons into small pieces, put them in 2 litres of warm water and add 4 spoonfuls of honey. Strain the infusion and drink at intervals during the day.

STOMACH UPSETS, INDIGESTION, CHOLERA, NAUSEA AND VOMITING Dissolve the juice of a lemon in a large glass of cold boiled water. Add half a teaspoon of sodium bicarbonate or ordinary table salt (sodium chloride). Drink this mixture at least 3 times a day. In the case of cholera, add a teaspoon of sugar or honey as well. For nausea, headache or vomiting (particularly in the case of travel or sea sickness), it is helpful to lick a piece of fresh lemon sprinkled with salt and dry ginger powder. For indigestion and stomach pain, add a pinch of salt to a mixture of a teaspoon of fresh lemon juice and a teaspoon of fresh ginger, and take twice daily after meals for 5 days.

SKIN PROBLEMS (ACNE, SCARS, DRY SKIN AND OTHER BLEMISHES) Rub a slice of lemon onto the affected areas and leave for 2–3 hours. Then wash off with warm water. Repeat the treatment twice a day until blemishes disappear. To treat dry itch caused by dry skin, rub on a mixture consisting of equal quantities of lemon juice and olive oil.

NERVOUSNESS, INSOMNIA, PALPITATIONS AND MIGRAINE Add 30g of pounded fresh leaves to a litre of water. Sweeten with honey and drink 3 cups of the infusion daily for 3 days.

HERPES LABIALIS LESIONS Apply the peel of a squeezed lemon directly to the herpes lesion or – if this is found to be too painful – add a drop of vegetable oil.

LOW BLOOD PRESSURE, SWOLLEN LEGS, OEDEMA, VARICOSE VEINS, HAEMORRHOIDS AND THROMBOSIS Squeeze the juice of a fresh lemon into 500ml of cold boiled water. Sweeten with honey and drink twice a day for a week before or after meals.

> ⚠ **WARNING!** Keep lemon juice (especially the peel of fresh unripe fruit) away from the eyes. Sour lemon juice can affect dental enamel, so direct contact with the teeth should be kept to a minimum.

PHARMACOLOGY AND CHEMISTRY

PHARMACOLOGICAL PROPERTIES

The essential oils in lemon peel have shown a dermatitis-producing effect when applied externally on humans.[P156, P203] Other findings in studies of these oils have shown antibacterial,[P79] antifungal,[P204] anti-obesity,[P205] anti-amoebic,[P206] anticellulite,[P205] and antivenin[P207] activities. In vivo studies showed the antiolytic effect of *Citrus limon* on mice.[P208]

COMPOUNDS REPORTED

Both lemon and orange flowers are rich in volatile oils, the principal components of which are limonene[P156] and 1-linalol. Other terpenic hydrocarbons are present in lesser proportions. All these compounds have sedative, antispasmodic and mildly somniferous properties.[P17] Lemon flowers contain flavonoids such as limocitrin.[P156, P209] A high vitamin C content gives lemons and oranges[P156] strong antidyspeptic and antiscorbutic properties.[P209] Bitter orange and lemon juice and their rind are rich in flavonoid glycosides (e.g. naringine, hesperidine, neohesperidin)[P17, P156] whose action is similar to that of vitamin PP[P17] in countering thrombosis, arteriosclerosis and blood circulation dysfunction.[P156]

Limonene   Ascorbic acid   Limocitrin

Indigenous

Common names Commiphora, African Myrrh • **Local names** Ammess (Bor.), Chibambara (Dig.), Hammeessa (Gab.), Musishwi (Gir.), Kitungu / Ndungu (Kam.), Arupiny / Arupien (Luo), Chotwa (Mar.), Mundorotwo (Pok.), Komper (Orm.), Lcheningiro (Sam.), Hammes-sagara (Som.), Mbambara / Mkororo (Swa.Ken.), Mwagori / Mwagari (Tai.), Ekadeli (Tur.), Osilalei (Aru., Maa.), Msomvugo (Gogo), Niimo (Goro.), Msagasi (Nyam.), Muhuju (Nyat.), Idaki (Ran.), Mturituri (Swa.Tan.), Mawezi (Zin.), Ekadeli / Etopojo (Ate.)

Description and ecology

Spiny, low-branching, deciduous shrub or small tree 3–6(–10)m tall, with a short cylindrical bole and dense rounded crown, from near the base usually beset with horizontal spiny branches. **Bark** green-grey, peeling in shiny reddish-brown or grey scrolls, showing green inner parts, yellowish gum dripping out when cut. **Leaves** soft, hairy, bright green, fragrant when crushed, compound with 3 leaflets, edges wavy, central leaflet much longer than the other two. **Flowers** small, red, in tight axillary clusters of 4–10. **Fruit** pink-red, soft, 0.6–1cm, pointed, ovoid, with stony seed inside. Common in all the driest areas of East Africa, especially in *Acacia–Commiphora* bushland, open savanna, desert and both coastal and northern areas, at 300–1,900m.

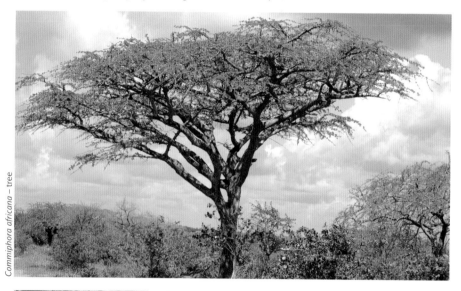

Commiphora africana – tree

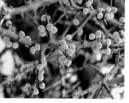

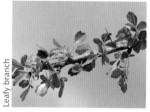

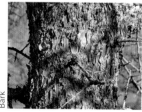

Fruit & thorns

Leafy branch

Bark

PARTS USED Root, stem bark, resin/gum and fruits.
TRADITIONAL MEDICINAL USES Roots are used to soothe stomach pain and to treat swollen testicles. Powdered bark is mixed with porridge and taken for malaria.[M89] Bark and roots are used in steam baths in the treatment of coughs, colds and fever,[M1, M4] as well as to treat snakebite.[M89] Sap from fresh bark is used as a disinfectant for wounds and also for treating toothache.[M40, M70] Fruits are used to treat typhoid fever,[M89] stomach problems, ulcerated gums and toothache.[M3, M40, M89] Root and bark decoctions are taken as a remedy for constipation. Poultices of dry leaves or bark powder are used for covering and healing wounds.[M4, M70]

PREPARATION AND DOSAGE
STOMACH PAIN AND CONSTIPATION Boil a handful of fresh bark or roots in a litre of water for 10 minutes. Filter and drink the decoction at intervals during the day. Chewing pieces of fresh stem bark, and swallowing the juice, will help to relieve constipation and abdominal pain.
COUGHS, COLDS AND FEVER Boil a handful of fresh stem bark and roots in water. Inhale the steam or use as a steam bath.
DISINFECTING OPEN WOUNDS Apply sap from fresh bark directly to an open wound or dress with a poultice of dry leaf or bark powder.
SNAKEBITE Fresh bark is chewed or pounded, then mixed with tobacco and applied on the snakebite.
PAINFUL GUMS AND TOOTHACHE Fresh fruits are chewed or pounded and used as a remedy for toothache and diseases of the gum.

PHARMACOLOGICAL PROPERTIES
Sap or resin from dried bark and dried leaves has shown antibacterial activity and antiseptic effects,[P210] helpful in disinfecting and healing wounds and for treating toothache. The roots have triggered strong antigiardiasic activity.[P211]

COMPOUNDS REPORTED
The volatile oil in the leaves of *Commiphora africana* contains several monoterpenoids, such as α-pinene,[P212] and also some sesquiterpenoids, such as aromadendrene.[P212] Some flavonoids (e.g. phellamurin) have been isolated from stem bark.[P213] The pentacyclic triterpene commafric A isolated from *C. africana* showed antiproliferative activity against a lung cancer cell line (A549). Similarly, a co-metabolite, α-amyrin, was weakly active against ovarian cancer (A2780), pancreatic cancer (MIA-PaCa-2) and stomach cancer (SNU638).[P214]

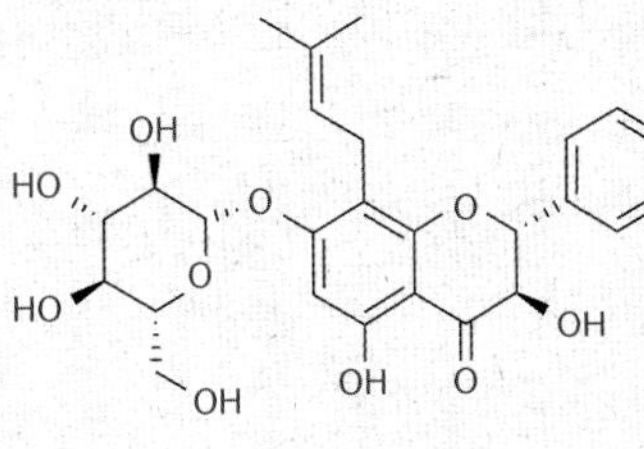

Phellamurin

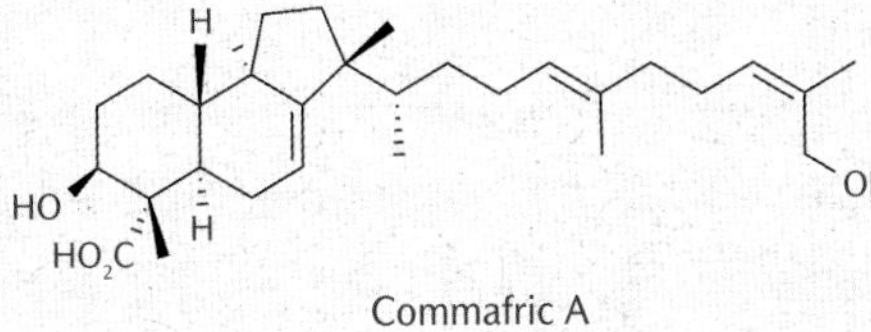

Commafric A

a. *Cordia africana* Indigenous

Common names Large-leaved Cordia, East African Cordia • **Local names** Wandesi (Bor.), Muvutu (Kam.), Muringa (Emb., Kik., Mer.Ken.), Omokobokobo (Kis.), Mukamari / Kumukomari (Luh.), Samutet (Nan.), Chibulukwa (Sam.), Makobokobo (Swa.Ken.), Muringaringa (Tai., Tav.), Samut (Tug.), Mringaringa (Chag.), Sei (Goro.), Mrungurya (Pare), Mbapu / Msinzizi (Lugu.), Mringaringa (Mer.Tan.), Mfufu / Mzingazinga (Samb.), Mringamringa (Swa.Tan.), Mukebu, (Lug.), Chichikiri (Lugi.), Hinghobe (Luny.), Akoiyi (Luo-J), Mujugangoma (Ruki., Runy.), Muzugangoma (Runyan.), Mutumba (Ruto.), Mugengere (Sebei)

Description and ecology

Large, deciduous forest tree, heavily branched, with a rounded spreading crown and often a crooked trunk, up to 15m tall but sometimes reaching 25m. **Bark** pale brown, rough and fissured with age. **Leaves** simple, alternate, oval, up to 16cm long, with pointed apex and rounded or heart-shaped base, dull dark green, leathery and sandpapery above, paler below, with prominent veins. **Flowers** white, showy and very attractive, funnel-shaped, 2.5cm across, sweetly scented, borne in bunches. **Fruit** a yellow or orange, round or oval drupe, 1–1.2cm in diameter, with sweet pulp containing 4-angled stone with 1 or 2(–4) creamy white, oval, flattened seeds. *C. africana* prefers moist, well-drained soils but can also grow on rocky slopes. Common in wooded grassland, open forest and riverine forest, edges and clearings in montane forest, at 1,200–2,200(–2,400)m.

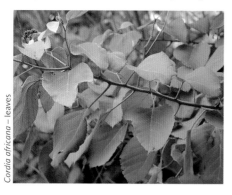

Cordia africana – leaves

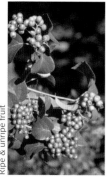

Ripe & unripe fruit

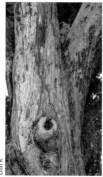

Bark

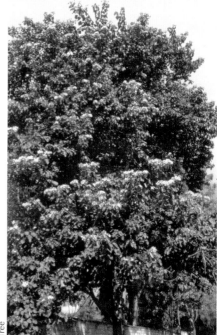

Tree

PARTS USED Root, bark, leaves and fruits.
TRADITIONAL MEDICINAL USES Fresh bark is applied to fractures, and bark extracts are taken against fatigue.[M90] Eating fresh or dried fruits helps to relieve a dry cough.[M70] Fresh bark juice is applied locally to help treat broken bones.[M1, M70] Leaf decoctions are drunk to treat headache, nose-bleeding, dizziness and vomiting during pregnancy and to get rid of intestinal worms.[M90] Root decoctions are taken to treat jaundice and schistosomiasis.[M90]

PREPARATION AND DOSAGE
HEADACHE, VOMITING AND INTESTINAL WORMS Boil a handful of fresh leaves or 5g of dry leaf powder in a litre of water for 10–15 minutes. Filter and drink at intervals during the day.
JAUNDICE AND SCHISTOSOMIASIS (BILHARZIA) Boil a handful of fresh roots or 5g of dry root powder in a litre of water for 10–15 minutes. Cool, filter and drink a cup an hour after a meal 3 times a day.

b. *Cordia monoica*   Indigenous

Common names Sandpaper Tree, Saucer-berry • **Local names** Qotte (Bor.), Kithei / Muthei (Kam.), Muthigi / Mukuo / Mukuu (Kik.), Nogirwet (Kip.), Oseno (Luo), Kumukhendie (Luh.), Oseki / Olseki (Maa.), Ikuo / Mukuo (Mer.), Araba (Orm.), Toperewo / Toporewo (Pok.), Se'eki / Lamantume (Sam.), Marergom / Marer-girgir (Som.), Msasa (Swa., Ran.), Entuntun / Elkaisekiseki (Tur.), Oseki (Aru.), Mdawi (Gogo), Bagharimo (Goro.), Mlembu (Nyam.), Mongoongo (Nyat.), Mshasha (Pare), Mshasa / Magamoi (Samb.), Nembu / Mnyage (Suk.), Edomel (Luo-L), Mukebu (Luso.)

Description and ecology

Multi-stemmed shrub 3–4m tall or small tree up to 6m, occasionally reaching 12m, with a rounded, spreading crown. **Bark** yellow to ash-grey, thin and fibrous, smooth or peeling in strips. **Leaves** alternate, broadly oval to almost round, 5–8cm long, upper surface very rough like sandpaper but softly hairy below, with prominent veins and slightly toothed margin. Branchlets, leaf and flower stalks densely covered with rusty hairs. **Flowers** pale yellow or cream, turning brown on drying, fragrant, in dense terminal or rarely axillary panicles 1.5–5(–7)cm long. **Fruit** ovoid or ellipsoid, 9–20mm long, pointed, yellow-orange, soft when ripe, single-seeded and with jelly-like edible pulp. Found in varied habitats, from *Acacia–Euphorbia* bush and wet riverine forest to woodland and grassland, even in dry thickets, at 0–2,100m.

PARTS USED Roots, bark, leaves and fruits.
TRADITIONAL MEDICINAL USES Juice from the roots is given to children to treat vomiting and malaria.[M3, M40] A leaf extract is given to women to drink after childbirth to help remove a retained placenta.[M3] Leaf juice is used for eye inflammation.[M70, M91] Roots are applied as poultices to pus-filled wounds.[M1, M70] Leaves and stem bark can be used in treatments for leprosy.[M70, M91] Men eat fresh fruits to maintain the consistency of seminal fluid and also to treat spermatorrhoea.[M70]

PREPARATION AND DOSAGE
LEPROSY Add some fresh leaves to boiling water and use initially to steam-bath the body. Wash the body with the warm decoction. Then rub a paste, made from 5–10g of dry bark powder mixed with a little boiled water, on affected areas of the body.
EYE INFECTIONS Add a few drops of fresh leaf juice to a tablespoon of boiled water and apply as eyedrops.

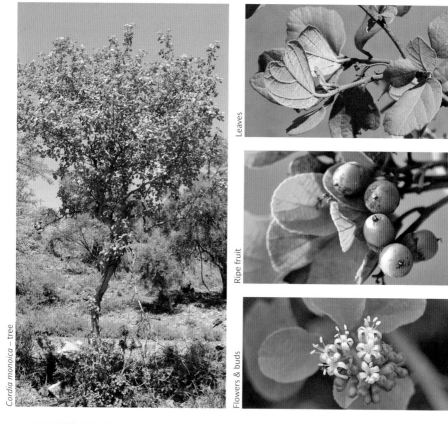

Cordia monoica – tree

Leaves

Ripe fruit

Flowers & buds

c. *Cordia sinensis*

Indigenous

Common names Grey-leaved Cordia, Grey-leaved Saucer-berry • **Local names** Harores / Mader-boor / Madee'r (Bor.), Mad'eera (Gab.), Mderia / Mkayukayu (Gir.), Kithea / Muthei-munini / Kithia (Kam.), Nokirwet (Kip.), Ol-durgo / Ol-dorko / Ol-olgot (Maa.Ken.), Odomoyon (Mar.), Mader (Orm.), Adomeyon / Adomeon / Muhale / Muhali / Mtale (Pok.), Gaer / Gayer (Ren.), Dorgo / Igueita / Igweita-orok (Sam.), Mareer / Marer (Som.), Adumewa / Edoma (Tug.), Edome (Tur.), Mdawi (Gogo), Hanarmo (Goro.), Ol dorko / Ol-olfot (Maa.Tan.), Mochocho (Mbug.), Mlembu / Mnerabu (Nyam.), Mdumwa-kiguu (Nyat.), Mpololo (Pare), Mnembu (Ran.), Mkamasi / Nyamate (Swa.)

Description and ecology

Leafy, compact, multi-stemmed, deciduous shrub 4–6m tall, rarely a small tree up to 12m, often with drooping branches. **Bark** smooth, brown to grey-white, later yellow-brown to black, sometimes finely longitudinally fissured. **Leaves** opposite, smooth or slightly rough, grey-green, narrow, up to 9cm long, with rounded or notched tip, stalk about 1cm long.

Flowers cream, in terminal clusters, fragrant, on branched hairy stalks. **Fruit** ovoid with a long tip, up to 2cm long, green at first but orange-red when mature, cupped in the persistent remains of the calyx, with sticky, edible, orange-red pulp. Widespread in hot, drier areas including dry riverine forest, open bushland and bushed or scattered tree grassland, at 0–1,400m.

PARTS USED Roots and fresh ripe fruits.

TRADITIONAL MEDICINAL USES A decoction of roots can be used to treat malaria.[M91] Chewing fresh roots is said to induce abortion.[M1, M91] Fruits are eaten as a remedy for dry coughs, dysentery and spermatorrhoea as well as to stop premature ejaculation.[M40, M70] A decoction of root and bark may help to treat stomach disorders.[M91]

PREPARATION AND DOSAGE

SPERMATORRHOEA Eat 2 or 3 fresh ripe fruits twice a day for a week.

INDUCED ABORTION Chewing about 3 pieces of fresh root, the size of a finger, is said to be sufficient for this purpose.

MALARIA Boil a handful of fresh roots or 5g of dry root powder in a litre of water for 10–15 minutes. Cool, filter and drink a cup an hour before a meal 3 times a day.

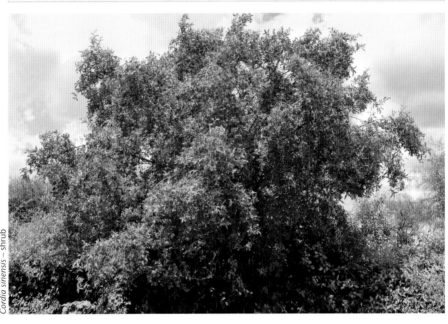

Cordia sinensis – shrub

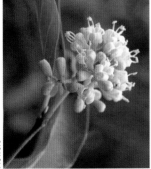

Flowers

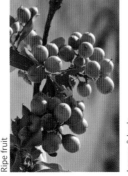

Ripe fruit

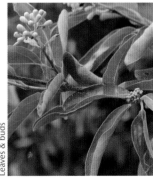

Leaves & buds

PHARMACOLOGY AND CHEMISTRY

PHARMACOLOGICAL PROPERTIES

Some species of *Cordia* have shown anti-inflammatory and analgesic activities.[P215] Stem bark extracts of *C. africana* showed antimicrobial activity against two Gram-positive bacterial strains, two Gram-negative bacterial strains and two fungal strains.[P216]

COMPOUNDS REPORTED

The presence of sesquiterpenes (e.g. trichotomol) and terpenoid benzoquinones (e.g. cordiachrome C) has been reported for some species of *Cordia*,[P217] including *C. monoica*.[P218] Six known compounds – oleanolic acid, 3-β-lup-20(29)- en-3-ol, stigmast-5,22-dien-3β-ol, 2-(2Z)-(3-hydroxy-3,7-dimethylocta-2,6-dienyl)-1,4-benzenediol, 4-hydroxy-3-methoxy-benzaldehyde and 7-hydroxy-4'-methoxyisoflavone – were isolated from a root bark extract of *C. africana*, while stem bark yielded oleanolic acid (1), 3-β-lup-20(29)-en-3-ol, ubiquinone-8 and 1-octacosanol. Among these, oleanolic acid showed moderate antibacterial activity against the bacterium *Enterococcus faecium*.[P219]

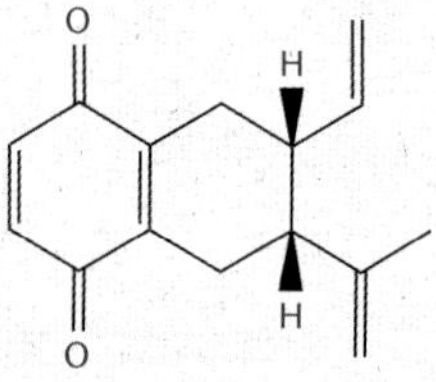

Cordiachrome C

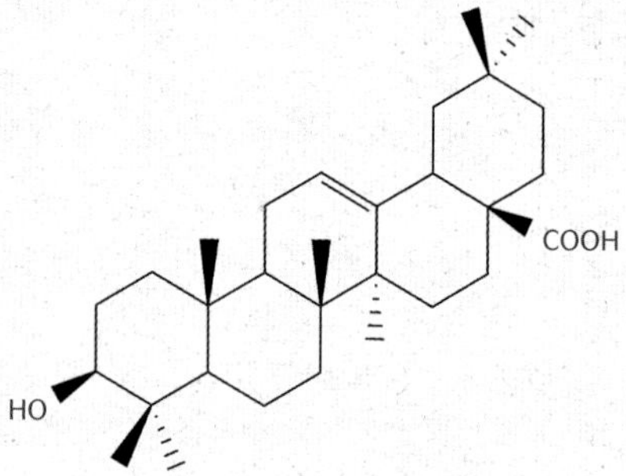

Oleanolic acid

Native to southern Europe, western Mediterranean and southwestern Asia

Common names Coriander, Dhania, Cilantro, Indian Dhania • **Local names** Dhania (Hind., Punj., Swa.), Dhana / Kotimiri (Guj.)

Description and ecology

Very small, soft, herbaceous plant 30–60cm high. **Leaves** of variable shapes, broadly lobed at the base of the plant, slender and feathery at the top of the flowering branches. **Flowers** white or pale pink, in small umbels. **Fruit** a beaked, finely ribbed, light brown, round, dry schizocarp, aromatic when crushed, 3–5mm in diameter. On account of the distinctive smell, both fresh leaves and dried seeds are widely used around the world as a seasoning herb and a spicy ingredient used in cooking, especially in Indian dishes. Today it has also become part of East African cuisine (specially used in curries and soups). Grows in moist soils from low to high altitudes and requires a moderate temperature.

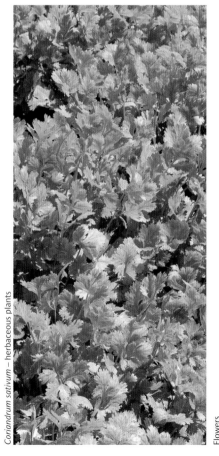

Coriandrum sativum – herbaceous plants

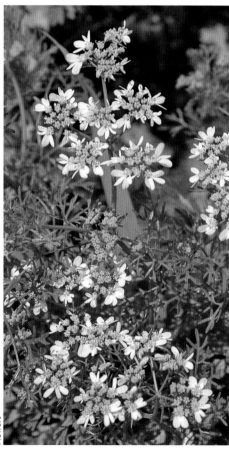

Flowers

USAGE AND TREATMENT

PARTS USED Dry fruits.

TRADITIONAL MEDICINAL USES Dhania fruits are used as an aid to digestion and for stopping diarrhoea caused by indigestion.[M7, M9] Dhania may be taken orally as a remedy for gastritis and relieving stomach bloating and flatulence,[M92] while also serving as an appetite stimulant and a remedy for headache.[M9, M25] Fruits are also taken to overcome dizziness and vertigo, and are used in

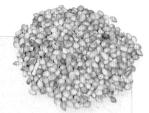

Coriandrum sativum – dry fruits

treatments for passing of blood in stools following dysentery or diarrhoea.[M7, M70] Coriander seed is used to treat digestive and respiratory disorders and diseases of the urinary system as it has diaphoretic, diuretic, carminative and stimulant effects.[M92]

PREPARATION AND DOSAGE

DIGESTIVE DISORDERS (GASTRITIS, FLATULENCE) AND TO STIMULATE THE APPETITE Chew a tablespoon of dry dhania fruits 3 times a day after meals.

HEADACHE AND VERTIGO Add a tablespoon of sifted dhania powder to a tablespoon of sugar. Take this to dispel dizziness, particularly when it is experienced while convalescing from other illnesses.

DIARRHOEA, DYSENTERY AND THE PASSING OF BLOOD IN STOOLS Chew a tablespoon of dry dhania fruits after a meal 3 times a day. To fortify the stomach after protracted dysentery or chronic diarrhoea, add a tablespoon of sifted dhania powder to half a cup of plain yogurt and drink 2 or 3 times a day. To help arrest the passing of blood in stools, add a tablespoon of ground dry dhania fruits to a cup of cold boiled water, stir and strain, then drink the infusion 3 times a day.

PHARMACOLOGY AND CHEMISTRY

PHARMACOLOGICAL PROPERTIES

The eupeptic and carminative[P156, P220] properties of *Coriandrum sativum* are associated with the monoterpene linalool.[P156] In small doses, this acts as a mild invigorator of the nervous system.[P221] The essential oils and other extracts from coriander have shown antibacterial, antioxidant, antidiabetic, anticancer and antimutagenic activities.[P222] Extracts from seeds have shown contraceptive, antidiabetic, antihyperlipemic, antioxidant, hypotensive and anthelmintic activities.[P223]

COMPOUNDS REPORTED

The fruit of *C. sativum* contains a volatile oil that is rich in the monoterpene linalool.[P156] Distilled oil (coriander oil BP) contains 65–70% of (+)-linalool (coriandrol) and α-pinene.[P17] A number of isocoumarins have been isolated from the plant as a whole.[P220] The essential oil from leaves of *C. sativum* showed antibacterial activity against Gram-positive (*Staphylococcus aureus, Bacillus* spp.) and Gram-negative (*Escherichia coli, Salmonella typhi, Klebsiella pneumonia, Proteus mirabilis* and *Pseudomonas aeruginosa*) bacteria, as well as antifungal activity against the pathogenic fungus *Candida albicans*. From the oil, the major constituents were identified as 2E-decenal, decanal, 2E-decen-1-ol and n-decanol.[P224]

Linalool

α-Pinene

Coriandrone A

a. *Croton dichogamus*   Indigenous

Common names Orange-leaved Croton, Orange-leaved Bush • **Local names** Mokhof (Bor.), Mookofe (Gab.), Mulinduri (Kik.), Muthiani (Kam.), Kelelwet (Kip.), Racher (Luo), Ol-logerdangai (Maa.), Lakingdrirgat / Lageridingai (Sam.), Gobole (Som.), Kekelwa (Tur., Pok.), Girigirmu (Mbu.)

Description and ecology
Multi-stemmed shrub or small tree usually 2–4m high but can reach 7m, with symmetrical or pyramidal and sometimes straggling crown. **Leaves** alternate, regularly spaced along slender branches, lanceolate or elliptic, up to 6cm long, margin entire, silvery below, turning orange before falling, aromatic. **Flowers** small, white, inconspicuous, few, on short terminal spikes. **Fruits** 3-lobed capsules up to 1cm across, in small terminal clusters. Common in dry forest, dry bushland, especially in rocky soils, lava, limestone and porous soils and in thickets in *Acacia–Euphorbia* woodland as well as along dry upland forest edges and in disturbed and grazed areas, at 550–2,100m.

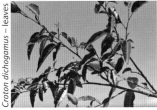

Croton dichogamus – leaves

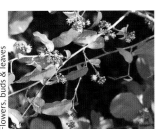

Flowers, buds & leaves

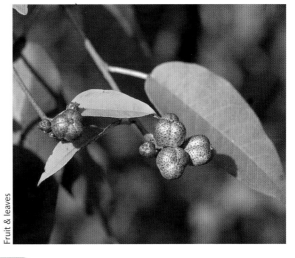

Fruit & leaves

USAGE AND TREATMENT

PARTS USED Leaves, bark and roots.
TRADITIONAL MEDICINAL USES Leaves are used to treat stomach ailments.[M70] Decoctions of roots or bark are taken for stomach ache and as a remedy for intestinal worms.[M1] Root decoctions are also taken as a tonic.[M93] Leaves are used in the treatment of chest afflictions, fever, a cough and sore throat.[M70] Roots and sometimes leaves are used in traditional medicine to treat colds, fever, tuberculosis and syphilis.[M112, M115]

PREPARATION AND DOSAGE
CHEST AILMENTS, FEVER, COUGHS AND SORE THROAT Burn some dry leaves and inhale the fumes. Alternatively, either chew some fresh leaves or roll dry leaves into a cigarette that can be smoked for relief from chest afflictions. An infusion, made by boiling a handful of fresh leaves in a litre of water, can be taken 2 or 3 times a day.

b. *Croton macrostachyus* Indigenous

Common names Broad-leaved Croton, Woodland Croton • **Local names** Mukanis (Bor.), Mutundu / Kitundu (Kam.), Mutundu / Mutundu wa njora (Kik.), Tebesuet (Kip.), Ngong'ngong (Luo), Ol-keparke (Maa.), Omosocho (Kis.), Musutsu / Omuswitswi (Luh.), Mutuntu (Mer.), Taboswa (Mar.), Tebesuet (Nan., Tug.), Mfirifiri (Tai., Tav.), Olobiago / Ololyapiyapi (Aru.), Mfurufuru (Chag., Mer.Tan.), Meali (Goro.), Muhugu / Muvulugu (Hehe), Livuluku (Nyak.), Mfurifuri (Pare), Mshunduzi (Samb.), Muhuwa (Zin.), Musogasoga (Lug.), Ofunze (Lugb.), Guyi / Gwihihi / Iwihihi (Lugi.), Muchwichwi (Lugw.), Mwiyo (Lugwe.), Nahingunya (Luny.), Ekwanga / Ekwanga (Luo-A), Epoli (Luo-J), Ekwango (Luo-L), Muyemba (Luso.), Murangari (Ruki.), Mulangara (Runyan.), Muhoti (Ruto.), Toboswa (Sebei)

Description and ecology

Deciduous tree with a rounded, open crown and large, spreading branches, 25(–30)m tall, with a cylindrical bole up to 100cm in diameter. **Bark** grey or grey-brown, fairly smooth when young but finely fissured and cracked when old. **Leaves** simple, alternate, up to 15cm long, heart-shaped, soft, with prominent veins and irregularly toothed margin, turning orange before falling. **Flowers** creamy yellow to white, sweetly scented, clustered in erect spikes up to 25cm long and borne all over the tree. **Fruits** grey, pea-sized capsules, 8–12mm in diameter and slightly 3-lobed, hairy, on drooping spikes. **Seeds** ellipsoid, flattened, cream-coloured. Grows on moist or dry evergreen upland forest edges, in riverine forest or woodland and in wooded grassland or bushland, at 1,100–2,500m.

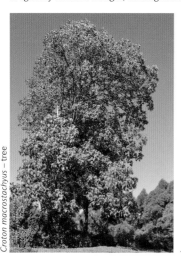

Croton macrostachyus – tree

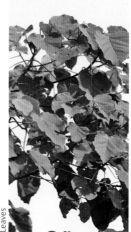

Leaves

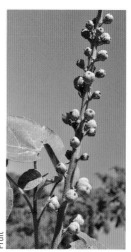

Fruit

USAGE AND TREATMENT

PARTS USED Roots, leaves, bark and seeds.

TRADITIONAL MEDICINAL USES Decoctions of roots are taken as a remedy for stomach worms (including tapeworm), venereal diseases[M94] and malaria, and have also been used as a purgative.[M4, M70] A decoction of leaves may help to treat a cough and sore throat. Leaf juice can serve as a clotting aid in the healing of wounds and additionally may be taken as an anthelmintic. Stem and root bark decoctions are applied to a skin rash on a newborn baby.[M1, M70] Pounded fresh leaves are used as a poultice to treat haemorrhoids, skin sores, warts and ringworm.[M94] A mixture of crushed leaves and seed in water is drunk as a remedy for tapeworm.[M94]

c. *Croton megalocarpus*   Indigenous

Common names Silvery-leaved Croton, Kenya Croton • **Local names** Nyapo (Bor.), Mukinduri (Emb., Kik., Mer.), Nyaap'po (Gab.), Muyama (Gir.), Muthulu / Nthulu (Kam.), Mukinduri (Kik., Mer.), Musine (Luh.), Ol-mergoit (Maa.Ken.), Taboswa (Mar.), Masineitet (Nan.), Ortuet (Tug.), Mkigara (Tai.), Marakuet (Sam.), Mbali / Lali / Mlalai / Mlandee (Chag.), Meali (Goro.), Muhihi (Haya), Ol-mergoit / Ol-margait / Ol-marbait (Maa.Tan.), Muhande (Pare), Nkulumire (Lug.), Mutakura / Muyuni (Ruki.), Mutungunda (Runyan.), Munyabakuru / Mwenyabakikuru (Ruto.)

Description and ecology
Large, hardy, fast-growing, deciduous tree 15–35m tall, monoecious or dioecious, with a distinctive layering of spreading branches and a flat crown. **Bark** dark grey, rough and cracking. **Leaves** variable, long, oval and pointed, up to 12cm long, often much smaller, dull green above, silvery below, stalked. **Flowers** unisexual, pale yellow, in clusters on erect hanging spikes 16–20cm long, short-lived. **Fruits** conspicuous grey, woody capsules, ovoid-ellipsoid, very numerous, 2.5–3.3cm long. **Seeds** rounded-oval, grey-brown. Common in dry upland evergreen or semi-deciduous forest, in moist upland forest, dense riverine woodland and scattered-tree grassland, at 900–2,400m.

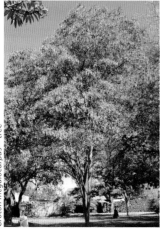
Croton megalocarpus – tree

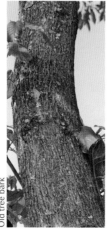
Old tree bark

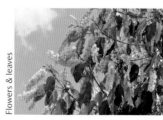
Flowers & leaves

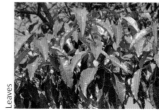
Leaves

USAGE AND TREATMENT

PARTS USED Roots, leaves and bark.
TRADITIONAL MEDICINAL USES Decoctions of roots and stems are used as a remedy for intestinal worms and also as a purgative.[M70, M93] Leaves are used as a remedy for whooping cough and throat infections.[M4, M70] Bark is used to treat chest complaints, rheumatism and indigestion. A bark decoction is taken as a vermifuge and can also be used in the treatment of whooping cough, pneumonia, stomach ache, fevers such as malaria, and abdominal complaints associated with gall bladder and spleen problems.[M93] Juice from leaves and young twigs is applied to wounds.[M93]

PREPARATION AND DOSAGE
WHOOPING COUGH AND THROAT AILMENTS Boil a handful of fresh leaves or fresh pounded stem bark in a litre of water for 10 minutes. Drink a cup of the decoction twice a day. Chew 2 or 3 fresh leaves, swallowing the leaf juice for relief from coughing.
PURGATIVE AND FOR TREATING INTESTINAL PARASITES Add a handful of pounded fresh root or stem bark or 2.5g of dry root or stem bark powder to a litre of boiling water. Leave for 20 minutes, stirring intermittently. Take this mixture before breakfast in the morning.

 WARNING! Overdosing can be very harmful, as most species of *Croton* contain poisonous compounds.

PHARMACOLOGY AND CHEMISTRY

PHARMACOLOGICAL PROPERTIES
Croton bark has shown mitogenic activity.[P225] Oven-dried leaves and stems have shown molluscicidal activity.[P226] Some diterpenoids[P26] in species of *Croton* are toxic irritants of the skin and mucosas,[P96] and these compounds may be the cause of a burning sensation in the throat and mouth.

COMPOUNDS REPORTED
The anti-ulcerogenic effects of *C. cajucara* bark (not described here) has been ascribed to the presence of crotonin and related Nor-clerodane diterpenes.[P227] Compounds isolated from species of *Croton* include several alkaloids, flavonoids, cardenolides, saponins, monoterpenoids and diterpenoids.[P228] Nor-clerodane diterpenes such as crotonin are the most common metabolites.[P227] Triterpenes such as betulin[P229] are found in *C. megalocarpus* stem bark. Phenylpropanoids in the bark include ferulic acid, and a trans-hexacosyl ester is also reported from this plant.[P230] Among diterpenes isolated from roots of *C. dichogamus*, 10-epi-maninsigin D showed cytotoxicity against Caco-2 cell line.[P231]

Crotonin

Betulin

Native to Indian subcontinent and Southeast Asia

Common names Turmeric, Asian Turmeric • **Local names** Bizari / Manjano (Swa.), Haldi (Urd., Hind., Punj.), Hardar (Guj.)

Description and ecology

Small, perennial, rhizomatous herb 0.5–1m tall and growing from yellow to orange underground tubers or stems, with warm, bitter, peppery taste. **Leaves** 5–10, large, with long stalk and oblong-lanceolate blade pointed near the base.

Flowers white or yellowish green, sometimes tinged reddish purple. Prefers humid conditions, temperatures of 20–30°C and rich loamy soils. Widely grown in East Africa, as in tropical Asia and America. A key ingredient in Indian cooking, turmeric is also widely used medicinally.

USAGE AND TREATMENT

PARTS USED Underground rhizomes.

TRADITIONAL MEDICINAL USES Turmeric is a remedy for indigestion, flatulence[M6, M95] and appetite loss[M9] as well as for bronchial coughs,[M6] colds and stomach ailments. It is used as an anthelmintic to kill intestinal worms.[M7] Its also said to relieve swelling, bruises and pains suffered in accidents.[M7, M70] A strained infusion applied as eyedrops is used as a remedy for sore red eyes.[M7] Turmeric acts as an astringent in arresting haemorrhages and bleeding from wounds. It is used to treat painful boils full of pus and also helps in the treatment of rheumatic arthritis.[M7, M70]

PREPARATION AND DOSAGE

ARTHRITIS, BODY SWELLINGS, BRUISING AND OTHER INJURIES Add 1g of powdered turmeric to a cup of warm milk. Drink 3 times daily after meals. Or mix equal parts of turmeric and sundried or oven-dried lime (citrus) powder with warm water to make a paste. Apply to affected areas.

INTESTINAL WORMS Boil 1–2g of turmeric and 1–2g of dry ground ginger in half a cup of water. Drink 3 times a day before meals. Alternatively, add 15–20g of fresh turmeric to a litre of boiled water, leave for 10–15 minutes and drink a cup 3 times daily with meals.

BRONCHIAL COUGHS, COLDS AND A RUNNY NOSE Add 1–2g of turmeric powder to a cup of warm milk. Drink twice a day (morning and night) after meals. Inhaling the smoke from burning turmeric powder for a few minutes at a time can also be helpful. To treat bronchial coughs, mix 1g of turmeric, 1g of ginger and 1g of clove powder with a tablespoon of honey and take 3 times a day. Or add 1–2g of finely ground, dry, roasted turmeric to a cup of lukewarm water and drink twice daily for a few days.

PAINFUL BOILS AND BLEEDING WOUNDS Mix a tablespoon of fresh turmeric powder in half a cup of brown wheat flour and make a warm poultice. Place it over the boil and cover with a bandage. Apply a fresh poultice 3 times a day. After cleaning a wound, sprinkle some fresh turmeric and cinnamon powder on the wound for relief from pain and as a healing aid.

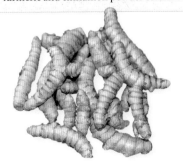

Curcuma longa – fresh rhizomes

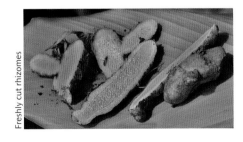

Freshly cut rhizomes

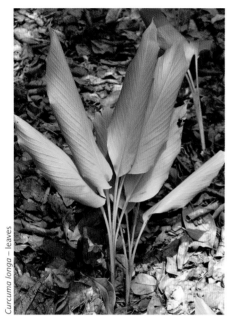

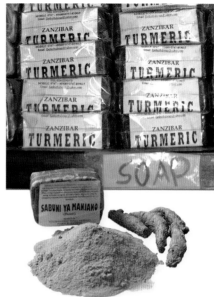

Curcuma longa – leaves

Curcuma longa – soap, dry rhizomes and powder form

PHARMACOLOGY AND CHEMISTRY

PHARMACOLOGICAL PROPERTIES

Curcuma longa has both cholagogue (enhancing the emptying of the gall bladder) and carminative properties; it is helpful in gastritis and hypochloridia, and increases the production of gastric juices, thereby easing digestion.[P84] Its curcuminoids, including curcumin, produce antioxidant, anti-inflammatory, antiviral and antifungal activities.[P232] Curcumin has been shown to be safe in six human trials.[P232]

COMPOUNDS REPORTED

Turmeric's colouring is a result of the presence of curcuminoids, principally curcumin (or diferuloyl methane).[P17, P84, P156] The volatile oil contains sesquiterpenes (e.g. zingiberene), alcohols, ketones and monoterpenes. The rhizome contains arabinose, fructose and glucose as well as abundant zingiberaceous starch grains.[P17] Curcumins I, II and III isolated from *C. longa* showed anticancer activity against leukaemia, colon, CNS, melanoma, and renal and breast cancer cell lines. These compounds also showed antioxidant and anti-inflammatory activities.[P233]

Curcumin I

Zingiberene

a. *Cyphostemma adenocaule*   Indigenous

Common name Cyphostemma • **Local names** Mwengele (Swa.), Mwenjere (Dig.), Mutumutua (Kik.), Mwengere (Zig.)

Description and ecology

Climbing, scrambling, trailing, herbaceous perennial plant. Stems 1.5–7.5m long, produced from a tuberous rootstock, scrambling over the ground, climbing into surrounding vegetation with the support of tendrils. **Leaves** 3–5-foliolately compound, the elliptic to broadly ovate leaflets glabrous to densely hairy, with toothed margins and pointed apices. **Flowers** small, cream or greenish yellow, borne in cymes 3–15cm long. **Fruits** ellipsoid berries with a pointed apex, green at first but turning to red or purple, 10–14 × 6–9mm. Seeds ellipsoid. Common in dry bushland, especially riverine thickets, throughout East Africa, at 0–2,500m.

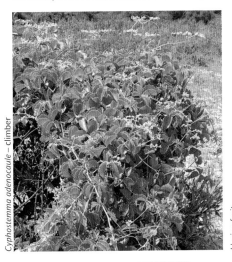

Cyphostemma adenocaule – climber

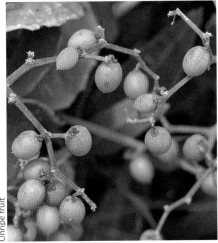

Unripe fruit

USAGE AND TREATMENT

PARTS USED Roots, leaves and tubers.

TRADITIONAL MEDICINAL USES A warm decoction made by boiling the entire plant is used to wash and heal wounds.M31 A fresh leaf poultice is used on body swellings and placed over the chest as a treatment for pneumonia.M1, M31 Leaf infusions are taken as a purgative and may help to treat a swollen abdomen.M96 A poultice made from the tubers is used to reduce swellings and abscesses.M70 A decoction of tubers may help to treat syphilis, abdominal pain during pregnancy, and to give relief from knee, shoulder and joint pains and swellings.M31, M70 A decoction of roots is taken orally for a hernia, appendicitis and uvulitis, while root powder is used in oral treatments for an enlarged spleen, stomach ache, migraine, mental disease and syphilis.M32, M70 A root decoction also helps to prevent miscarriage (abortion) and to treat malaria.M96 A decoction of dried roots, mixed with root bark of *Albizia anthelmintica* and *Harrisonia abyssinica*, is drunk on the first day of menstruation to help with possible sterility.M30 A root infusion is taken against tapeworms.M96

b. *Cyphostemma serpens* {style="float:left"} Indigenous

Common name Cyphostemma • **Local names** Bwombwe (Luo), Ol kilenyei (Maa.)

Description and ecology

Erect, thick, compact, herbaceous plant with or without tendrils, growing close to the ground from a tuberous taproot. **Leaves** palmate, the 3–7 leaflets linear and elliptical, very hairy below. **Flowers** pale greenish yellow. **Fruits** green, round or oval berries covered with hairs, turning to bright red when ripe. Commonly found in bushed grassland, at 1,200–2,200m.

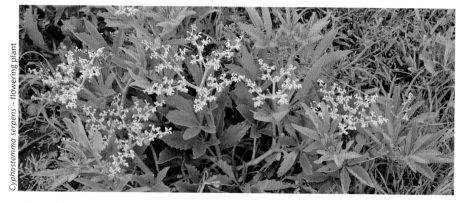

Cyphostemma serpens – flowering plant

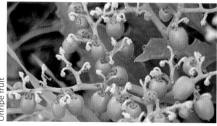

Unripe fruit

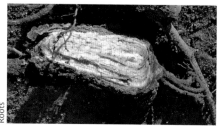

Roots

USAGE AND TREATMENT

PARTS USED Leaves, tuberous roots and green fruits.
TRADITIONAL MEDICINAL USES Decoctions of the tuberous roots are given to children as a tonic. The green fruit is also eaten as a tonic[M1, M70] and is a good source of vitamin C. Decoctions of pounded fresh leaves are applied to abscesses and boils, and a boiled root decoction can be taken for gonorrhoea and syphilis.[M1, M70]

PREPARATION AND DOSAGE
ABSCESSES AND BOILS Boil a handful of fresh leaves in a litre of water for 10 minutes. Use the warm decoction to clean the afflicted areas. A poultice of pounded fresh leaves can also be applied to the affected area.
CHILDREN'S TONIC Boil some fresh green berries in water until they are soft and pulpy, then add milk and give the mixture to children to eat. The tuberous roots can also be boiled in this way until soft and then served to children as a tonic.

PHARMACOLOGY AND CHEMISTRY

PHARMACOLOGICAL PROPERTIES
Cyphostemma adenocaule is a non-cultivated vegetable eaten in most countries in Africa.[P234] Ethanolic extracts of leaves, stem and roots of *C. adenocaule* showed antioxidant activity in a DPPH radical scavenging assay.[P234] Extracts of leaves and roots also possess appreciable anti-inflammatory potential.[P234] Leaves of this plant have been used as an insecticide.[P234]

COMPOUNDS REPORTED
Triterpenoids, including cyphostemmic acid, and steroids, including β-sitosterol and its glucoside, have been reported from *C. adenocaule*.[P235] The compound 3β,28-dihydroxy-30-norlupan-20-one isolated from this plant exhibited antiplasmodial activity against the chloroquine-sensitive strain 3D7 of *Plasmodium falciparum*.[P235]

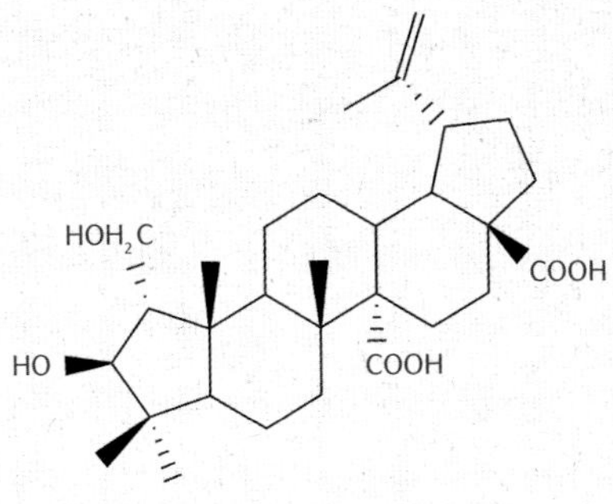

Cyphostemmic acid

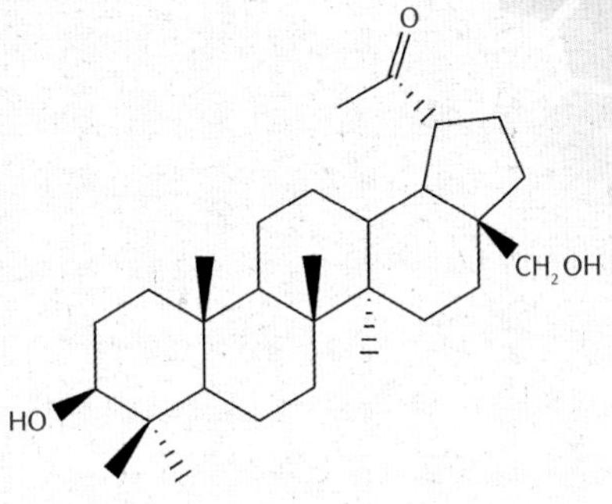

3β,28-Dihydroxy-30-norlupan-20-one

35 *Datura stramonium* SOLANACEAE

Native to tropical America

Common names Datura, Common Thorn Apple, Devil's Apple, Devil's Trumpet • **Local names** Mranaa (Swa.), Barutu / Chemogong' (Kip.), Mwalola (Tai.), Silulu (Buk.), Dhatoria (Guj.), Dhatura (Hind., Urd.)

Description and ecology

Erect, annual, bushy plant 0.6–1.5(–2)m tall, with stout, green to purplish stems. **Leaves** ovate, 8–20cm long, smooth, soft, dark green above, light green below, margin dentate, stems and leaves with unpleasant smell when crushed. **Flowers** white to creamy or bright blue, trumpet-shaped, 6–9cm long. **Fruit** an ovoid, erect capsule densely covered with prickles, 3.5–6.5 × 2–5cm, splitting at and between divisions when dry. **Seeds** numerous, dark brown to black, flat, kidney-shaped, 3–4 × 2–3mm. Grows as a weed throughout the world, in East Africa found mainly in disturbed areas, at 0–2,300m.

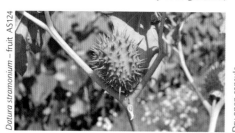

Datura stramonium – fruit AS124

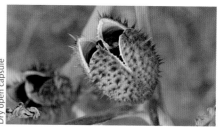

Dry open capsule

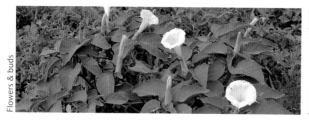

Flowers & buds

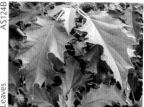

AS124B

Leaves

USAGE AND TREATMENT

PARTS USED Leaves, green fruits and seeds.

TRADITIONAL MEDICINAL USES Leaves of *Datura stramonium* are used to treat coughs, asthma and bronchitis.[M6, M70, M97] Warm fresh leaves are a trusted remedy for rheumatism,[M1, M2, M9] boils, abscesses and gout. Fresh leaves are used for dressing wounds and treating insect bites, and the seeds are used in treatments for ringworm and other fungal afflictions.[M6, M70] Leaves, pounded and boiled, are applied to burns to prevent infection and to ease pain. Fresh green fruit can be used for toothache and tonsillitis. Seeds are administered for spermatorrhoea, premature ejaculation and tenuous semen; they are also used to treat diabetes and to stop sweating from the palms and soles,[M7, M97] a condition for which the leaf paste is also used. Seeds can also be used as a remedy for intestinal spasm, digestive disorders,[M9] colic pain, gastric ulcers and Parkinson's disease.[M2, M7] The leaf juice can treat head lice on the scalp and in the hair. The fruit juice is applied to the scalp for treating falling hair and dandruff, and the juice is also applied onto painful wounds and sores.[M97]

PREPARATION AND DOSAGE

SWEATING FROM THE PALMS AND SOLES Grind some leaves into a fine powder. Add water to make a paste for rubbing on the palms and soles.

RHEUMATISM, JOINT SWELLINGS, BOILS, ABSCESSES AND GOUT Warm a few fresh leaves over a fire and use them to make a poultice. Apply directly to affected areas. In the case of joint pain and rheumatism, cover the poultice with a bandage or warm cloth.

DRESSINGS FOR WOUNDS Pound 3 fresh leaves and add 50g of ghee or regular Vaseline® (non-scented). Mix thoroughly. Rub this ointment on the wound. Even severe wounds can be dressed in this way.

INSECT BITES, FUNGAL INFECTIONS AND RINGWORM Swab the affected area with fresh sap from some leaves. An ointment made from ground dry seeds mixed with ghee can also be applied to affected areas of the skin.

COUGHS, ASTHMA AND BRONCHITIS Pound some dried leaves. Roll into a cigarette or insert into a pipe and smoke the burning leaves, inhaling deeply. A mixture comprising 1g of dried datura leaves, 2g of dried eucalyptus leaves and 5g of dried paw-paw leaves, all crushed together, can also be smoked for relief from asthma and bronchitis.

BURNS Boil some fresh leaves for 3 minutes. Pound them and apply directly to burns to reduce the pain and prevent bacterial infection.

 WARNING! Datura is a highly toxic, hallucinogenic plant. Prolonged internal use in high doses can trigger mental disorders as well as hallucinations.

PHARMACOLOGY AND CHEMISTRY

PHARMACOLOGICAL PROPERTIES

Datura stramonium is highly toxic. Its poisonous alkaloids include atropine and hyoscine, which can cause hallucinations, insomnia, confusion and mental disorders.[P84, P96] Atropine's antispasmodic properties help to relax the muscles of the digestive tract, of the bronchi and of the urinary and bile ducts,[P84, P156] while reducing saliva, sweat and other bodily secretions. The plant has depressant, sedative, analgesic, antitussive and anti-asthmatic properties.[P84]

COMPOUNDS REPORTED

This plant contains atropine and other antispasmodic alkaloids,[P84, P159] especially the seeds, which have a constant 0.4% alkaloid content, the main components of which are atropine = (±)-hyoscyamine[P84, P96, P156, P159, P236] and (-)-hyoscine (-)-scopolamine.[P84, P156] These compounds act on the autonomic nervous system.[P84] Over 60 compounds, including scopoline, have been identified from the seeds of this plant.[P236] The alkaloids found in this plant are used clinically as anticholinergic agents. Extracts of leaves and seeds could be used to manage the two-spotted spider mite. *D. stramonium* was once used to cure cancer but there were side effects.[P236] In a chronic toxicity study, the alkaloids atropine and scopolamine administered intraperitoneally did not produce death. However, diarrhoea and hypoactivity were observed.[P236] The plant also contains citric and malic acids as well as tannins and essential oils.[P84]

Atropine = (±) Hyoscyamine

Scopoline

Malic acid

Indigenous

Common names Sickle Bush, Tangle Pod • **Local names** Msingoni (Bon.), Jirime (Bor.), Mkingiri (Gir.), Muvilisya (Kam.), Ruitie (Kik.), Okiri (Luo), Mukingili (Sam.), Ditar (Som.), Dungui (Tai.), Etiral (Tur.), Endundulu (Aru.), Mtundulu (Gogo, Suk.), Mtunduru (Ngu.), Mutunduu (Nyam., Nyat.), Mdabiri (Ran.), Mkulagembe / Msigino / Mvunja shoka (Swa.), Mchelegembe / Mjerejele (Zig.), Etira / Etirai (Ate.), Muwanika (Lug.), Okiro / Okito (Luo-A), Atila / Okutu-ipeti (Luo-L), Luburyango (Luso.), Kalemanjovu (Runyan.)

Description and ecology

Bushy, thorny, semi-deciduous shrub or small tree with an open crown, reaching 2–7m, occasionally 12m. **Bark** grey-brown, rough and fissured, branches hairy, with alternate thorns up to 8cm long. **Leaves** bipinnately compound, up to 15cm long, feathery like *Acacia* leaves, with tiny leaflets in 9–41 pairs. **Flowers** fragrant, in pendulous, cylindrical, bicoloured spikes 6–8cm long, the basal half (closest to point of attachment) pink or mauve, the apical half (at the tip) yellow. **Fruits** in clusters of flat, strangely twisted or contorted pods up to 10cm long, green when young but later brown or black, containing 3 or 4 dark brown, rounded seeds. Found in varied habitats throughout East Africa. Confined mainly to wooded grassland, various types of bushland, riverbanks and rocky hillsides down to coastal plains and in disturbed areas, at 0–1,700m.

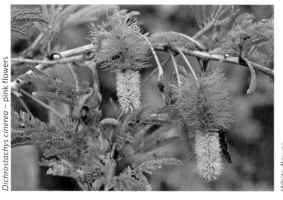

Dichrostachys cinerea – pink flowers

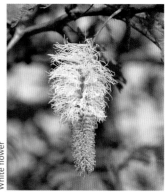

White flower

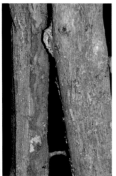

Bark

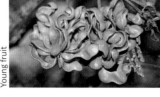

Young fruit

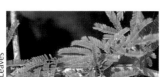

Leaves

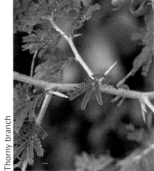

Thorny branch

PARTS USED Bark, roots and leaves.
TRADITIONAL MEDICINAL USES Roots are used as an astringent for scorpion bites and may help to counter poison from snakebite. They are also used as an aphrodisiac.[M70] The leaves can serve the same purpose and are also used as a local anaesthetic and for treating ulcers and gonorrhoea.[M4] The bark serves as an astringent and vermifuge in the treatment of dysentery, headache and toothache.[M98] Leaf extracts are taken for stomach ache and conjunctivitis.[M1, M40] Steam from fresh roots, leaves and bark, all boiled together, is inhaled to soothe coughs. A root decoction is anthelmintic, purgative and strongly diuretic, and a decoction of leaves is used as a diuretic and laxative.[M98] Stem bark of *Dichrostachys cinerea* is used by the Maasai in Tanzania to treat suspected malaria.[M127]

PREPARATION AND DOSAGE

APHRODISIAC Mix a handful of fresh roots, washed and crushed, into a bowl of porridge or boil in water and drink warm twice a day.
SCORPION BITE AND SNAKEBITE Boil a handful of fresh or dry roots in half a litre of water for 10–15 minutes. Apply the warm decoction directly to the bite. A poultice of pounded fresh leaves can also be applied.
STOMACH ACHE AND CONJUNCTIVITIS Add 2 or 3 crushed fresh leaves to a cup of cold boiled water, together with a quarter teaspoon of salt. Stir the infusion. Filter and drink twice a day for relief from stomach pain. Administer as eyedrops to treat conjunctivitis.

PHARMACOLOGICAL PROPERTIES

Both the fruits and leaves have shown antibacterial activity against different organisms.[P237] Extracts of stem bark showed very significant antimalarial activity in albino mice.[P238]

COMPOUNDS REPORTED

Triterpenes (e.g. friedelin), steroids (e.g. sitosterol) and fatty acid derivatives (e.g. octacosanol) have all been isolated from this plant.[P239] A novel flavan, (-)-mesquitol, with a potent radical scavenging activity has been isolated from stem wood.[P240] The crude extract and the triterpene betulinic acid, obtained from bark, showed anticancer activity against nine multifactorial drug-resistant cancer cells.[P241]

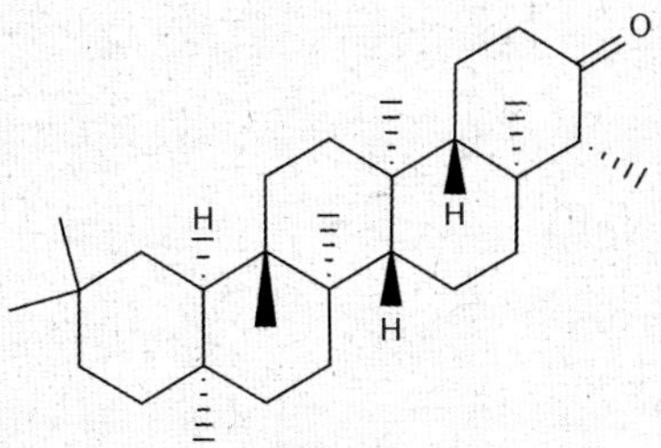

Friedelin

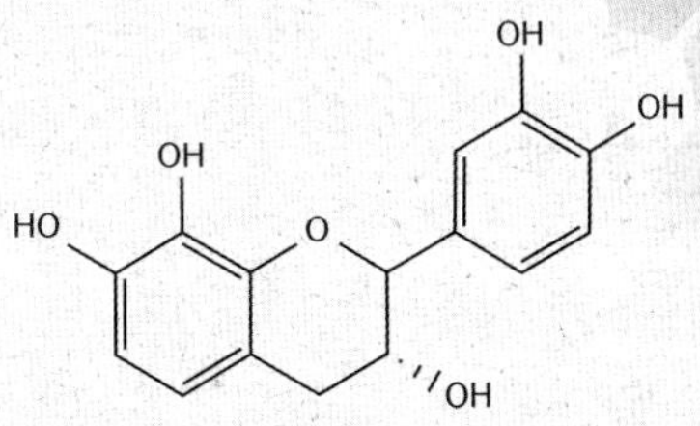

(-)-Mesquitol

37 *Dodonaea viscosa*
(Dodonaea angustifolia)
SAPINDACEAE

Indigenous

Common names Dodonaea, Hopbush, Sand Olive • **Local names** Hidesa (Bor.), Kithongoi / Muthongoi (Kam.), Ol-geturai / Oltuyesi (Maa.), Murema-muthua (Kik.), Muendu (Luh.), Oking (Luo), Tabilikuet (Tug.), Mkaa-Pwani (Swa.Ken.), Msidu (Tai.), Tombolokwo (Pok.), Ol-getinai (Aru.), Berimi (Goro.), Luhahi / Lunyahi (Hehe), Kiganhihangi / Mhangehange (Lugu.), Iwuwu (Mer.), Mgwiti / Mnjitwe (Pare), Muberimo (Ran.), Mzutu / Mzutwe (Sam.), Mkengeta (Swa.Tan.), Musamba (Ruki.), Mushambya / Omusamba (Runyan.), Tombolokwa (Sebei)

Description and ecology
Slender, multi-stemmed, evergreen shrub 1–4m tall, rarely a small tree up to 9m, with an open, shallow crown. **Bark** light grey, grooved and peeling, branches red and sticky. **Leaves** simple, alternate, obovate or lanceolate, 4–7cm long, glossy, thin, sticky with resin, stiffly erect, tapering to a stalk. **Flowers** small, yellow-green to orange-red, in panicles up to 2.5cm long, male and female flowers separate.

Fruits distinctive capsules with 2 or 3 papery wings, sometimes inflated, greenish to red, resembling blossoms, turning light brown when dry. The wind-dispersed fruits render *D. viscosa* a pioneer species where forests are colonising grassland and it is well known as drought and wind resistant. Widespread throughout East Africa where it grows in a variety of habitats from riverine forest to rocky areas, at 0–2,800m.

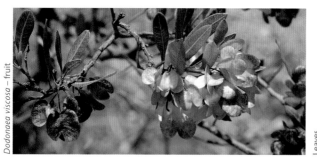

Dodonaea viscosa – fruit

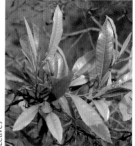

Leaves

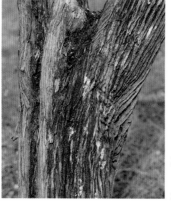

Bark

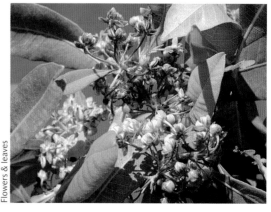

Flowers & leaves

USAGE AND TREATMENT

PARTS USED Roots, leaves and twigs.
TRADITIONAL MEDICINAL USES Root decoctions are given to nursing mothers to stimulate lactation.[M4] Leaf infusions are taken as a remedy for diarrhoea or are applied locally as a haemostatic (to stop bleeding).[M1, M70] 8Fresh leaves and twigs are taken in decoctions for colds, influenza, pneumonia, tuberculosis,[M99] stomach pain and even arthritis.[M70] Gargling with these decoctions is a treatment for a sore throat, while their external application to a skin rash acts as an anti-itching agent.[M2, M4, M70, M116] Leaf extracts are used as a mild purgative and for rheumatism, a sore throat and haemorrhoids.[M99] A leaf decoction is given for influenza and colds and also to induce sweating. It helps to relieve a cough and the congested feeling typical of influenza.[M116]

PREPARATION AND DOSAGE
DIARRHOEA Add 5g of pounded fresh leaves to half a litre of cold boiled water. Stir. Strain the extract after half an hour and drink in small quantities during the day.
BLEEDING WOUNDS Dry some fresh leaves and grind them into a powder. Mix with water and apply to fresh wounds, adding some freshly squeezed leaf juice.
FEVER, COLDS, INFLUENZA, PNEUMONIA, TUBERCULOSIS, STOMACH PAIN, SORE THROAT AND SKIN RASHES Steep half a cup of crushed fresh leaves and twigs in a litre of water for 20 minutes. Stir intermittently. Filter and drink or gargle (for a sore throat) the infusion twice daily or apply externally (to stop itching caused by a skin rash).

PHARMACOLOGY AND CHEMISTRY

PHARMACOLOGICAL PROPERTIES
Leaf extracts of *Dodonaea viscosa* have produced anti-inflammatory activity, with no toxicity or mortality in mice.[P242] The crude leaf extract shows antibacterial activity against *Streptococcus pyogenes* and *Staphylococcus aureus* and strong activity against Coxsackie virus B3 and influenza-A virus.[P243] No antifungal activity has been reported, however.[P244] Leaves exhibit analgesic and antipyretic activities.[P244]

COMPOUNDS REPORTED
Many flavonoids, such as santin,[P245, P246] and structurally similar diterpenoids[P245] (e.g. dodonic acid, hautriwaic acid) and steroids such as ß-sitosterol, stigmasterol, along with a glycoside of ß-sitosterol[P247] have been reported from different species of *Dodonaea*. The substance 5,7,4'-trihydroxy-3,6-dimethoxyflavone has been identified as the major compound in the leaves.[P245] In an antimicrobial assay, the diterpene hautriwaic acid lactone and the flavonoid catechin isolated from *D. viscosa* were the most active compounds.[P248]

Santin

Dodonic acid

a. *Dombeya burgessiae*   Indigenous

Common names Dombeya, Pink/White Dombeya • **Local names** Mukeu (Kik.), Silibwet (Kip.), Muvau (Kam.), Mukusa (Luh.), Owich (Luo), Ol-subukioi (Maa.), Monde (Mer.), Kilipehet (Nan.), Ilporowai (Sam.), Epongoi (Tur.), Omukarabo (Nyan.)

Description and ecology

Multi-stemmed, much-branched shrub or small tree 2–4(–7)m tall, branching from low down, branches densely hairy. **Bark** outer bark brown, inner bark tough and fibrous. **Leaves** simple, alternate, broadly ovate, heart-shaped, up to 15 × 15cm, 3–5-lobed or entire, hairy both sides, margin finely dentate. **Flowers** white or pink, in long-stalked bunches (umbels), stalks up to 10cm long. **Fruit** an ovoid to globose capsule 0.5–1.5cm in diameter, brown, hairy. **Seeds** triangular, rough, dark brown to black, 3–4 × 2mm, very hairy. Commonly found in all the region's drier upland forest edges, riverine and lakeshore vegetation, on rocky sites in semi-evergreen bushland and in lightly wooded grassland, at 750–2,400m.

USAGE AND TREATMENT

PARTS USED Bark, roots and leaves.

TRADITIONAL MEDICINAL USES Dry root powder is used as a cough medicine. Infusions of roots are taken to relieve stomach pain.[M4, M70, M112, M115] A leaf decoction is drunk for leprosy, and pounded fresh leaves are applied to the sores.[M112, M115] The bark, either chewed or taken in decoctions, is used as both an aphrodisiac[M112, M115] and a treatment for indigestion.[M1, M4, M70]

PREPARATION AND DOSAGE

STOMACH PAIN AND INDIGESTION Steep a handful of crushed fresh roots in a litre of water for 10–15 minutes. Stir, drain and drink the resulting infusion at intervals during the day.

COUGHS Burn some dry root powder and inhale the smoke. Use the burned residue as snuff.

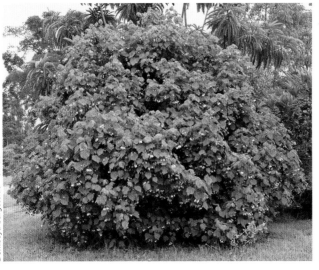

Dombeya burgessiae – shrub

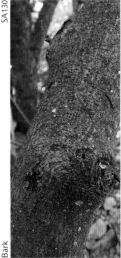

SA130

Bark

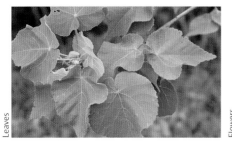
Leaves

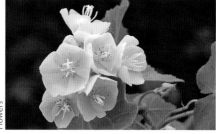
Flowers

b. *Dombeya rotundifolia*　　　　　　　　　　　Indigenous

Common name Round-leaved Dombeya • **Local names** Mtoo (Kam.), Mutoo (Kik.), Olawuo (Maa.), Mtorobwe (Swa.), Mugeriswa (Pok.), Porowet (Tug.), Ndowa (Tai.), Ebolis (Tur.), Mringaringa (Chag.), Mtati (Gogo), Gwaata-aati (Goro.), Mkangatowo (Hehe), Mlwati / Msoto / Mswayu (Lugu.), Mutogotogho (Nyat.), Mtogo (Nyir.), Msagusa (Nyam.), Mchakay (Ran.), Mluati / Mlwati (Zig.), Mukole (Lug.), Mufudufu (Lugw.)

Description and ecology
Small and much-branched, deciduous tree 4–6(–9)m tall, with a rounded crown and single well-defined trunk. **Bark** dark brown or blackish, rough and corky. **Leaves** simple, alternate, broad, oval to almost round, 6–18cm across, rough and sandpapery above, often very hairy below, stalked, with toothed margin, crispy and hard when dry. **Flowers** 15–20mm diameter, abundant, usually white but occasionally pale pink in clusters (umbel-like cyme), sweetly scented, attracting bees; leaves and flower buds densely covered in stellate hairs. **Fruits** small, round, hairy capsules. **Seeds** triangular, 3 × 2.5mm, brown. Usually confined to open or wooded grasslands in dry areas, often near termite mounds and rocky places, at 900–2,250m.

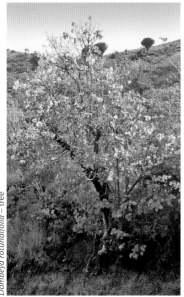
Dombeya rotundifolia – tree

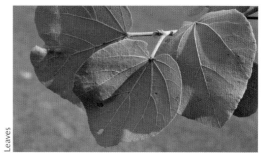
Leaves

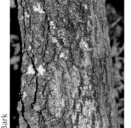
Bark

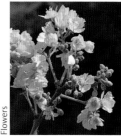
Flowers

PARTS USED Bark and roots.

TRADITIONAL MEDICINAL USES Root decoctions are used to treat rheumatism and are given to children suffering from diarrhoea and stomach pain.[M1, M4, M112, M115] Boiled roots are applied externally to treat rheumatism.[M112, M115] An infusion of the root is drunk as a possible treatment for syphilis and infertility.[M100] A bark decoction is drunk against dizziness and meningitis.[M100] Decoctions of fresh roots of another *Dombeya* species found in East Africa, *D. kirkii*, are used for abdominal pain, while a decoction of bark of *D. goetzenii* is taken as a remedy for indigestion after feasting on meat. In South Africa, bark decoctions are used for chest ailments and also to hasten the onset of delayed labour. Bark infusions are taken, orally or as enemas, for haemorrhoids, diarrhoea, stomach ailments and internal ulcers.[M2, M112, M115] Bark decoctions are also taken for nausea and headache in expectant mothers.[M2] Dry root powder is burned and the smoke inhaled to soothe coughs and chest pain. Burned root powder is taken as snuff.

PREPARATION AND DOSAGE
DIARRHOEA IN CHILDREN Steep half a cup of pounded fresh roots in a litre of water for 15 minutes. Stir and filter the mixture. Drink at intervals during the day.
COUGHS AND CHEST PAIN Dry some fresh roots in the sun or in an oven at low heat, then crush and make into a powder. Burn the powder, inhaling the smoke. Use the burned powder as snuff.

PHARMACOLOGICAL PROPERTIES
Strong anti-inflammatory and antibacterial activities have been detected in *Dombeya rotundifolia* leaf and young shoot extracts.[P249, P250] The aqueous and ethanolic leaf extracts of *D. rotundifolia* showed antihypertensive activity, corroborating its traditional use.[P250] The extracts were not toxic to Vero cells.[P250]

COMPOUNDS REPORTED
Phytochemical screening has found saponins in *D. rotundifolia* bark, while detecting cardiac glycosides in leaves, young shoots and bark material.[P249] Cardiac glycosides, fatty acids, flavonoids, iridoids, phenolics, saponins, steroids, tannins, and terpenoids have been isolated from leaf extracts of *D. rotundifolia*.[P250] The triterpene lupeol and the steroid β-sitosterol have been reported from a stem bark extract, while ethanolic leaf extracts produced the fatty acids lauric acid 3, myristic acid 4, palmitic acid 5 and stearic acid.[P250]

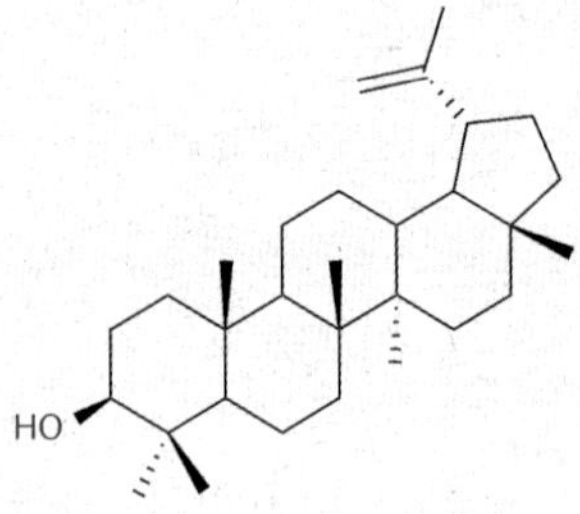

Lupeol

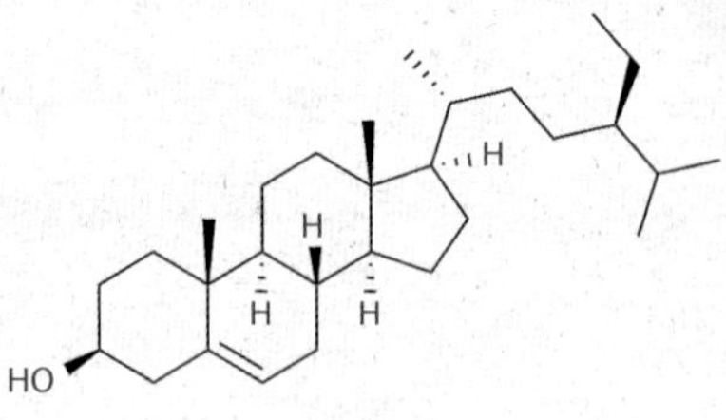

β-Sitosterol

Indigenous

Common names Ekebergia, Dogplum, Mountain Ash • **Local names** Mrongoleh (Bon.), Mukongu (Kam.), Araruet (Kip.), Omonyamavi (Kis.), Mununga (Kik.), Manuki-masi (Tai.), Ol-subukiai / Osongoroi (Maa.Ken.), Muchogomo (Mer.Ken.), Teldet (Nan.), Bumet (Sebei), Arariet / Ternwa (Tug.), Eng'amwo (Tur.), Tido (Luo), Ol-mukuma / Olmukuna (Aru.), Mfuare / Mfyahi / Msisi (Chag.), Mvumba (Gogo), Musimbi (Haya), Olmukuna / Osongoroi (Maa.Tan.), Mkuna / Olmkuna / Olmkuno (Mer.Tan.), Mnu / Mtarima (Ran.), Monko (Samb.), Umuyagu (Zin.), Musalamumali (Lugi.), Mufumba (Ruki.), Bumet (Sebei)

Description and ecology
Medium-sized to large tree reaching 8–30m, evergreen or sometimes semi-deciduous, with a large spreading crown and a straight or sometimes crooked bole which is fluted or has short buttresses at the base. **Bark** grey-brown and rough, cracking and splitting with age, branches dotted with prominent creamy white pores or lenticels. **Leaves** compound, up to 30cm long, crowded at ends of branches, leaflets thin, glossy green, in 5–7(–8) pairs plus a terminal one, pointed at bases and apices. **Flowers** small, up to 5mm in diameter, greenish white tinged with pink, in loose sprays 8–10cm long, sweetly scented. **Fruit** a rounded drupe, 1.5cm across, thin-skinned, fleshy, orange-yellow to deep red when ripe, on long stalks, with 2–4 stones, each stone containing 1 seed. Widespread in various habitats from lowland scrub, woodland and wooded grassland to dry highland forest, especially *Podo–Olea* forest, riverine forest and forest edges, at 0–2,600m.

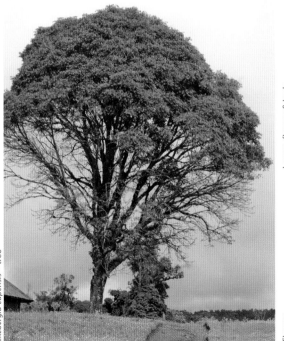

Ekebergia capensis – tree

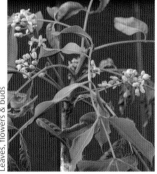

Leaves, flowers & buds

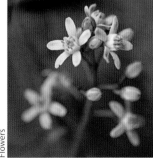

Flowers

PARTS USED Bark, roots and leaves.

TRADITIONAL MEDICINAL USES Decoctions of leaves are taken as a remedy for intestinal worms, especially hookworms and tapeworms.[M70, M71, M101] Bark is used to treat dysentery, heartburn and as an emetic. The roots are diuretic and expectorant and a root decoction is used to treat chronic coughs, heartburn, respiratory problems, dysentery and scabies.[M2, M70, M101, M116] Bark and root infusions are taken for relief from headache and gastritis. Leaf and bark decoctions are used as a vermifuge.[M116] Poultices of powdered bark are applied externally to fungal infections, skin rashes, acne, boils and abscesses.[M2, M70, M71, M101] Bark is also used as an astringent. Decoctions or infusions are taken to treat several conditions including gastritis, heartburn, dysentery, epilepsy and gonorrhoea.[M101]

PREPARATION AND DOSAGE

SKIN RASHES, FUNGAL INFECTIONS, ACNE, BOILS AND ABSCESSES Dry some fresh bark and grind it into a powder. Add a tablespoon of the powder to half a litre of water. Leave for 20–30 minutes, stirring intermittently. Filter and apply the infusion directly to the affected areas. A paste made by mixing the bark powder with a small quantity of water can also be rubbed on the affected areas.

DYSENTERY, INTESTINAL WORMS AND GASTRITIS Boil half a cup of pounded fresh leaves or bark in a litre of water for 10 minutes, stir and filter the mixture. Drink at intervals during the day.

PHARMACOLOGICAL PROPERTIES

Crude extracts of the plant have been reported to possess antiplasmodial, anti-inflammatory, hypotensive, uterotonic and antituberculotic activities.[P251]

COMPOUNDS REPORTED

The limonoid ekebergin[P252] has been isolated from the seeds. Analysis of the bark and stems has found no limonoids, however.[P252] Oleanonic acid isolated from root bark of *Ekebergia capensis* possessed high toxicity against the 4T1 and HEp2 cancer cell lines, while displaying low toxicity against the normal Vero cells. The plant also elaborates other triterpenoids that showed comparable cytotoxicity towards 'normal' (Vero) and tumour cells. The metabolites of this plant have also showed moderate in vitro antiplasmodial activity against the D6 and W2 strains of *Plasmodium falciparum*.[P251]

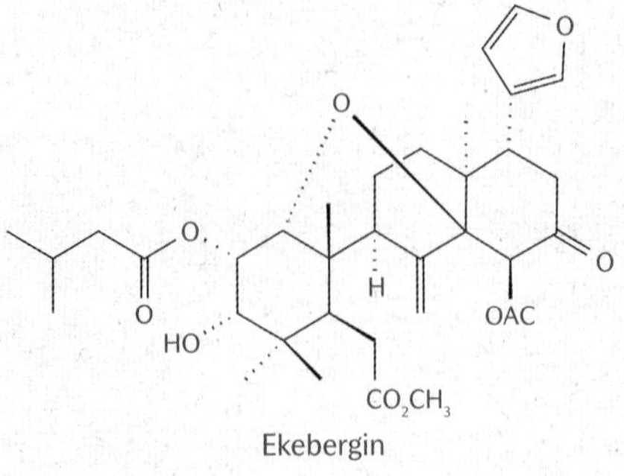

Ekebergin

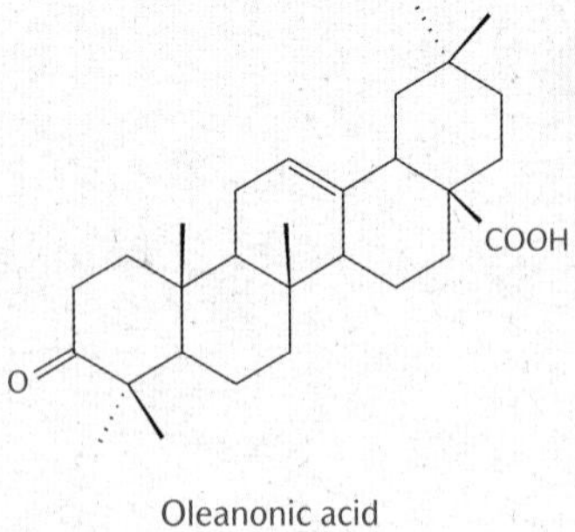

Oleanonic acid

a. *Entada abyssinica*   Indigenous

Common name Tree Entada • **Local names** Musembe / Kumusembe (Luh.), Osembe (Luo), Katutet / Mushembut (Nan.), Musiembu (Sebei), Aere-desu (Goro.), Mugelagela (Hehe), Mvutambula (Lugu.), Mfutambula (Nyam.), Msaningala (Nyir.), Ijwejwe (Ran.), Mfutamula (Suk.), Mfufumasimba (Zig.), Musangisangi (Zin.), Mwolola / Musambamazzi (Lug.), Musembe (Lugi.), Mukozia (Lugw.), Mujengejenge (Luny.), Oberipangala (Luo-J), Musambamadhi (Luso.), Kisangi (Ruki.), Muyora (Runyan.)

Description and ecology

Thornless deciduous shrub or small, low-branching tree 3–10m tall, with a spreading, flat or rounded crown. **Bark** grey-brown, smooth or rough, slightly fissured, flaking off in irregular patches. **Leaves** compound, feathery, with 2–20 pairs of pinnae, each bearing 15–45 pairs of tiny *Acacia*-like leaflets that are linear-oblong and up to 1cm long. **Flowers** small, creamy white fading to yellow, fragrant, in fluffy spikes 7–15cm long and in groups of 1–4. **Fruits** very long, broad pods, 15–35 × 3–8cm, brown, margins wavy, often remaining on the tree for long periods. **Seeds** oval, flat, 10–12 × 7–10mm, papery winged. Widespread across East Africa in woodland, wooded grassland, riverine forest and moist forest edges, at 450–2,200m.

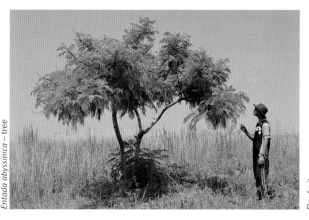

Entada abyssinica – tree

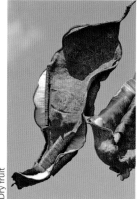

Dry fruit

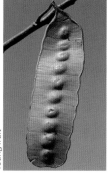

Young fruit

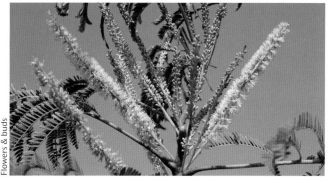

Flowers & buds

PARTS USED Roots, leaves and stem bark.
TRADITIONAL MEDICINAL USES A decoction of roots is used as a treatment for rheumatic pain[M1, M40, M70] and as an aphrodisiac. Root infusions are taken internally as a remedy for snakebite.[M1] Leaves are applied externally for fungal infections, and stem bark is used to heal wounds, boils, abscesses and burns.[M40, M70] A bark decoction is used in the treatment of colds, stomach pain and bronchial problems.[M112]

PREPARATION AND DOSAGE
RINGWORM AND OTHER FUNGAL INFECTIONS Mix some powdered dry leaves in water to form a paste. Rub on the affected areas.
WOUNDS, BOILS, ABSCESSES AND BURNS Dry some fresh stem bark and grind it into a fine powder. Add a tablespoon of the powder to half a litre of water and leave for 20–30 minutes, stirring the infusion intermittently. Filter and apply the infusion directly to the wound or mix it with flour and apply as a poultice.

b. *Entada leptostachya*

Indigenous

Common name Climbing Entada • **Local names** Hundad (Bor.), Mwaitha (Kam.), Kobagor (Som.), Mgambari (Swa.), Ldalampo (Sam.)

Description and ecology
Climbing shrub 6–10m long, with glabrous branchlets. **Bark** smooth, grey. **Leaves** compound, with 2–4 pairs of pinnae, each with 7–10 pairs of leaflets, narrowly oblong, 9–25mm long. **Flowers** creamy yellow, in 1–3 spikes 3–8cm long. **Fruits** very large pods, 16–22 × 4–8cm, green at first then turning brown, straight or slightly curved. **Seeds** oval, flat, 11–14 × 9mm. Common in dry *Acacia–Commiphora* bushland or woodland, at 100–1,500m.

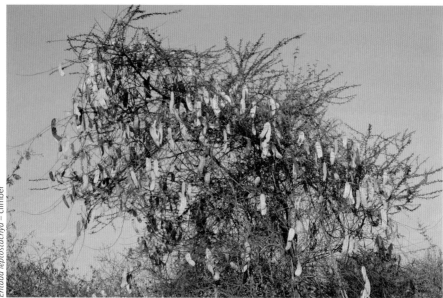

Entada leptostachya – climber

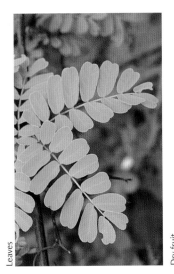

Leaves

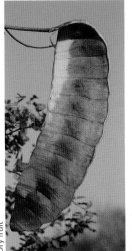

Dry fruit

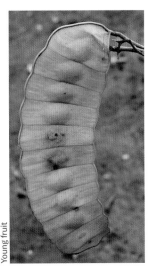

Young fruit

PARTS USED Roots.
TRADITIONAL MEDICINAL USES A decoction of boiled roots is taken as an aphrodisiac.[M40] An infusion of roots is used in the treatment of snakebite,[M33] chest pain and tuberculosis.[M1, M40, M70]

PREPARATION AND DOSAGE
No reliable information on precise dosages for this plant has been found.

PHARMACOLOGY AND CHEMISTRY

PHARMACOLOGICAL PROPERTIES
Entada abyssinica leaves have been found to show anti-inflammatory[P253] and antifungal[P254] activities. Dried roots have shown antitrypanosomal activity,[P255] while dried stem bark has exhibited antibacterial activity[P256] against different organisms. The leaves of *E. abyssinica* have proved highly active against the Semliki Forest virus.[P257]

COMPOUNDS REPORTED
Diterpenoids have been isolated from stem bark of *E. abyssinica*.[P258] The flavonoids entadanin and quercitrin, isolated from leaves and stem bark of this plant, showed good activity against *Salmonella typhimurium*, with minimum inhibitory concentration (MIC) values of 1.56 and 3.12µg/mL, respectively.[P258]

Entadanin

Quercitrin

a. *Erythrina abyssinica*   Indigenous

Common names Red-hot-poker Tree, Flame Tree, Lucky Bean • **Local names** Muvuti (Kam.), Muthuti (Kik.), Kogoruet (Kip.), Omotembe (Kis.), Mwembe (Luh.), Orembe (Luo), Olepangi (Maa.Ken.), Muuti (Mer.), Kagaruet (Nan.), Kokorwo (Pok.), Garacha (Sam.), Mwamba-ngoma (Swa.Ken.), Mulungu (Tai.), Olowani (Aru.), Miriri (Chag.), Mlinzi (Haya), Muhemi (Hehe), Ol-ngaboli / Ol-obani (Maa.Tan.), Msiviti (Nyat.), Mhalalwanhuba / Mkalalwankuva (Nyam.), Muungu (Pare), Kichumbichumbi (Ran.), Murungu (Samb.), Mkalalwanhuba / Pilipili (Suk.), Mjafari (Swa.Tan.), Mtasa (Zin.), Engosorot (Ate.), Lucoro (Ach.), Muyirikiti (Lug.), Oluo / Olugo (Lugb.), Cheroguru (Lugi.), Mutembetembe (Lugwe.), Lochoro (Luo-A), Koli (Luo-J), Ewilakot (Luo-L), Olawu (Madi), Muko / Kiko (Ruto.), Kaborte (Sebei)

Description and ecology

Deciduous tree 6–12(–15)m tall, with a short trunk, thick, spreading branches and a rounded crown. **Bark** yellowish brown, thick, corky and fissured, often with woody spines, branches twisted, twigs armed with strong curved prickles, initially densely hairy, later glabrous. **Leaves** alternate, 3-foliolately compound, leaflets broadly ovate, round, wider than long, leaf stalk 6–20cm long, often prickly. **Flowers** red to scarlet red, in strong, sturdy, dense heads 5–6cm long at the ends of branchlets, with thick stalks. **Fruits** hairy, woody pods, straight or curved, light brown, 4–14 × 1–2.5cm, prominently constricted between the seeds. **Seeds** 1–10 per pod, bright red with a black patch. Common in open savanna woodland, grassland and scrubland in East Africa (in all but very dry or colder areas), at 0–2,300m.

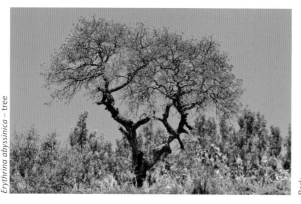

Erythrina abyssinica – tree

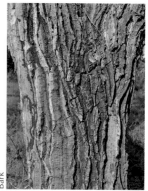

Bark

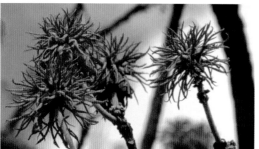

Flowers

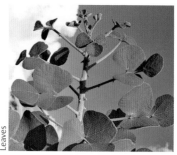

Leaves

PARTS USED Bark, roots, leaves and flowers.

TRADITIONAL MEDICINAL USES The bark of roots and stems is used in remedies for trachoma, malaria[M70, M71] and syphilis.[M37, M36] The bark is also used to treat gonorrhoea, hepatitis, anthrax and abdominal pain.[M4, M70] Powdered bark is applied to burns and general body swellings and is also used to treat rheumatism and arthritis.[M1, M4, M70] Roots are used in treatments for malaria,[M4, M71] syphilis, epilepsy, schistosomiasis[M102] and snakebite. An infusion of pounded dried flowers is used to treat syphilis[M38] and dysentery.[M102] An extract of dried leaves is used for the treatment of leprosy,[M39] fever[M40] and dysentery.[M41] Juice from fresh green bark is taken as an anthelmintic and to relieve abdominal pain.[M70, M71] A leaf decoction is consumed as an emetic and as a treatment for diarrhoea. The liquid from ground leaves is applied externally to wounds and to painful joints.[M102]

PREPARATION AND DOSAGE

BURNS, BODY SWELLINGS, ARTHRITIS AND RHEUMATISM Roast some dry bark and crush into a powder. Mix with water to form a paste and apply directly to burns or rub on body swellings 3 times a day. Alternatively, pound a handful of fresh roots, steep in a litre of boiling water for 10 minutes and apply the warm decoction externally.

INFLAMMATION OF THE EYELIDS (TRACHOMA) Bind some crushed green bark in a piece of fine cloth and squeeze. Collect the liquid that seeps out, dilute with boiled water and apply twice daily as eyedrops.

ABDOMINAL PAIN AND AS AN ANTHELMINTIC Squeeze the fresh young stems and collect the juice. Drink a tablespoon before meals to relieve abdominal pain.

MALARIA AND FEVER Boil a tablespoon of powdered root or bark in a litre of water for 10 minutes. Drink at intervals during the day.

b. *Erythrina lysistemon*   Native to South Africa

Common names Lucky-bean Tree, Common Coral Tree

Description and ecology

Very attractive small to medium-sized, deciduous tree 6–10(–12)m tall with spreading crown, branches thick and thorny, generally smaller than *E. abyssinica*. Bark pale grey-brown, smooth, not thickly corky, hooked thorns scattered on the trunk and branches. **Leaves** 3-foliolately compound, leaflets pointed and up to 17 × 18cm, with hooked thorns on leaf stalk and midrib. **Flowers** scarlet red, in short, dense heads about 9cm long, very showy, in elongated clusters. **Fruits** black, cylindrical pods, up to 15cm long, tightly constricted between the seeds, hanging in clusters and bursting open on the tree, thus releasing shiny, scarlet-and-black seeds resembling lucky beans. Widely cultivated as an ornamental in gardens, parks and along avenues in East Africa.

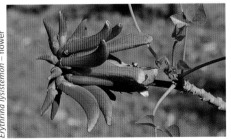

Erythrina lysistemon – flower

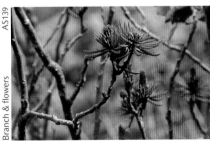

AS139

Branch & flowers

PARTS USED Bark, leaves and roots.

TRADITIONAL MEDICINAL USES Although quite common as an ornamental tree in East Africa, *Erythrina lysistemon* has not been widely used medicinally in the region. In its native South Africa, however, the bark is applied as a poultice for treating wounds, abscesses and arthritis;[M2, M70, M112, M116] infusions of the leaves are used as eardrops to relieve earache; and decoctions of the roots are applied to relieve painful injuries and sprains.[M2, M70, M116] Crushed leaves placed on a maggot-infested wound are said to clear the maggots.[M112, M116]

PREPARATION AND DOSAGE

No reliable information on precise dosages for this plant has been found.

Erythrina lysistemon – leaves

Bark

PHARMACOLOGY AND CHEMISTRY

PHARMACOLOGICAL PROPERTIES

Various pharmacological effects have been reported for species of *Erythrina*. Dried bark has produced antibacterial,[P168] antidiarrhoeal[P259] and antiviral[P254] activities. Dried root bark has shown antibacterial and antifungal effects against some bacteria and fungal organisms.[P118, P260] *Erythrina* alkaloids, found in the seeds and flowers, are known to be highly toxic.[P96] *E. abyssinica* roots have produced potent antiplasmodial[P261] and antimicrobial[P260] activities.

COMPOUNDS REPORTED

Compounds isolated from *E. abyssinica* include pterocarpans (e.g. phaseollin)[P260] from the roots, flavanones (e.g. abyssinone II) from the roots[P260] and stem bark,[P261] and erythrinaline alkaloids (e.g. erysodine)[P262] from the seeds and flowers. A number of erythrinaline alkaloids, flavonoids and isoflavonoids have been reported from the seeds of *E. lysistemon*[P263] and other species of *Erythrina*.[P261, P263] Pterocarpans isolated from stem bark of *E. abyssinica* could be considered as new anticancer agents.[P264]

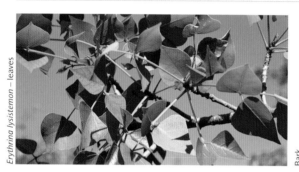

Phaseollin

Abyssinone II

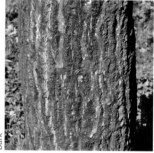

Erysodine

a. *Eucalyptus citriodora*   Native to northeastern Australia

Common names Spotted Gum, Lemon-scented Gum, Lemon-scented Eucalyptus •
Local names Makaratusi (Swa.), Mbanyi (Chag.)

Description and ecology

Medium-sized to very tall tree reaching 20–40(–45)m, with drooping foliage and a rounded crown, easily identified by the strong lemon scent of the leaves that perfume the air, especially after rain. **Bark** smooth, pale grey, with cream or pink patches, powdery and flaking. **Leaves** alternate, lance-shaped, 6–16cm long, pale green, veins parallel to the edges, with strong lemon scent when crushed. **Flower** buds borne in leaf axils on a branched peduncle, each branch with 3, rarely 7, buds, flowers creamy white, in groups of 3(–7). **Fruits** woody, urn-shaped or cup-shaped capsules, often warty, green when young, turning to blackish brown when dry, 8–15mm long, in clusters. Grows well in a variety of climates, both dry and wet, at higher altitudes.

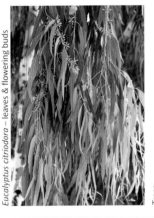

Eucalyptus citriodora – leaves & flowering buds

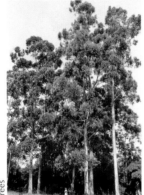

Trees

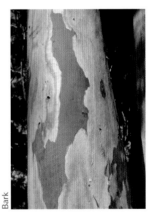

Bark

USAGE AND TREATMENT

PARTS USED Leaves and essential oil.
TRADITIONAL MEDICINAL USES Fresh leaves are used for colds, coughs, influenza and asthma. Infusions of dried leaves are taken orally for diarrhoea, coughs, anaemia, urinary tract infections, diabetes and dental care.M42, M70 Leaf infusions are applied locally to infected wounds and fungal infections.M42, M70 Oil from the leaves is applied to the skin as a medicine for skin rashes and fungal infections, and as an insect/mosquito repellent.M103 Lemon eucalyptus oil is used for treating muscle spasms, toenail fungus and osteoarthritis and other joint pain. It is also an ingredient in chest rubs used to relieve congestion.M103

PREPARATION AND DOSAGE
COLDS, COUGHS, INFLUENZA, BRONCHITIS AND ASTHMA Add a few drops of the essential oil (citronellal) from the leaves to very hot water and inhale the steam. Alternatively, boil a handful of pounded leaves, fresh or dry, in a litre of water and inhale the steam for 15 minutes.
INFECTED WOUNDS Crush a handful of fresh or dry leaves and boil in water for 15 minutes. Filter and use the warm infusion for washing infected wounds. Prepare a fresh infusion every time.

b. *Eucalyptus globulus*

Native to southeastern Australia

Common names Tasmanian Blue Gum, Eucalyptus Tree • **Local names** Makaratusi / Kalafulu (Swa.), Mbanyi (Chag.)

Description and ecology

Very tall, slender tree growing to 30–45m, with a rounded, open crown and long, straight, cylindrical bole up to 200cm in diameter. **Bark** white to cream or blue-grey, smooth. **Leaves** oval, thin, juvenile leaves whitish blue, arranged in opposite pairs, elliptic to egg-shaped, without a stalk, older leaves glossy green to dark green on both sides, arranged alternately, lance-shaped or slightly curved, stalk 1.8–6mm long, smelling of camphor when crushed, tip sharp. **Flowers** white, 1 or 3 in leaf axils. **Fruit** a woody, conical or half-sphere capsule with valves close to rim level, rough, 3cm across, without a stalk. Generally grows in cooler, wetter conditions, including highlands, at altitudes above 1,800m.

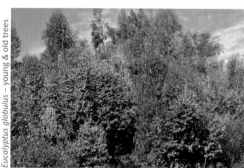

Eucalyptus globulus – young & old trees

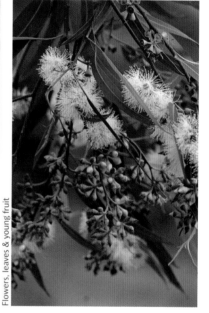

Flowers, leaves & young fruit

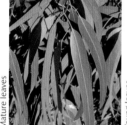

Mature leaves

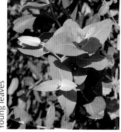

Young leaves

USAGE AND TREATMENT

PARTS USED Leaves, twigs, bark and essential oil.

TRADITIONAL MEDICINAL USES Leaves are used to treat coughs, colds, influenza, tuberculosis, asthma, bronchitis, rheumatism, dysentery and urinary tract infections.[M6, M70] Leaf infusions or oil are applied externally as a remedy for fungal infections, wounds and abscesses.[M6, M25] Soft twigs are used as toothbrushes for dental hygiene. Fresh leaves are chewed as a remedy for a sore throat.[M70] Leaves and bark are used for treating inflammation of the skin, colitis, intestinal fermentation (causing bad breath) and diarrhoea,[M9] or as an antidote to bacterial food poisoning.[M9] The essential oil found in the leaves is a powerful antiseptic and is used all over the world for relieving coughs and colds, a sore throat and other infections.[M9, M70] The oil can be used externally, applied to cuts and skin infections; it can also be inhaled in steam for treating blocked nasal passages and can be gargled for a sore throat.[M9]

PREPARATION AND DOSAGE

COUGHS AND SORE THROAT Boil a handful of pounded fresh or dry leaves in a litre of water for 5 minutes and filter. Drink in portions during the day to soothe a cough or to supplement tuberculosis treatment regimens. Alternatively, steep 20 dried leaves in a cup of boiling water for an hour and filter. Adults take half a cup and older children a quarter cup 2 or 3 times a day.

Young children can be given a eucalyptus cough syrup, made by adding a cup of sugar to the above mixture and bringing to the boil briefly. Children aged 7–10 can be given a teaspoon of the cool mixture 3 times a day. Younger children, aged 4–7, should be given half this dose, i.e. a quarter of a teaspoon 3 times daily. Intake is not recommended for children under two years of age.

For a sore throat and cough, chew half a fresh leaf for a few hours 3 times daily. For a chronic cough, add 100g of crushed dried leaves to a mixture of 700ml plain 95% alcohol and 300ml of boiled water. Leave for a week. Then press and remove the leaves. Adults and older children can take half a teaspoon of this mixture 3 times a day. Children aged 4–10 should be given a quarter of a teaspoon 3 times daily.

For relief from bronchitis and a severe throat infection, add 2 teaspoons of honey and 3 or 4 drops of eucalyptus oil to a cup of warm water and mix thoroughly. Adults can drink 3 or 4 cups daily (children 2 cups).

COLDS, ASTHMA AND BRONCHITIS Boil a handful of crushed dried or fresh leaves in half a cup of vegetable oil for 2 minutes. Leave for an hour to cool. Filter and massage onto the chest 2 or 3 times daily. Cover the massaged area with a warm blanket. Add a handful of fresh or dried leaves or 4 or 5 drops of essential oil (extracted from the leaves) to a litre of boiling water in a bowl. Inhale the steam vapour for 10–15 minutes 3 or 4 times a day, under a covering towel to ensure maximum penetration.

INFECTED WOUNDS, ABSCESSES AND FUNGAL INFECTIONS Boil a tablespoon of chopped dried leaves in a cup of water for 10 minutes. Filter and then wash the infected area with the warm infusion 3 times a day, preparing a new mixture every time. Alternatively, heat a handful of crushed dried leaves in half a cup of vegetable oil for 10 minutes. Leave for an hour to cool. Then rub on the affected areas.

A paste can be made for treating inflamed skin by burning 100g of mixed dried leaves and bark until you are left with a charcoal-like powder. Mix a tablespoon of this powder in water to form a paste and apply gently to affected areas.

FOOD POISONING, COLITIS, INTESTINAL FERMENTATION (CAUSING BAD BREATH), DYSENTERY AND DIARRHOEA Burn 100g of mixed dried leaves and bark. Grind the charcoal-like residue into a powder. Add 5–10g of powder to half a cup of water and stir. Drink 3 or 4 times a day or, in an emergency, eat pieces of the charcoal itself.

c. *Eucalyptus maculata*
(*Corymbia maculata*)

Native to Eastern Australia

Common names Spotted Gum, Gum Tree, Eucalyptus Tree • **Local names** Mkaratusi (Swa.), Kalitunsi (Lug.)

Description and ecology

A medium-sized to very tall tree with a distinctive spotted stem, up to 30m tall, sometimes reaching 40–60m. **Bark** smooth, mottled, jigsaw patterned, flaking into patches of bluish grey or pinkish grey, older bark smooth, greyish white. **Leaves** narrow, lance-shaped or curved, 0.8–2.2cm long, with many thin veins parallel to the margin, stalk 10–25mm long. **Flower** buds borne in leaf axils on a branched peduncle 3–20mm long, each branch with 3, rarely 7, buds on pedicels 1–8mm long, flowers white, in groups of 3–7. **Fruit** a woody, bell-shaped or slightly urn-shaped capsule, 9–14mm long, 8–13mm wide, with the valves enclosed in the fruit. Very common in upland areas of East Africa, at 1,200–2,400m.

PARTS USED Leaves and essential oil.

TRADITIONAL MEDICINAL USES Fresh leaves are used to treat colds and coughs. Infusions are applied to infected wounds.[M70] The essential oil is used to treat fungal infections. Leaves are also a remedy for a sore throat and urinary tract infections.[M70] A bark decoction is taken internally as a treatment for dysentery, and can also be used as a gargle and mouthwash.[M104] A warm bark decoction, applied externally as a wash, is an effective styptic and can be used to treat cuts and skin problems.[M104]

PREPARATION AND DOSAGE

COLDS, COUGHS AND SORE THROAT Add 3 or 4 drops of leaf oil to half a litre of boiling water or boil a handful of pounded fresh or dried leaves in a litre of water. Inhale the steam vapour for 15 minutes.

FUNGAL INFECTIONS AND WOUNDS Boil a handful of crushed fresh or dry leaves in a cup of water for 10 minutes and filter. Use the warm infusion to wash infected wounds, preparing a fresh infusion every time. Alternatively, heat a handful of crushed dried leaves in half a cup of vegetable oil for 10 minutes. Leave for an hour to cool, then filter and rub on the affected areas.

 WARNING! Do not exceed recommended internal dosage (of extract or oil), as it may trigger adverse gastric, blood and urinary reactions.

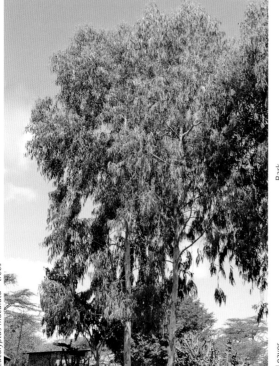

Eucalyptus maculata – trees

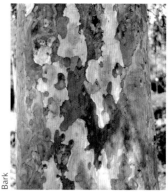

Bark

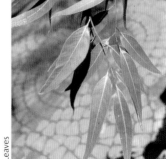

Leaves

PHARMACOLOGY AND CHEMISTRY

PHARMACOLOGICAL PROPERTIES

Terpenoids, such as eucalyptol, in the essential oils of species of *Eucalyptus* produce pharmacologically important expectorant, antiseptic,[P159] bronchodilatory, sudorific and balsamic effects,[P159, P206] particularly helpful in treating bronchial and pulmonary afflictions. These oils also show antibacterial, antifungal[P265] and anti-amoebic[P206] activities.

COMPOUNDS REPORTED

Species of *Eucalyptus* contain terpenoids, particularly in their volatile oils, where the active components are concentrated. Monoterpenes (e.g. borneol,[P266] terpinen-4-ol[P267]), terpene hydrocarbons (pinene), sesquiterpenes (aromadendrene),[P267] triterpenes (betulonic acid)[P268] and phenolic compounds have all been reported. From *E. maculata*, some flavanones (e.g. sakuranetin[P269]) have been isolated. The leaf essential oil of *E. maculata* and its major compound, 1,8-cineole, showed antibacterial activity against fish pathogenic bacteria *Aeromonas hydrophila* and *A. jandae*, which cause wound infections in immunocompetent and immunocompromised humans exposed to freshwater sources.[P270]

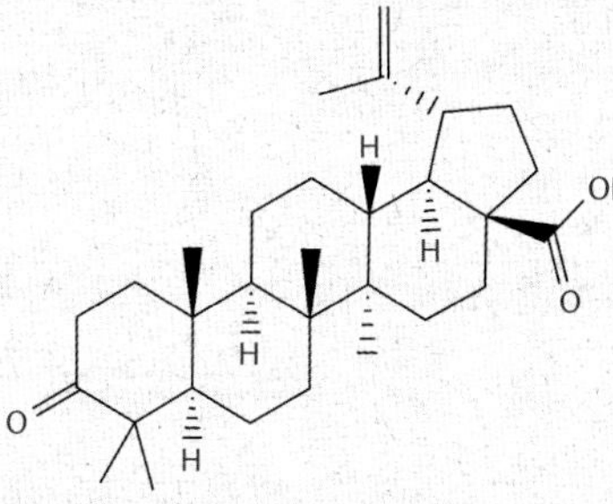

Betulonic acid

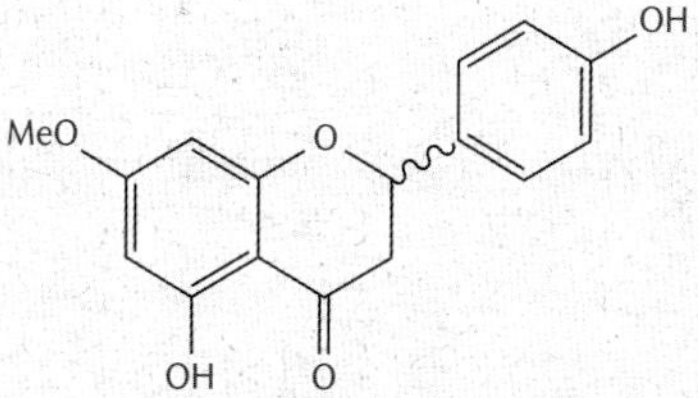

Sakuranetin

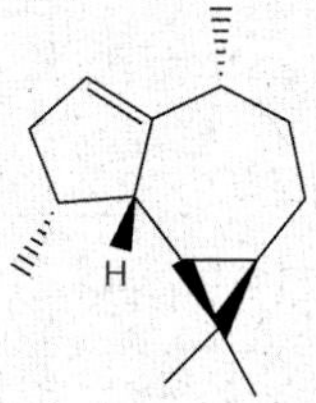

Aromadendrene

Indigenous

Common names Euclea, Diamond-leaved Euclea, Magic Guarri • **Local names** Mukinyai / Mukuthi (Kam.), Mukinyai / Mukinyei (Kik.), Usuet / Uswet (Kip., Nan., Tug.), Shiendet (Sebei), Kanerape (Tug.), Ol-kinyei / Ilkinyei (Maa.), Kumuchanjaasi / Muswa (Luh.), Ochol / Akado / Ochond radoho (Luo), Mukiinyei / Mukiinyi (Mer., Mbe.), Chetuya (Pok.), Ilchinge / Shinghe / Lchinge (Sam.), Mmbuku (Tai.), Mukonde (Tha.), Olkinye (Aru.), Iwaruka / Mkenye (Chag.), Sinyanyi (Goro.), Musikizi (Haya), Mhekele (Hehe), Mhekela / Mhekele (Lugu.), Ekeni / Ikeng (Mer.Tan.), Mudaa (Nyat.), Mbanjiru (Ran.), Mdaa (Swa.Tan.)

Description and ecology

Evergreen multi-stemmed shrub or small single-stemmed tree 3–5m high, occasionally reaching 10m, with much-branched, rounded crown and dense foliage. **Bark** ash-grey-brown to black, rough, cracking and flaking longitudinally with age, young stems smooth and pale grey with rusty granules. **Leaves** opposite or subopposite, shiny, olive-green, stiff, leathery, narrow, up to 8cm long, with blunt tip, broad in the middle, margin conspicuously wavy, leaf stalk up to 6mm long. **Flowers** white to creamy yellow, sweetly scented, borne on short and dense branched sprays arising from the axils of leaves, short-lived, male and female on separate trees. **Fruit** round, small, 5–7mm in diameter, single-seeded and fleshy, green, turning purple-black when ripe. Widespread on dry forest margins, along streams and rivers in bushland or forest and in bushy grassland from sea level to 2,400m.

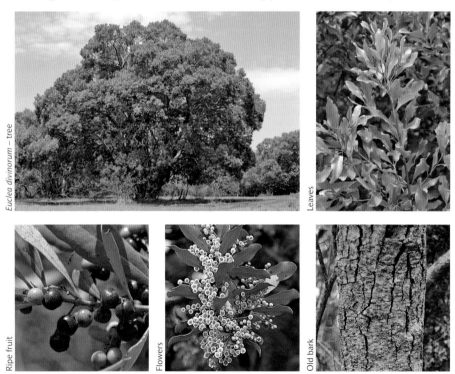

Euclea divinorum – tree

Leaves

Ripe fruit

Flowers

Old bark

PARTS USED Bark, roots, leaves and fruit.

TRADITIONAL MEDICINAL USES A hot-water extract of dried roots and bark is taken orally as a purgative or an anthelmintic.[M4, M30, M70] Root and bark decoctions are taken as a tonic. A root decoction is used for treating gastrointestinal ailments and stomach pain.[M3, M28] A paste of dried root powder is applied externally to treat ulcers, leprosy, wounds, arthritis, snakebite, headache, toothache and gonorrhoea.[M112, M115] A boiled root infusion is taken for stomach ache, diarrhoea and headache. Roots are chewed as a remedy for toothache.[M3] A decoction of roots of *Euclea divinorum* and *Croton megalocarpus*, boiled together, is used for treating chest pain, pneumonia and internal body pain.[M1, M3, M70] Bark infusions serve as an appetiser. A decoction of a root mix of *E. divinorum*, *Carissa spinarum* (*C. edulis*) and *Carica papaya* is taken orally to treat venereal diseases.[M26, M70] A leaf decoction is taken for malaria, leprosy, gonorrhoea, syphilis and tapeworm, and a root bark decoction to treat diarrhoea and skin problems.[M105] Root bark is also used as a toothbrush, or the dry powder is rubbed on the teeth for dental care.[M105] The fruits are taken as a mild laxative, but can also have a strong purgative effect.[M112, M115]

PREPARATION AND DOSAGE

PURGATIVE AND ANTHELMINTIC Add a tablespoon of mixed dried root and bark powder to a cup of hot water, stir and leave for 10 minutes. Filter and drink twice a day, after breakfast and supper.

DIARRHOEA, GASTROINTESTINAL AILMENTS AND STOMACH ACHE Add a tablespoon of dried root powder to a cup of hot water, stir and leave for 10 minutes. Filter and drink twice a day, after morning and evening meals.

CHEST PAIN, PNEUMONIA AND INTERNAL BODY PAIN Boil 5g of pounded fresh roots of *E. divinorum* with 5g of pounded fresh roots of *Croton megalocarpus* in a litre of water for 15 minutes. Drain when cool and drink a quarter of a cup 3 times daily for 2 days.

TOOTHACHE AND CLEANING THE TEETH Chew fresh root bark or make a powder after drying and apply directly on affected teeth.

PHARMACOLOGICAL PROPERTIES

Activities ascribed to the naphthoquinones in *Euclea divinorum* include antischistosomal[P271] and antibacterial[P272] effects. Antimicrobial activity towards oral micro-organisms has been reported for this plant.[P273] The antitumour and antileishmanial[P274] activities of some of the naphthoquinones have also been documented.

COMPOUNDS REPORTED

The most common metabolites are the naphthoquinones (e.g. 5,8-dihydroxy-2-methyl-1,4-naphthoquinone). Flavanones such as aromadendrin-3-O-L-arabinopyranoside[P275] and triterpenes such as betulin[P276] have also been reported. The naphthoquinone 7-methyljuglone and the pentacyclic triterpene 3b-(5-hydroxyferuloyl)Lup-20(30)-ene isolated from *E. divinorum* showed cytotoxicity against some cancer cell lines.[P276]

5,8-Dihydroxy-2-methyl-1,4-naphthoquinone

Aromadendrin-3-O-L-arabinopyranoside

44 *Eugenia caryophyllata*
(*Syzygium aromaticum*)
MYRTACEAE

Native to the Southeast Asian islands and the
Moluccas in Indonesia

Common name Clove Tree • **Local names** Makonyo / Karafuu (Swa.), Loving (Guj.), Long (Urd., Punj.)

Description and ecology

Attractive pyramidal evergreen tree 5–12(–20)m
tall, much-branched with a bushy conical crown.
Bark brown, rough and fissured with age. **Leaves**
pink when young, large, ovate-oblong, 10 × 5cm,
smooth, shiny, aromatic, tip pointed. **Flowers**
crimson or pale purple, small, in terminal clusters,
scented. Cloves are the unopened flower buds,
pink or brilliant crimson at first, turning reddish
brown on drying in the sun, strongly aromatic.

Fruits oblong-ellipsoid, 2–2.5cm long, 1-seeded.
The clove tree was introduced into Zanzibar and
Pemba islands in 1818 and rapidly became the
major export, in the past accounting for over 80%
of the world's supply of cloves (the sun-dried
flower buds) and clove oil. Widely grown in East
Africa and in Asia, especially China. Cloves are
an indispensable ingredient of many spicy Indian
dishes and are also popular as a tea spice (in
tea masala).

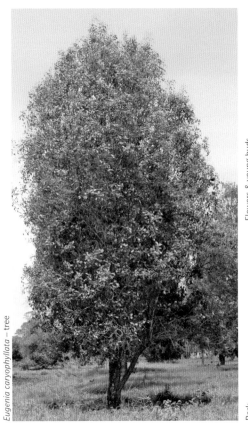

Eugenia caryophyllata – tree

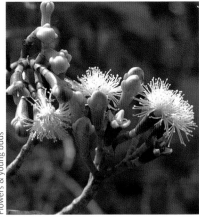

Flowers & young buds

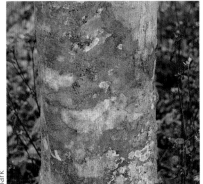

Bark

PARTS USED Dried flower buds and volatile oil.

TRADITIONAL MEDICINAL USES Dried cloves or clove oil offers quick relief from toothache and is helpful in reducing gum inflammation.[M7, M9, M25, M70] Clove infusions stimulate the appetite and act as a carminative in expelling intestinal gas.[M7, M9, M25] Drops of clove oil are used as a mouth freshener, a disinfectant for the mouth and a treatment for coughs and colds.[M70] Applied externally in embrocations, clove oil helps to relieve neuralgic pain and rheumatism.[M25] Flower buds are chewed to freshen breath or ease toothache.[M111] Dried flower buds and oil are used to treat skin ulcers, bruises, burns, bronchitis, asthma and colic.[M111]

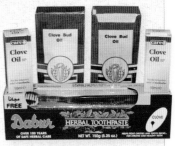

Eugenia caryophyllata – oil and toothpaste products

PREPARATION AND DOSAGE

TOOTHACHE Place a piece of a clove or a drop of clove oil on the aching tooth.

MOUTH ELIXIR Add 2 or 3 drops of clove oil to a cup of warm water. Use this mixture to rinse and disinfect the mouth.

APPETISER AND CARMINATIVE Add 3 or 4 cloves to a cup of water, add a pinch of ginger powder and boil for 10 minutes. Cool and filter the mixture. Drink a cup with every meal.

COUGHS Mix 1g each of turmeric, ginger and clove powder in a tablespoon of honey. Drink in water 3 times a day.

WARNING! In high doses, cloves can cause irritation of the digestive system and may also cause stomach ache and nausea. People suffering from abdominal ulcers or gastritis should avoid using cloves, both medicinally and as a spice.

PHARMACOLOGICAL PROPERTIES

The bioactivity of cloves emanates from the presence of eugenol in the volatile oil. It acts as an oral antiseptic and analgesic, also as a stimulant and appetiser.[P17, P156] A methanolic extract of the cortex of *Eugenia caryophyllata* has shown strong inhibiting activity of PGE2 production (implicated in cases of inflammation and carcinogenesis). Eugenol has been found to be the active principle.[P277]

COMPOUNDS REPORTED

Cloves contain 14–21% of volatile oil. This oil is highly aromatic, due mainly to eugenol and the presence of small amounts of gallotannic acid, acetyleugenol and cariophilene.[P156] Both tannins and terpenoids[P277] have also been reported. Eugenol (68.9%), trans-caryophyllene (12.6%) and eugenol acetate (12.4%) were identified as the main constituents of the essential oil from buds of *E. caryophyllata*, which showed antimicrobial and free-radical scavenging activities.[P278]

Eugenol

trans-Caryophyllene

Flueggea virosa PHYLLANTHACEAE

Indigenous

Common names White-berry Bush, Snowberry Tree • **Local names** Mkwamba (Dig., Swa., Gir.), Kaera / Kagena / Odok (Luo), Mukuluu / Mukururu (Kam.), Esarara (Kis.), Mukururu (Mbe., Tha.), Getaruwet (Kip.), Kisasari (Luh.), Segeteti (Maa.), Kororo (Orm.), Kptarpotich / Chepochepkai (Pok.), Ikirebuk (Sam.), Elakis / Kkalis (Tur.)

Description and ecology
Deciduous, multi-stemmed, fast-growing bushy shrub 2–3m tall, rarely a small spreading tree up to 4m high, with many erect or arching thorn-like branches. **Bark** reddish brown to brown. **Leaves** simple, alternate, entire, obovate, 2–4(–6)cm long, non-hairy, base rounded, stalk 3–6mm long and narrowly winged. **Flowers** yellow-green or cream,1–few together in sparse or dense axillary groups, pedicels up to 6mm long. **Fruit** a fleshy, slightly 3-lobed, globose capsule, white, 2–3 × 4–5mm. **Seeds** ovoid, 2–3mm long, shiny, yellowish brown. Found in various habitats such as deciduous woodland, riparian areas, rocky bushland, bushed and wooded grassland, forest margins and in black cotton soils, at 0–1,800m.

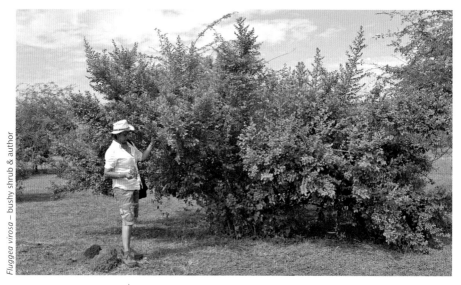

Flueggea virosa – bushy shrub & author

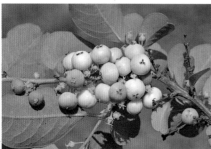

Ripe fruit

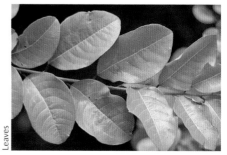

Leaves

PARTS USED Roots, twigs, leaves, fruits and seeds.

TRADITIONAL MEDICINAL USES Root decoctions are used to treat chest pain, schistosomiasis[M3, M4] and intestinal worms.[M43] Fresh twigs are used as toothbrushes. Pounded leaves can serve as an insect repellent, while dried leaves are used for treating chronic headache[M43] and malaria.[M4, M70] Dried roots are used for treating venereal diseases, wounds, diarrhoea, ulcers, stomach ache, earache and skin diseases.[M44, M70] Dried seeds are used to treat conjunctivitis[M43] and as a contraceptive for women. The fruits are used as a remedy for itching skin. A leaf extract mixed with leaves of *Lantana trifolia* is given to children with diarrhoea.[M3, M70] Root decoctions have been taken for the treatment of schistosomiasis, stomach ache and dysmenorrhoea.[M106] The leaves are considered to be an aphrodisiac and laxative, and are used to treat fever, venereal disease and constipation.[M106] A leaf macerate is added to baths and applied as a stimulant during massage in the treatment of fatigue and stiffness; a leaf decoction is also used in baths for treating fever.[M106]

PREPARATION AND DOSAGE

HEADACHE AND MIGRAINE Crush a handful of dry leaves and mix with a cup of olive oil. Leave for a few hours. Rub the mixture on the forehead and insert a drop into each nostril. Repeat this treatment until the pain abates.

WOUNDS AND SKIN DISEASES (ECZEMA, ABSCESSES, FURUNCLES) Pound a few fresh leaves and apply directly to affected areas of the skin. Repeat 2 or 3 times daily while symptoms last. Alternatively, steep a handful of dried root powder in half a cup of vegetable oil and leave for a week, then rub on the affected areas.

DYSMENORRHOEA, SCHISTOSOMIASIS (BILHARZIA) AND STOMACH ACHE Crush and pound a quarter of a cup of fresh roots and mix in half a litre of boiled water. Leave it for an hour, sieve and drink a cup 3 times a day.

PHARMACOLOGICAL PROPERTIES

Antifungal activity against *Candida albicans* has been reported for stems of *Flueggea virosa*.[P279] Leaf and bark extracts of *F. virosa* showed significant anthelmintic activities comparable to the standard piperazine citrate.[P280]

COMPOUNDS REPORTED

Two C-C linked dimeric indolizidine alkaloids, flueggenine A and B, have been isolated from this plant.[P281] Three new indole alkaloids (e.g. flueindoline A) along with nine known alkaloids have been reported from the fruits of *F. virosa*.[P282]

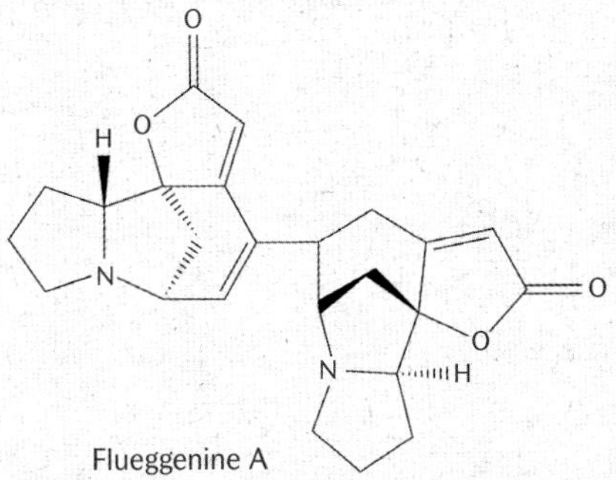

Flueggenine A

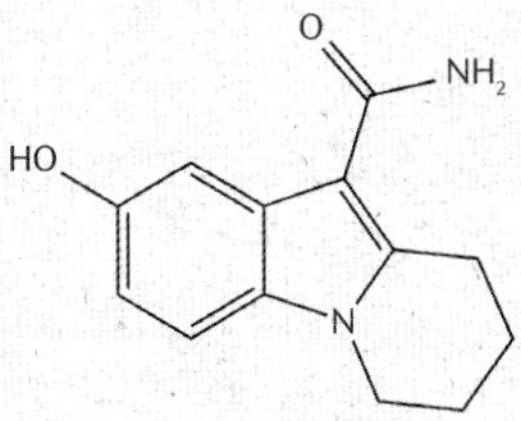

Flueindoline A

Native to Mediterranean countries

Common names Fennel, Sweet Fennel • **Local names** Kibeti (Gir.), Ndungu (Luh.), Saunf (Hind., Urd., Punj.), Veryali (Guj.)

Description and ecology

Erect, multi-stemmed, aromatic, perennial herb 1–2m high with thick, hollow, greenish-blue stems. **Leaves** alternate, decompound, divided into fine needle-shaped leaflets, with a distinctive aroma. **Flowers** small, yellow, in terminal compound umbels (clusters) 10–15cm in diameter, sometimes smaller, the flower stalks of equal length emerging from one point. **Fruit** a small, ovoid-cylindrical, slightly curved, dry schizocarp, light green to yellowish brown, 3–8 × 2–2.5mm, divided into two segments. Grown in most parts of East Africa, thriving in rich, well-drained soils.

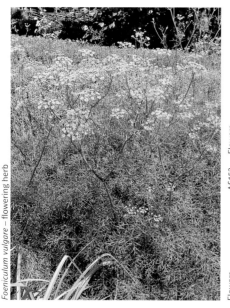

Foeniculum vulgare – flowering herb

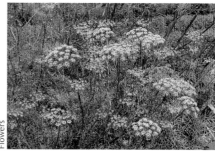

Flowers   AS152

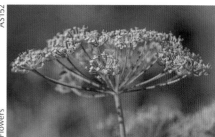

Flowers

USAGE AND TREATMENT

PARTS USED Fruits, occasionally leaves and roots as well.

TRADITIONAL MEDICINAL USES Well known for its carminative properties,[M107] fennel helps to treat stomach disorders, facilitating removal of intestinal gas from a bloated stomach[M7, M70] while acting as a mild laxative.[M9, M70] Boiled or roasted roots are used to treat gonorrhoea.[M1] Dry fennel fruits boost lactation in breast-feeding mothers.[M107] An infusion or decoction of pounded roots has a diuretic effect, increasing urine flow.[M7, M9] Fennel is given to children with flatulence and indigestion.[M2, M25] It is also used to stop diarrhoea and to fortify the stomach. Extracts of fennel seeds are used for irritation of the eyes in cases of chronic conjunctivitis,[M7] for glaucoma and as a diuretic and a potential drug for the treatment of hypertension.[M107] It is also a remedy for colds and bronchial coughs.[M70]

PREPARATION AND DOSAGE

FLATULENCE AND INDIGESTION Soak 40g of dry fruit in a litre of boiling water for 2 hours, shaking the mixture intermittently. Sieve and then drink half a cup of the decoction after every meal for 3 days, preparing a fresh mixture every day. Children aged 4–7 years should be given half the adult dose, while very young children need to be fed only half a teaspoon of the decoction 3 times daily after meals. Alternatively, add a teaspoon of dry fruit to a cup of boiled water. Leave for half an hour. Adults and children can drink a cup of the infusion after every meal, totalling 3 cups a day and making a fresh infusion every time.

Another option is to mix a teaspoon of powdered fennel fruit with half a teaspoon of brown sugar or honey and to take this before every meal.

COLDS AND BRONCHIAL COUGHS Add a teaspoon of dry fruit to a cup of boiled water. Add a teaspoon of honey and then leave for half an hour. Drink 3 or 4 cups of the infusion daily after meals, preparing a fresh infusion every time.

EYE IRRITATION AND CHRONIC CONJUNCTIVITIS Add a teaspoon of dry fruit to a cup of boiled water. Wash the eyes with the warm mixture 3 or 4 times a day, preparing a fresh mixture every time.

PHARMACOLOGY AND CHEMISTRY

PHARMACOLOGICAL PROPERTIES

The use of fennel oil is mainly for treating the digestive and respiratory systems.[P17] The aromatic oil produces carminative, expectorant and antispasmodic effects.[P17, P156] It also has a galactogenic effect, increasing milk production in breast-feeding mothers.[P96] The essential oil and monoterpenoid compounds in fennel produce acaricidal activities against house dust mites.[P283] An ethanol extract of fruits has a strong apoptotic effect on leukaemic cell lines.[P284] The prolonged intake of *Foeniculum vulgare* tea is believed to cause premature thelarche, a disorder characterised by breast development in infancy amid no other signs of puberty.[P285] Estrogenic activity of the seed extract has also been reported.[P96] It has been reported that cream containing extracts of fennel can be used to manage the symptoms of vaginal atrophy in postmenopausal women, without side effects.[P286]

COMPOUNDS REPORTED

The whole fennel plant, especially the fruit, contains an essence rich in phenylpropanoids (e.g. anethol and estragol) and monoterpenes (e.g. fenchone).[P17, P96, P156] The fruit also contains flavonoids and coumarins.[P156] The composition of the essential oils (which may be bitter or sweet, depending on the variety of the fennel) determines the medicinal properties of the plant.[P17, P156]

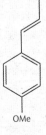

OMe

Anethol

OMe

Estragol

O

Fenchone

Indigenous

Local names Aremo (Luo), Pirirwob-sot / Birirwob-sot (Kip.), Kalaku (Kam.), Kimamuo (Chag.), Oloito-doraik (Maa.)

Description and ecology

Erect, branching, faintly aromatic herb or woody subshrub, stems arising from a branched fibrous rootstock or thin rhizome, branched above, often woody below, with long or short white hairs. **Leaves** opposite, oval, 0.8–3.3cm long, hairy, covered with tiny red gland dots that stain the fingers red when rubbed, margin toothed, stalk 2–10mm long. **Flowers** white, with hairy calyx, on very long 1- or 2(–4)-flowered racemes. **Fruits** brown, ovoid nutlets, 1.5mm long. Common in shallow grassland soils, often on volcanic soil, at 900–2,500m.

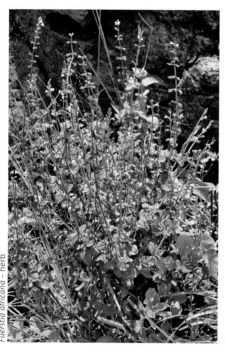

Fuerstia africana – herb

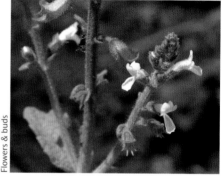

Flowers & buds

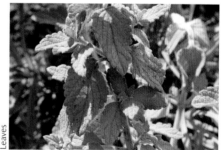

Leaves

USAGE AND TREATMENT

PARTS USED Leaves, roots, bark and young twigs.
TRADITIONAL MEDICINAL USES A leaf decoction is said to enhance fertility in women; it is also used as a treatment for malaria, as a purgative and as an anthelmintic, particularly against tapeworm.[M1, M70] The leaf juice is administered as drops for inflammation of the eyes. Leaves and young twigs are used as a remedy for stomach and tongue ulcers.[M1, M70] Hot-water extracts of leaves, roots and bark are used as a galactagogue to stimulate lactation in mothers[M17] and are also used to treat malaria.[M1]

PREPARATION AND DOSAGE

STOMACH ULCERS, STOMACH WORMS AND MALARIA Add a handful of pounded fresh leaves and young twigs to a litre of water. Boil for 10 minutes and drink the decoction 3 times daily for 3 days, preparing a fresh decoction every day.

EYE INFLAMMATION Squeeze juice from fresh leaves and add a few drops of boiled water. Apply as eyedrops for relief from ophthalmia.

PHARMACOLOGY AND CHEMISTRY

PHARMACOLOGICAL PROPERTIES

A hot-water extract of dried leaves has shown weak molluscicidal activity.[P226] The plant as a whole also shows some antimalarial activity.[P287]

COMPOUNDS REPORTED

A diterpene, fuerstione, has been isolated from the leaves of *F. africana*.[P26, P288] Ferruginol, an abietane diterpene, has been identified as the antiplasmodial active principle of the plant.[P287] Antitumour, antioxidant and antihypertensive activities of ferruginol have also been reported.[P287]

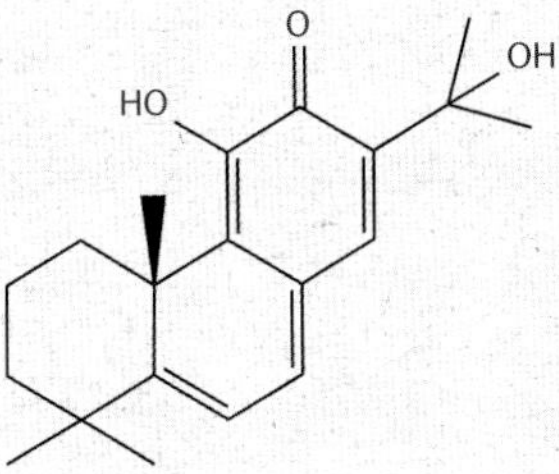

Fuerstione

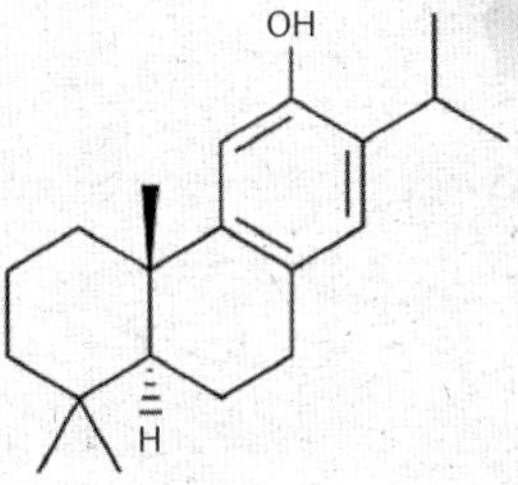

Ferruginol

Indigenous

Common names Wild Gardenia, Jove's Thunder Gardenia • **Local names** Kimwemwe (Swa.), Kurkoi (Bon.), Mukumuti (Kam.), Siuma (Luh.), Onduongi (Luo), Geninyet (Maa.), Odwong' (Ach.)

Description and ecology

Evergreen, multi-branched savanna shrub or small tree 2–6(–8)m tall, usually stunted and twisted in appearance, bole up to 20cm wide, with a broad crown. **Bark** greenish pale grey or yellowish brown, smooth, powdery, dotted with breathing pores. **Leaves** extremely variable, obovate-elliptic or oblong-obovate, spoon-shaped, opposite or in whorls of 3 or 4 on short, rigid side branchlets, glossy, dark green, leathery, 4–12cm long, with rounded apex, stalk 0–5mm long. **Flowers** white, turning yellow when fading, solitary at the end of branchlets, funnel-shaped, fragrant. **Fruit** hard, grey-green or yellow-brown, ellipsoid, ovoid or lemon-shaped, warty, up to 7 × 3.5cm. **Seeds** 3.5–4 × 2–3mm, chestnut-coloured, flattened, ellipsoid. Common in wooded grassland and riverine woodland, at 0–2,100m.

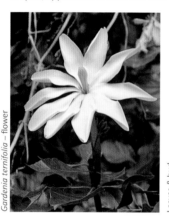

Gardenia ternifolia – flower

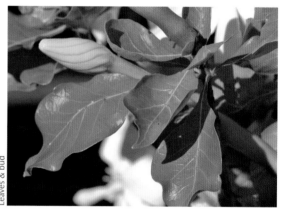

Leaves & bud

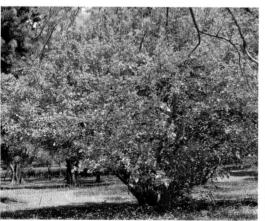

Shrub

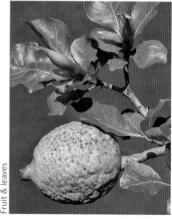

Fruit & leaves

USAGE AND TREATMENT

PARTS USED Root bark, roots, stem bark and fruits.

TRADITIONAL MEDICINAL USES *Gardenia ternifolia* is mainly used in the treatment of malaria, hypertension, diabetes, coughs, asthma, rheumatism, diarrhoea, tooth problems, leprosy, a hernia, haemorrhoids and cancer.[M108] A decoction of fruits is used to treat malaria and is taken as a purgative[M4, M70] and as a remedy for eye complaints. A hot-water decoction of roots or bark is applied as an antiseptic to heal infected wounds.[M70] A warm decoction is taken orally to kill intestinal worms.[M70] A root infusion is taken for snakebite.[M1] The bark has emetic properties.[M33] An infusion or a decoction of roots is used as laxative and vermifuge[M108, M112] and in the treatment of stomach ache and kwashiorkor.[M112]

PREPARATION AND DOSAGE

SNAKEBITE (EMETIC) Add a tablespoon of root powder to half a litre of boiled water. Leave for 10 minutes, stirring intermittently. Drink in 3 portions during the day – vomiting will follow but will help to alleviate the effects of the poisoning.

INFECTED WOUNDS Add a tablespoon of root or stem bark powder to half a litre of boiled water. Stir, filter and wash the wound with the warm mixture.

STOMACH ACHE, LAXATIVE AND VERMIFUGE Add a tablespoon of root powder or pounded fresh roots to half a litre of boiled water. Leave for 10–15 minutes, stir and filter. Drink in 3 portions during the day before or after meals.

PHARMACOLOGY AND CHEMISTRY

PHARMACOLOGICAL PROPERTIES

Leaves of *Gardenia ternifolia* have shown bronchodilator and hypotensive activities,[P289] but no anthelmintic or molluscicidal activities have been reported.[P290] Roots have shown several pharmacological activities such as antimalarial, antioxidant, anticancer and antimicrobial effects.[P291] However, more extensive toxicological and pharmacological tests are necessary in order to establish the therapeutic potential of this plant.

COMPOUNDS REPORTED

Phytochemical investigations on the leaves, fruits and roots of this plant revealed the presence of saponins, reducing compounds, sterols, triterpenes and polyphenolic substances such as tannins, flavonoids, coumarins and anthocyanins.[P291] Triterpenes reported in the root bark of *G. ternifolia* included hederagenin.[P292]

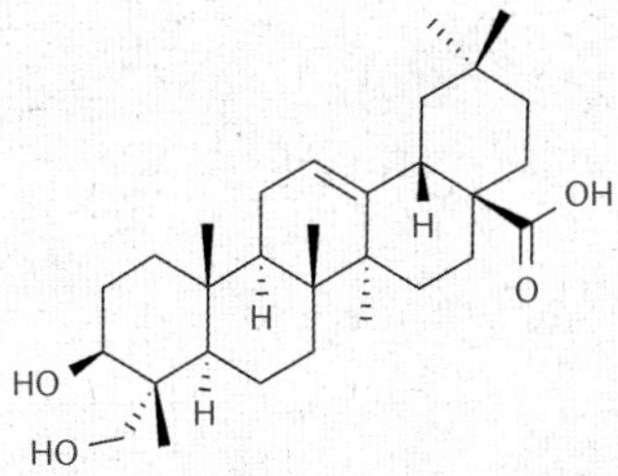

Hederagenin

Indigenous

Common names Flame Lily, Climbing Lily, Creeping Lily, Tiger's Claw, Cat's Claw •
Local names Mkalamu (Swa.), Kemagugu (Mar.), Datavo (Som.)

Description and ecology
Deciduous climber up to 1.5m, with fleshy tuberous roots or bulbs or rhizomes and slender upright to scrambling stems, can reach 4m. **Leaves** alternate, shiny, bright green, lance-shaped, 13–20cm long, stalkless, tipped with a tendril that allows the plant to climb into anything it touches.

Flowers spectacular, brilliant red, often striped yellow or with yellow at the base, borne on long stalks on the upper parts of stems after good rains. **Fruit** a large fleshy 3-valved capsule, changing from green to brown over time, 6–12cm long. **Seeds** red, round, 4–5mm in diameter. Common in dry lowland areas and upland forest, at 1,200–2,500m.

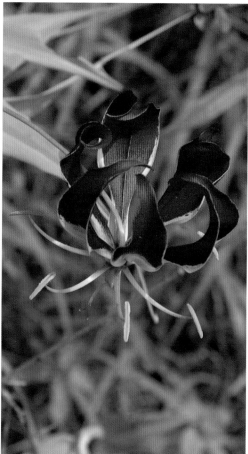

Gloriosa superba – flower

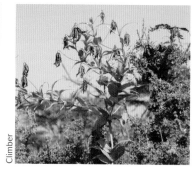

Climber

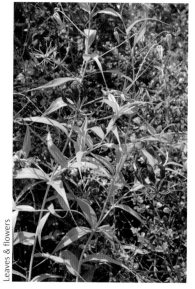

Leaves & flowers

USAGE AND TREATMENT

PARTS USED Corm or bulb, tubers only.

TRADITIONAL MEDICINAL USES A decoction of the corm is used as a laxative, anthelmintic, purgative and also for treating indigestion and stomach ache.[M70] A tuber infusion is taken to induce abortion and for abdominal disorders.[M70, M109] The anthelmintic properties of the tuber, fruits and leaves make these plant parts useful for the treatment of stomach worms, including roundworm, tapeworm and liver fluke, and for dealing with schistosomiasis.[M109] Soup made from sap of leaves or tubers is given to women suffering from sterility, delayed puberty, delayed childbirth or menstrual problems.[M109]

PREPARATION AND DOSAGE

SCHISTOSOMIASIS (BILHARZIA), STOMACH WORMS, INDIGESTION AND AS A PURGATIVE Wash a quarter of a cup of fresh bulb/corm, pound and mix it in a litre of boiled water. Leave it for an hour, stir, filter and drink the warm mixture before a meal 3 times a day.

 WARNING! The bulbs/tubers contain toxic alkaloids, so care should be taken in the case of internal use. Excessive intake may cause vomiting, diarrhoea and hypotension.

PHARMACOLOGY AND CHEMISTRY

PHARMACOLOGICAL PROPERTIES

Toxic alkaloids in fresh corms/bulbs/tubers may cause vomiting, diarrhoea, delirium and hypotension.[P293] No part of the plant has shown any analgesic activity.[P6] The alkaloid colchicine isolated from the tuber of *Gloriosa superba* is used clinically to treat rheumatism and gout.[P294]

COMPOUNDS REPORTED

Several isoquinoline compounds (e.g. S-(+)-floramultine) have been isolated from corms of *G. superba*.[P295]

MeO
HO
MeO
MeO
OH
NMe
H
S-(+)-Floramultine

50 *Grewia* species TILIACEAE

a. *Grewia tenax* Indigenous

Common names Grewia, Small-leaved White Raisin, White Cross-berry • **Local names** Deka / Deeka (Bor., Ilw.), D'eeka (Gab.), Mkone-kilaa (Gir.), Oyirri / Oirri / Iri (Maa.), Toronwo (Pok.), Mulahanyo (Ren.), Irri / Ikarayoi / Ikogomi (Sam.), Damiek / Deka / Kamasha / Mared (Som.), Taran / Taronwet (Tug.), Eng'omo (Tur.)

Description and ecology

Small, much-branched, multi-stemmed shrub 2–3m high, generally a very slow-growing plant. Younger stems ash-grey with longitudinal streaks, young twigs hairy, older stems dark grey. **Leaves** alternate, small, papery, ovate-elliptic or obovate, 0.6–4.5 × 0.4cm, broader at the base and pointed at the tip, margin wavy and sharply dentate. **Flowers** white, solitary or rarely paired, 2cm across, on a hairy stalk. **Fruit** a drupe, 2–4-lobed, lobes 5–7mm in diameter, glabrous, green, turning orange-yellow with a reddish tinge when ripe. Found in *Acacia* bushland or bushed grassland, at 0–1,500m.

USAGE AND TREATMENT

PARTS USED Bark and roots.

TRADITIONAL MEDICINAL USES The bark yields a sticky gum that acts as an insect repellent.[M1, M70] It is also used to soothe wounds, burns, itching, eczema, boils and fungal skin infections.[M4, M70] Dried powdered roots are used to make a poultice to cover wounds and burns.[M111] Fresh stem bark is used to treat colds, chest complaints and typhoid.[M111]

PREPARATION AND DOSAGE

CUTS, BURNS, SORES, SKIN AILMENTS AND FUNGAL INFECTIONS Add a little boiled water to a teaspoon of dried powdered bark to form a paste, which can then be rubbed onto affected areas of the skin.

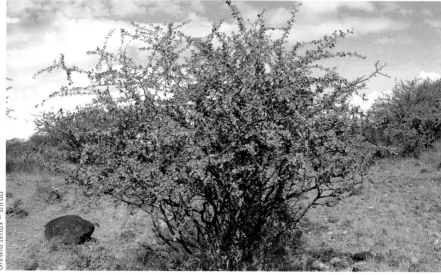

Grewia tenax – shrub

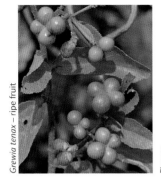
Grewia tenax – ripe fruit

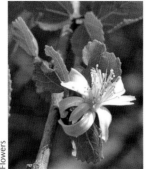
Flowers

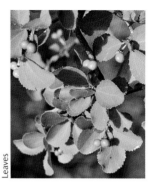
Leaves

b. *Grewia tephrodermis (Grewia bicolor)* Indigenous

Common names Grewia, Donkey Berry, White-leaved Raisin • **Local names** Hororessa (Bor.), Mulawa (Kam.), Setetit (Kip.), Lulala (Luh.), Powo (Luo), Olsitete (Maa.Ken.), Sitet (Pok.), Depi (Sam.), Debi / Debhi (Som.), Mkone (Swa.), Ekali (Tur.), Mkole (Gogo), Lomo (Goro.), Mpelemehe (Hehe), Esitete / Os-siteti (Maa.Tan.), Mkoma / Mkomalendi (Nyam.), Musuna-nu-kuu (Nyat.), Mduwau (Ran.), Mkole-ngoda (Samb.), Mkoma / Mukoma (Suk.), Mkomakoma (Zin.)

Description and ecology

Low, much-branched, fast-growing shrub or small tree growing to a height of 3–5m, occasionally reaching 9m. Bark smooth, grey, becoming dark grey, deeply fissured and peeling away in old trees, young branches velvety grey or brown. **Leaves** alternate, simple, oval to oblong, 1.5–9cm long, tip pointed and base rounded, edge finely serrate, glossy green above, almost white or silvery hairy below, leaf stalk 1–8mm long. **Flowers** bright yellow, sweetly scented, often in clusters (1–3 flowers in axillary cyme), borne at ends of branches, flower stalk 4–12mm long. **Fruits** round, fleshy drupes, green, hairy, becoming glossy orange-brown and black when ripe, unlobed or rarely deeply 2-lobed, the lobes then 4–8 × 5–8mm, sparsely hairy. Widespread in dry *Acacia* scrub, along riverine vegetation, bushed grassland and woodland, at 0–2,000m.

USAGE AND TREATMENT

PARTS USED Roots and bark.

TRADITIONAL MEDICINAL USES Bark is used as a vermifuge, diuretic and laxative, and to treat boils, sores, intestinal inflammation[M70] and syphilis.[M110] Root decoctions are used to treat diarrhoea.[M3] Roots are also used for treating chest pain, colds and snakebite. Bark is used for intestinal infestations and syphilis.[M4, M70] Pounded fresh bark is applied locally to body cuts, itches and other skin ailments.[M3, M4, M70] A cold infusion of the root is drunk for anaemia, chest complaints, colds, diarrhoea, snakebite, mental illness, a hernia and female infertility.[M110] A decoction of root or bark is taken as a tranquilliser.[M110] The juice or a decoction of root bark is applied on wounds and cuts.[M110]

PREPARATION AND DOSAGE

DIARRHOEA, COLDS AND CHEST PAIN Pound a handful of dry or fresh roots and immerse in a litre of cold boiled water. Stir and leave for 15 minutes. Drink the infusion twice a day for 3 days.

INTESTINAL WORMS, DIURETIC AND LAXATIVE Boil one and a half tablespoons of dry bark powder in a litre of water for 10 minutes. Leave to cool, then filter and drink an hour before breakfast for 2 days.

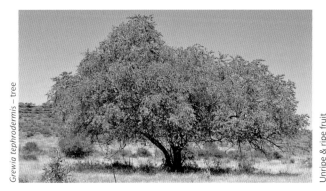

Grewia tephrodermis – tree

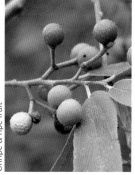

Unripe & ripe fruit

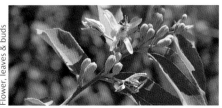

Flower, leaves & buds

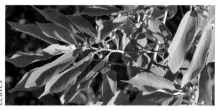

Leaves

c. *Grewia villosa*

Indigenous

Common names Round-leaf Grewia, Mallow Raisin • **Local names** Ogomdi / Buruudo (Bor.), Ogomdi (Gab.), Muvu / Mbu (Kam.), Ner powo (Luo), Olmankulai / Emankulai (Maa.), Mokoghio / Mokuwo / Makow (Pok.), Obhoob (Ren.), Ipupoi / Ipopoi (Sam.), Mukorobosho (Swa.), Shoshoti / Mshashote (Tai.), Mokuiwo (Tug.), Epong'ae / Epokoo (Tur.), Olmalungai (Aru.), Mumpembe (Nyat.), Msarasi (Suk.)

Description and ecology
Deciduous, much-branched shrub 1–3(–4)m tall, with spreading branches purple-brown, densely covered with villous hairs. Leaves large, broad, heart-shaped, coarse, hairy above, with prominent veins, margin serrate. Flowers brownish yellow or brownish, in clusters (in 2–10-flowered cymes). Fruit unlobed, subglobose, 1–1.6cm in diameter, green, turning copper-red or reddish brown when ripe, also covered with soft hairs. Common in dry *Acacia–Terminalia–Commiphora* bushland, thickets and often growing on rocky hills, at 0–1,550m.

USAGE AND TREATMENT

PARTS USED Roots and leaves.
TRADITIONAL MEDICINAL USES Pounded roots are used to treat diarrhoea. Boiled roots can relieve stomach ache and lower abdominal pain.[M3, M70] A boiled root extract is a remedy for aching bones and other body pain.[M111] A warm diluted solution of leaves and water is used for eyestrain (eyedrops) and spleen-related afflictions.[M70, M111] A decoction of roots, mixed with milk, is given to small children as a tonic.[M3] Powdered or fresh bark is applied as a poultice to treat wounds.[M111]

PREPARATION AND DOSAGE
STOMACH ACHE AND LOWER ABDOMINAL PAIN Boil a handful of fresh roots in a litre of water for 10–15 minutes. Filter the cool mixture and drink at intervals over 2 days, preparing a fresh mixture every day.

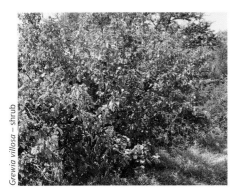
Grewia villosa – shrub

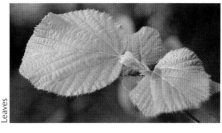
Leaves

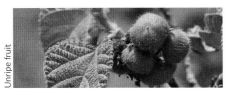
Unripe fruit

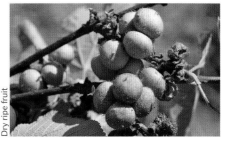
Dry ripe fruit

PHARMACOLOGY AND CHEMISTRY

PHARMACOLOGICAL PROPERTIES

Antibacterial[P296, P297] and antifungal[P298] activity is ascribed to the roots and the stem bark of some species of *Grewia*. Dried roots of *G. tephrodermis* (*G. bicolor*) have shown uterine stimulant effects,[P299] while aerial parts of the same plant have exhibited anti-inflammatory activity.[P300] Antioxidant, hepatoprotective, anti-inflammatory, anti-emetic, antimalarial, analgesic and antipyretic activities have also been reported for extracts of some *Grewia* species.[P296]

COMPOUNDS REPORTED

Species of *Grewia* contain a wide range of triterpenoids, such as betulin from the roots of *G. tephrodermis* (*G. bicolor*)[P299] and α-amyrin and other triterpenoids, and sterols from the whole plant of *G. tenax*.[P301] Steroids known from these species include stigmasterol from roots of *G. tephrodermis*[P299] and β-sitosterol from stem bark of *G. tenax*.[P302] Indole alkaloids, such as harman in roots of *G. tephrodermis*,[P299] and alkanols, such as triacontan-1-ol in stem bark of *G. tenax*,[P302] have also been reported. The alkaloids harman and harmine show a moderate antiproliferative activity towards human monocytes and a weak antileishmanial activity towards both promastigote and amastigote forms of this parasite.[P302]

Betulin

Harman

Harrisonia abyssinica

RUTACEAE

Indigenous

Common name No common name in English • **Local names** Raga (Bor.), Kidori / Chidori (Dig.), Mkithunga (Gir.), Mulilyyulu / Mukiliulu (Kam.), Gora (Ilw., Orm.), Pedo / Omindi (Luo), Mkidunya (Luh.), Kapkerelwa (Mar.), Mkidori / Msamburini (Swa.), Gora (Orm.), Mukurkona (Pok.), Lasaramai / Muruguti (Sam.), Eddih-chabel (Som.), Ekalale (Tur.)

Description and ecology

Spiny, scrambling evergreen shrub or small tree reaching 2–6m (sometimes climbing), with spreading drooping branches. **Bark** with conical corky protuberances up to 2cm, rarely unarmed, bole and larger branches with spines on short wart-like outgrowths 0.8–1.5mm long, usually in pairs and axillary, branchlets without or with hooked spines in pairs at base of leaf stalks, hairy or non-hairy. **Leaves** compound, often with 3–7 pairs of leaflets plus a terminal one, leaflets 4 × 2cm but usually smaller, without stalks, margins toothed. **Flowers** cream or yellow, in panicles 5–15cm long. **Fruit** 4–6-lobed berry, green at first, becoming red-black when ripe, fleshy, round, 4–8mm in diameter. Common along coastal forest margins and in riverine forest vegetation, dry bushland and wooded grassland, at 0–1,600m.

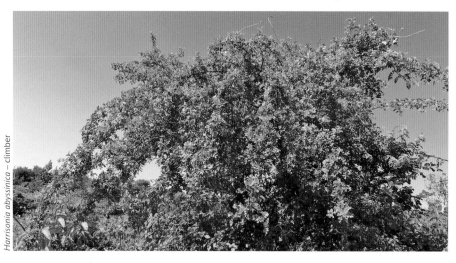

Harrisonia abyssinica – climber

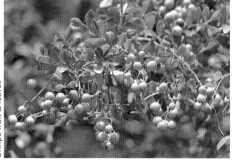

Unripe fruit & leaves

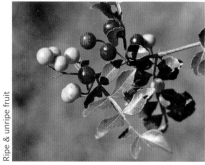

Ripe & unripe fruit

PARTS USED All parts.

TRADITIONAL MEDICINAL USES Root decoctions are taken for rheumatism, body pain, coughs, fever, a hernia, schistosomiasis, gonorrhoea and menorrhagia; the tea is also taken as a diuretic, an aphrodisiac and for body weakness, malaria,[M71] vomiting, nausea, ancylostomiasis, skin ailments, insomnia, tuberculosis, swollen testicles and diarrhoea.[M32, M47, M48, M51, M70, M112] The entire plant, dried, is used to treat malaria,[M71] stomach ache, abdominal pain, haemorrhoids and snakebite.[M46] A leaf extract, neat or mixed with roots, is also used for snakebite.[M1] A decoction of young leaves is taken as an aphrodisiac; a decoction of old leaves is taken as a remedy for menstrual pain.[M49, M70] Dried roots are used to quicken delivery in cases of prolonged pregnancy.[M50] A warm decoction of pounded roots or leaves is used to make a wash for disinfecting wounds and abscesses.[M112] Roots and bark are crushed, soaked in water and then drunk to purify the body, also serving as a body tonic.[M112]

PREPARATION AND DOSAGE

SCHISTOSOMIASIS (BILHARZIA), STOMACH ACHE AND ABDOMINAL PAIN Cut 6–8g of fresh roots into fine pieces and boil in a litre of water for 10 minutes. Drink the warm decoction twice daily for 2 days. Alternatively, boil a handful of fresh bark or a tablespoon of bark powder in a litre of water for a few minutes and drink the mixture twice a day.

RHEUMATISM AND TUBERCULOSIS Add a teaspoon of dry root powder to a cup of cold boiled water. Leave for 10–15 minutes. Then filter and drink twice daily for 3 or 4 days, preparing a new infusion every day. Alternatively, boil a tablespoon of mixed powder (comprising roots, leaves, twigs and bark of the whole dried plant) in a litre of water for a few minutes and drink the mixture twice a day.

MALARIA AND FEVER Add 3–4g of dry leaf powder to a litre of hot boiled water. Leave to cool, then strain and drink the infusion twice a day.

PHARMACOLOGICAL PROPERTIES

Both leaf and root extracts have shown antimalarial activity against some strains of *Plasmodium falciparum*.[P303] A root extract has shown weak activity against several bacterial, fungal and viral organisms.[P304]

COMPOUNDS REPORTED

Phytochemical analyses have resulted in the identification of triterpenes and limonoids (e.g. harrisonin) in *Harrisonia abyssinica* root bark,[P305] prenylated polyketides (e.g. aissatone) in stem bark,[P306] and a unique hydroperoxychroman, 8-acety-3a-hydroperoxy-2a-isohex-3-enyl-6-isopent-2-enyl-5-methoxy-2b-methylchroman in the plant as a whole.[P307] A new triterpene, cycloabyssinone, has been isolated from stem bark.[P308] Harronin I, a new prenylated acetophenone, was identified as one of the antifungal metabolites from ripe berries of *H. abyssinica*.[P309]

Harrisonin

Cycloabyssinone

52 *Hibiscus* species

a. *Hibiscus fuscus*
Indigenous

Common name Hibiscus • **Local names** Mukuma (Mer.), Esubukioi (Maa.), Mtakawa (Swa.), Kirundu (Chag.)

Description and ecology

Erect, sparsely branched, woody herb or shrub 1–3m high, with brownish-black hairs on the stem. **Leaves** simple, ovate, with a narrow tip and toothed margin, hairy. **Flowers** white, borne in the axils, usually solitary, 1.5–2.5cm in diameter, with a hairy flower stalk up to 6cm long, opening fully during the day, closing in the afternoon. **Fruit** a subglobose capsule, 10mm in diameter. **Seeds** with silky white or brownish hairs. Common in disturbed ground or in old cultivated fields as a short-lived perennial and in permanent grassland as a larger shrub, at 1,250–2,400m.

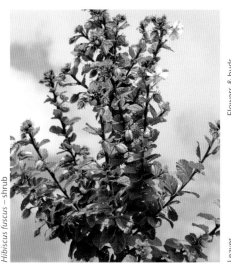

Hibiscus fuscus – shrub

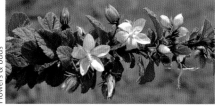

Flowers & buds

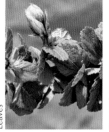

Leaves

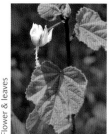

Flower & leaves

USAGE AND TREATMENT

PARTS USED Roots and leaves.

TRADITIONAL MEDICINAL USES Roots are used to soothe a cough and sore throat, and are also taken as an aphrodisiac and a general antidote to poisoning.[M1, M70] Leaves are used for treating skin ailments, including wounds, boils, abscesses, eczema and fungal infections.[M70] Another indigenous species, *Hibiscus flavifolius*, is used in a similar way. It has broadly ovate-rounded, hairy leaves and is commonly found in woodland and dry, rocky grasslands, at 750–2,100m.

PREPARATION AND DOSAGE

SKIN INFECTIONS (WOUNDS, ABSCESSES, ECZEMA AND FUNGAL INFECTIONS) Immerse some fresh leaves in boiling water. Use as a steam bath for 15 minutes to treat affected areas of the skin. A paste made by mixing a leaf powder with water can also be applied.

COUGHS AND SORE THROAT Chew some fresh roots, swallowing the juice.

b. *Hibiscus rosa-sinensis*　　　Native to tropical Asia (China)

Common names Hibiscus, Rose of China, China Rose, Chinese Hibiscus

Description and ecology

Magnificent bushy, evergreen, perennial shrub 2.5m high or small tree up to 5m if left unpruned, aerial stems woody, erect, green, cylindrical and branched. **Bark** grey-brown. **Leaves** simple, alternate, glossy green, oval, tip pointed, margin coarsely dentate, with a stalk. **Flowers** solitary, large, conspicuous, trumpet-shaped, 10cm in diameter, in a variety of colours from showy pink, red and white to yellow and orange. Makes a very attractive hedge and ornamental garden plant. Grown widely throughout East Africa at both low and high altitudes.

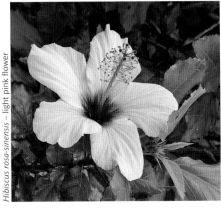

Hibiscus rosa-sinensis – light pink flower

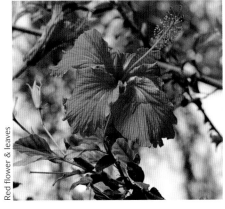

Red flower & leaves

WC167

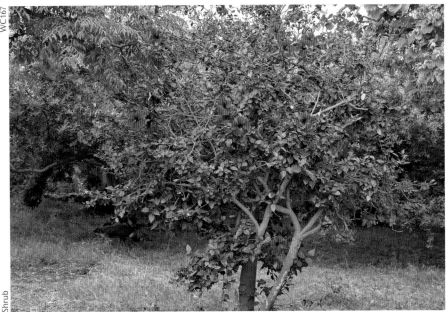

Shrub

USAGE AND TREATMENT

PARTS USED Flowers, roots and leaves only.

TRADITIONAL MEDICINAL USES The petals are used for treating fever, bronchitis, menstrual disorders and dysmenorrhoea[M10, M45, M70] and are also taken as an abortifacient.[M10] An infusion of flowers helps to treat eye infections. A decoction of the root is used to soothe sore eyes. A paste made from the root is used in the treatment of venereal diseases.[M112] Dried buds are eaten as a treatment for diabetes. Flowers and leaves are used for constipation and painful bowel movement.[M10] Another exotic species, *Hibiscus sabdariffa* (red sorrel, Indian sorrel), is native to India, Myanmar, Egypt and Guatemala. In East Africa, it is grown as a garden shrub, at 0–1,250m. A decoction of its leaves is drunk as a soothing cough remedy, and pounded fresh leaves are used as poultices on abscesses. Tea made from fresh ripe fruit and seeds of *H. sabdariffa* acts as a mild laxative, diuretic and tonic.

PREPARATION AND DOSAGE

FEVER, BRONCHITIS AND DYSMENORRHOEA Soak 3 or 4 of fresh flowers in half a cup of boiled water. Leave for an hour to cool and drink the water 2 or 3 times a day.

EYE INFECTIONS Wash the eyes with a cold flower infusion (prepared as above) 2 or 3 times daily.

DIABETES Chew or eat an unopened mature bud every morning before breakfast for up to 10 days. This is not a cure but it does help to reduce blood sugar levels.

PHARMACOLOGY AND CHEMISTRY

PHARMACOLOGICAL PROPERTIES

The leaves of *Hibiscus fuscus* have produced weak antiviral and antifungal activities.[P254] A wide range of antifungal, anti-inflammatory, antihypertensive, antipyretic, antispasmodic, antispermatogenic and antiviral activities, as well as analgesic, abortifacient, hypotensive and hypothermic effects, have been reported for *H. rosa-sinensis*.[P79] An aqueous and alcohol extract of *H. rosa-sinensis* leaves showed significant hypoglycaemic activity.[P310]

COMPOUNDS REPORTED

Friedelin and related triterpenes have been isolated from *H. tiliaceus*[P311] (not described here). A mixture of organic acids (citric, tartaric, oxalic and malvalic acids), hibiscus mucilage, β-sitosterol, glucose, fructose, heptacosan, N-heptacosane, hexacosan and other compounds are known from *H. rosa-sinensis*.[P79] Species of *Hibiscus* elaborate flavonoids, anthocyanins, terpenoids, steroids, polysaccharides, alkaloids, amino acids, lipids, sesquiterpene, quinones and naphthalene derivatives. Some of these compounds have been responsible for various activities in members of the genus.[P310]

Friedelin

a. *Jasminum floribundum* Indigenous

Common names Jasmine, Royal Jasmine • **Local names** Chepokiot (Kip.), Olopito / Olmainiyen (Maa.), Kongara (Mar.), Kaloyne (Pok.), Esthono (Tur.)

Description and ecology

Low, branched, evergreen or deciduous shrub, scrambler or climber reaching 0.6–3m, with slender, twig-like branches, glabrous. **Leaves** opposite, mostly 5-foliolately compound but leaflets sometimes up to 9 or as few as 3, non-hairy, 1.5–4.5 × 0.5–2.5cm, ovate to elongate-ovate, tips pointed, terminal leaflet larger than laterals. **Flowers** white, in terminal or axillary 3–7-flowered cymes, often streaked with pink or crimson outside, sweet smelling. **Fruit** black, globose,1- or 2-lobed, up to 8mm across. Found in savanna, upland evergreen bushland, bushed grassland and on rocky hillsides, at 1,200–2,400m.

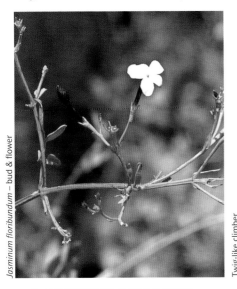

Jasminum floribundum – bud & flower

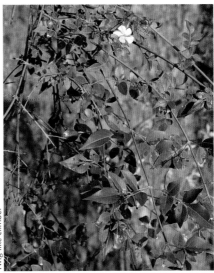

Twig-like climber

USAGE AND TREATMENT

PARTS USED Roots, leaves and flowers.
TRADITIONAL MEDICINAL USES A decoction of leaves is taken for stomach worms.[M33, M70] Leaves are chewed as a remedy for mouth ulcers and fresh juice of the plant is applied to corns.[M113] A root decoction is taken for liver ailments, diarrhoea and stomach pain.[M1] Fresh roots are chewed to treat tonsillitis.[M1] An infusion of flowers can relieve coughs and a flower infusion is applied externally to treat skin diseases.[M113] A mixture of pounded fresh leaves in butter is a treatment for infected wounds and a warm infusion of leaves is used for cleaning and sterilising ulcers.[M113]

PREPARATION AND DOSAGE
STOMACH WORMS Soak 2–3g of pounded fresh leaves in half a litre of water for 15–20 minutes. Drink the mixture before breakfast in the mornings.

b. *Jasminum fluminense*

Common names Jasmine, River Jasmine • **Local names** Mtunda ofu (Dig.), Uthui (Kam.), Moiywet (Kip.), Seke (Luo), Ollobito (Maa.), Epeloch / Manimani (Tur.), Mtanyeze (Suk.)

Description and ecology

Woody, evergreen, climbing or scrambling shrub or climber 4–6m long. Stems cylindrical, hairy, becoming non-hairy when mature, with numerous hairless or hairy lateral branches. **Leaves** opposite, 3–5-foliolately compound, leaflets broadly ovate or elliptic, 1.5–6 × 1–6cm, non-hairy to densely hairy, bases wedge-shaped or rounded, apices rounded or pointed, terminal leaflet larger than laterals. **Flowers** in terminal groups, numerous, white, often pink outside, sweetly scented. **Fruit** a purple or almost blue-black berry, shiny, globose or subglobose, 5mm in diameter, 1- or 2-lobed. Found in a variety of habitats, including evergreen bushland (coastal and inland), bushed grassland, thickets, woodland, forest edges and riverine forest, at 0–2,650m.

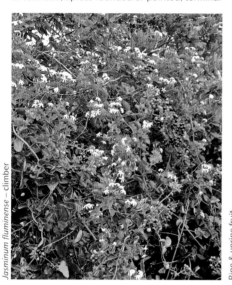

Jasminum fluminense – climber

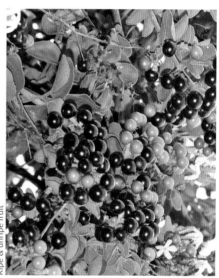

Ripe & unripe fruit

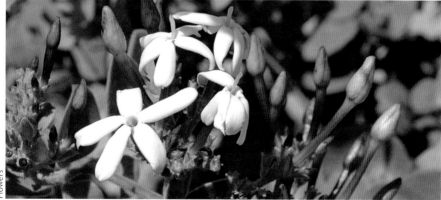

Flowers

PARTS USED Roots, leaves and fruit.
TRADITIONAL MEDICINAL USES Leaves are used to expel intestinal parasitic worms.[M70] Fruits are used to kill hair lice.[M33] A root extract is used for eye afflictions and also as a remedy for snakebite.[M1, M70] In Kenya, an infusion of dried leaves is used for treating *chira*, which is a local name for a disease characterised by 'thinning'/weight loss or impurity, associated with infertility in young women.[M26] Smoke from burned roots is inhaled to treat taeniasis.[M52]

PREPARATION AND DOSAGE
HAIR LICE Mix some ground fruit with mustard oil. Apply to the scalp and hair.
ANTHELMINTIC Soak 2–3g of pounded fresh leaves in half a litre of warm water for 15–20 minutes. Drink the infusion before breakfast in the mornings.
EYE AFFLICTIONS Add a teaspoon of dried root powder to half a litre of hot water. Stir, filter and use the warm mixture to wash the eyes.

PHARMACOLOGICAL PROPERTIES
Roots of *Jasminum* species have shown both taenicidal[P312] and anthelmintic activities.[P313] In a toxicity assessment test, a water extract of dried roots was found to be toxic to mice.[P312]

COMPOUNDS REPORTED
A flavone (cynaroside) has been isolated from *J. fluminense* leaves.[P314] From the root bark of some *Jasminum* species, oligomeric secoiridoid glucosides (e.g. craigosides C) have also been reported.[P315] GC-MS analyses of leaf extracts of *J. fluminense* identified several fatty acid derivatives and phenolics.[P316] It is reported that phenolics and flavonoids, which are major constituents of *J. floribundum*, are possibly responsible for anti-inflammatory and antioxidant properties of the plant.[P317]

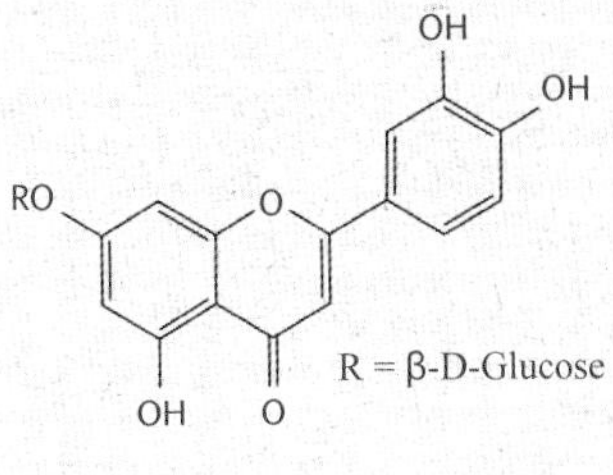

R = β-D-Glucose

Cynaroside

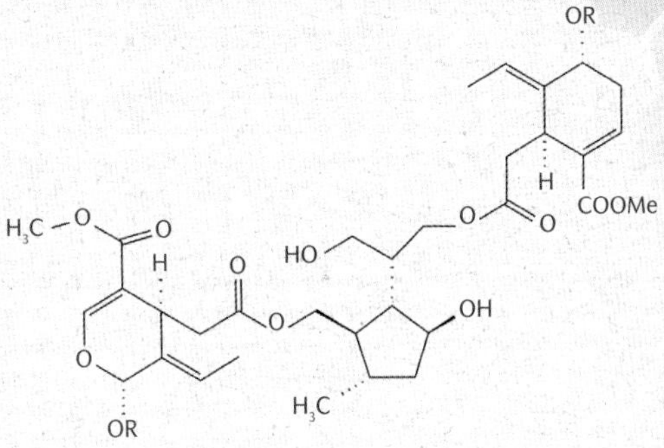

Craigosides C

Native to tropical America

Common names Physic Nut, Purging Nut, Pig Nut • **Local names** Mbogo-komo (Gir.), Kyaiki kyakyeni / Kya muunyi (Kam.), Jok (Luo), Kiryowa (Lug.), Kilowa (Luso.)

Description and ecology

Erect, semi-evergreen, stiffly branched, succulent shrub or small tree 3–4(–6)m tall. Stem and branches smooth, sparsely lenticellate. **Bark** thin, yellow-grey, papery, peeling, with unpleasant watery latex when cut. **Leaves** simple, green to pale green, alternate to slightly opposite, hairless, heart-shaped, usually with 3–5 shallow lobes up to 15cm long, stalk up to 16cm long. **Flowers** small, in greenish-yellow clusters (cymes) arising from leaf axils. **Fruits** round or egg-shaped capsules, slightly 3-angled, 2.5–3.5cm long, green when young, turning dark brown-black when ripe. **Seeds** 3 per fruit, black, oblong, 1.5–2cm long. Widely cultivated as a hedge plant, today growing wild both in bushland and along rivers, at 0–1,650m.

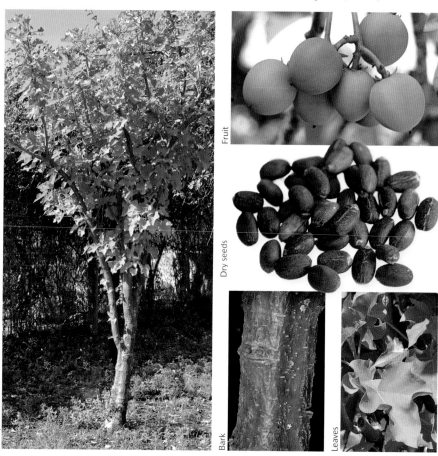

Jatropha curcas – tree

Fruit

Dry seeds

Bark

Leaves

PARTS USED Roots, stem bark, leaves and seeds/seed oil.
TRADITIONAL MEDICINAL USES Leaves, bark and seeds are used as a purgative.[M2] Fresh leaf or stem juice is applied to cuts, burns, ulcers, septic gums, boils, infected wounds, itchy and blistered skin, [M1, M10, M114] and ringworm.[M10] Roots are used as a remedy for chest and kidney ailments.[M1] The seeds are taken as an oral contraceptive. Hot-water extracts of seeds are drunk as an abortifacient or an anthelmintic.[M10, M114, M115] A decoction of dried or fresh roots is taken as a remedy for toothache and a sore throat,[M10] and for treating diarrhoea, dysentery and gonorrhoea.[M114] Crushed seeds and seed oil are used for eczema, wounds, skin diseases, rheumatic pain, arthritis and gout.[M114, M115]

PREPARATION AND DOSAGE

WOUNDS, CUTS, BURNS AND RINGWORM Apply squeezed juice from some leaves or stems to affected areas of the skin 3 times a day.
USE AS A PURGATIVE AND ANTHELMINTIC Swallow two crushed seeds in the morning before breakfast or boil 6–8g of fresh leaves or bark in a litre of water for 10–15 minutes and drink the warm decoction before breakfast.
TOOTHACHE AND SORE THROAT Boil 4g of dry root powder in half a litre of water for 10–15 minutes. Rinse the mouth with the warm decoction for toothache or gargle for a sore throat.

> **⚠ WARNING!** Do not exceed the number of seeds recommended in dosages for purgative and anthelmintic use as an overdose might result in severe diarrhoea, vomiting and abdominal pain.

PHARMACOLOGICAL PROPERTIES

Antibacterial, anticonvulsant, antifungal, antispasmodic, anti-inflammatory, antitumour and antiviral activities and hypoglycaemic, diuretic, cytotoxic cardiac and hypothermic effects have been ascribed to *Jatropha curcas*.[P79] Several diterpenoids with antimicrobial[P318] and antitumour[P318] activities are reported, including some with tumour-promoting effects.[P319] Owing to the presence of toxic proteins and diterpenoid irritants in the seed oil, high doses may cause severe diarrhoea and abdominal pain.[P320, P321] *J. curcas* showed anti-inflammatory activity upon topical application of root powder paste in TPA-induced ear inflammation in albino mice. A methanol extract of roots also exhibited anti-inflammatory activity in acute carrageenan-induced and formalin-induced rat paw oedema.[P322]

COMPOUNDS REPORTED

The seed oil contains diterpenoids (e.g. curcusone A, B, C and D).[P79, P318] A toxic protein, curcin, has been isolated from the seed oil.[P79, P322, P323] Activity of the seed oil is ascribed to the presence of curcanoleic acid, which is similar to ricinoleic acid from castor oil and to crotonoleic acid from croton oil.[P322, P323] Other compounds isolated include ß-amyrin, ß-sitosterol, jatrophone, jatropholone A, arabinose and ß-sitosterol-ß-D-glucoside.[P79]

Curcusone A

Jatrophone

Indigenous

Common name Sausage Tree • **Local names** Shelole (Bon.), Mobwoka (Gir.), Kiatine / Muatine (Kam.), Muratina (Kik., Mer.), Ratuinet (Kip.), Morabe (Luh.), Yago (Luo), Oldarpoi / Ortarboi (Maa.Ken.), Rotio (Mar.), Ratinuet (Nan.), Bogh (Orm.), Rotin (Pok.), Muum (Ren.), Imombi (Sam.), Bukorola (Som.), Mwegea / Mvungunya (Swa.), Mwaisina (Tai.), Mukisha (Tav.), Edot (Tur.), Oldaoboi (Aru.), Dati (Goro.), Mfumbi (Hehe), Muegea (Lugu.), Ol darboi (Maa.Tan.), Mvungwe (Ngu.), Msanghwa / Mdungwa / Mvungwa (Nyam.), Mungungu (Nyat.), Mulunzi (Nyir.), Musuva (Ran.), Ngwicha / Mgwicha (Suk.), Mwegea / Mwicha (Swa.), Mvungwe (Zig.), Mzingute (Zin.), Edodoi (Ate.), Mussa (Lug.), Odolo / Odologo (Lugb.), Lukulungu (Lugi.), Mwiago (Lugw.), Mujungwe (Luny.), Yago (Luo-Ug.), Muvunjudza (Luso.), Lado (Madi), Muikya / Mulolo (Runy.), Mwikya (Ruto.).

Description and ecology

Large, semi-deciduous tree with rounded crown and spreading branches, up to 9m tall in open woodland but reaching 18–20m along rivers. Bark grey-brown, smooth at first but flaking in round patches when old. Leaves crowded towards tips of branches, opposite or in whorls of 3, compound, with 7–11 large leaflets up to 10cm long, broadly oval, rough and rigid like sandpaper, often with sharp tips and wavy edges.

Flowers in pendulous panicles 40–120cm long, large, attractive, maroon or dark red with yellow veins, bell-shaped, velvety on the inside, with unpleasant smell. Fruit a large, woody, sausage-shaped berry 30–80cm long, grey-green or grey-brown, indehiscent, hanging down on long, rope-like stalks, containing numerous seeds embedded in the fibrous pulp. Widespread in East Africa in wooded grassland, shrubland, wet savanna, and along rivers in moist forests, at 0–3,000m.

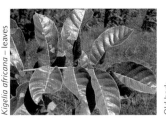

Kigelia africana – leaves

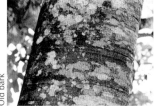

Old bark

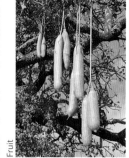

Fruit

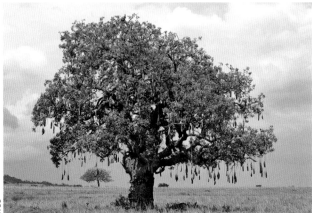

Tree

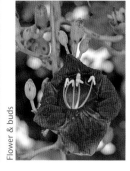

Flower & buds

PARTS USED Leaves, bark, fruits, roots, stems and twigs.

TRADITIONAL MEDICINAL USES A bark decoction is used as a remedy for headache and dysentery.[M4, M70] A leaf decoction is taken for malaria. Fruits are used as a remedy for measles in children,[M1] and are also taken as a purgative and to induce abortion.[M4] Roots, bark and ripe or unripe fruits are taken as a laxative or emetic, to treat chronic and acute digestive disorders and against gastric infections.[M115] Stems and twigs are also used to treat digestive disorders.[M115] Fruits, roots or leaves are said to treat sexual complaints such as poor libido, impotence and infertility; also, a small amount of unripe fruit is chewed or an infusion is prepared and taken orally as a sexual stimulant and aphrodisiac.[M115] In South Africa, a powder made from dried fruit is used as a dressing for ulcers, sores, syphilis and rheumatism; a mixed decoction of fruit and bark is taken orally or as an enema for stomach ailments.[M2, M70] A decoction of bark and leaves is administered as an abortifacient. Infusions of powdered bark, leaves, stems, twigs or fruits are used to clean and dress flesh wounds and open sores. A fruit decoction is used for oedema of the legs.[M115]

PREPARATION AND DOSAGE

MALARIA Boil 2g of dry leaf powder in half a litre of water for 10 minutes. Leave to cool, then filter and drink the decoction twice a day.

MEASLES IN CHILDREN Washing a child with a beer made from fermented fruit is reputed to be an excellent treatment for measles. (The beer is not to be consumed, however.)

PHARMACOLOGY AND CHEMISTRY

PHARMACOLOGICAL PROPERTIES

A water extract of *Kigelia africana* bark has shown antimicrobial activity.[P324] The presence of dihydroisocoumarins (e.g. kigelin) and their glycosides[P324, P325] may account for the beneficial effects of external use. An iridoid, verminoside, could be responsible for this plant's anti-inflammatory activity.[P326] Extracts from different parts of *K. africana* showed antibacterial activity against *Escherichia coli*, a blood glucose-lowering effect as well as antiplasmodial, anticonvulsant, antidiarrhoeal, diuretic, antioxidant and anticancer activities.[P327]

COMPOUNDS REPORTED

The major compounds of the roots and bark are the dihydroisocoumarin kigelin and the naphthoquinone lapachol.[P323, P325] Other compounds, such as kigelinone, pinnatal, isopinnatal, stigmasterol and ß-sitosterol, have also been isolated from *K. africana* bark.[P323]

Kigelin

Verminoside

Lapachol

a. *Lantana camara*
Native to tropical America

Common names Lantana Weed, Wild Sage, Tick Berry, Curse of India • **Local names** Mjasasa (Dig.), Kitavisi (Kam.), Mukigi / Mukenia (Kik.), Nyamrih / Magwagwa (Luo), Getipkamoskon (Tug.), Muwaha (Gogo), Luhongole / Lupebeta (Hehe), Mpugambu (Nyam.), Gigambu (Ran.), Mvuti (Samb., Swa.), Elantaana (Ate.), Owiny bilo / Abelwinyo (Lan.), Kayuukiyuuki (Lug.), Obwengere (Lugw.), Kapanga (Luso.), Omuhuki ogwamahwa / Omuhuuki / Omushkyera (Runyan.), Jerenga (Runy.)

Description and ecology
Evergreen, multi-stemmed, perennial shrub, 2–3(–5)m tall, with square or 3-angled prickly stems, covered with bristly hairs when young. **Leaves** simple, 3–8cm long, opposite or in threes, broader at base, pointed at apex, margin dentate, upper surface rough, strongly aromatic when crushed. **Flowers** multicoloured, may be red, orange, yellow, pink, white or cream, in flat rounded heads, up to about 1cm long. **Fruits** small, globose, green berries, up to 8mm across, deep blue or purple-black when ripe, in round heads. Forming extensive, dense thickets and often invading previously disturbed areas such as logged and cleared forests, the plant now occurs as a serious weed throughout East Africa, at 0–1,900m.

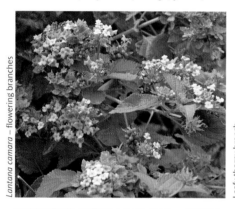

Lantana camara – flowering branches

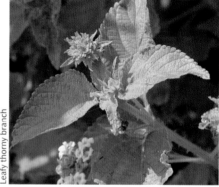

Leafy thorny branch

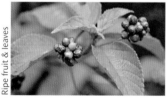

Ripe fruit & leaves

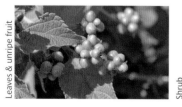

Leaves & unripe fruit

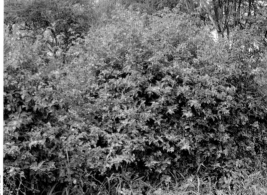

Shrub

PARTS USED Leaves, stem bark, roots.
TRADITIONAL MEDICINAL USES Leaves are used as a remedy for toothache, a cold and headache.[M4, M70] Ash of burned leaves, with a little added salt, is a remedy for a cough, sore throat, conjunctivitis and toothache.[M26] Leaves are used to treat leprosy, scabies,[M112] wounds, cuts,[M56] burns, eczema, boils, skin itches, fungal infections and ringworm.[M10] A decoction of dried leaves is taken as a remedy for malaria.[M55] A herbal tea made from leaves is taken as an emmenagogue and also as a carminative.[M56, M70] A hot-water extract of dried stems is used as an emmenagogue.[M10] A root decoction is taken for influenza, coughs, high fever, malaria, tuberculosis, asthma, toothache, headache, gonorrhoea and leucorrhoea.[M112] An infusion of leaves and flowering tops is used in the treatment of fever, constipation, tuberculosis, and bronchitis. Externally, leaves and stems are used as a wash to relieve dermatitis, eczema, measles and chickenpox rashes.[M112]

PREPARATION AND DOSAGE
TOOTHACHE Simply chew some fresh leaves.
HEADACHE, COLDS AND COUGHS Immerse some fresh leaves in boiling water and inhale the steam vapour 3 times a day.
WOUNDS, BURNS, SCABIES, LEPROSY AND FUNGAL INFECTIONS Apply a paste made from pounded fresh leaves as a poultice over the affected areas.
DERMATITIS, ECZEMA, MEASLES AND CHICKENPOX RASHES Pound 2 or 3 handfuls of fresh leaves and stems, boil in 2 litres of water for 10 minutes, sieve and use as a warm wash to treat the affected areas.

b. *Lantana trifolia* — Indigenous

Common names Lantana, Sage Bush, Three-leaved Lantana • **Local names** Kate (Bor.), Muvisavisi (Kam.), Mukenia (Kik.), Bek-ap-torit (Kip.), Esimenenua / Lumenenambuli (Luh.), Nyabend-winy / Magwaga (Luo), Ol magirigiriana / Ol makongora (Maa.Ken.), Chemosong / Kogumbosuwa (Mar.), Peptarit / Petiapteriet (Nan.), Sekechewo (Tug.), Mwemberi (Tai.), Luhongole (Hehe), Enkurma-onkayiok / Lukurman-oonkayiok / Ol magirigiriani (Maa.Tan.), Mpugambu (Nyam.), Msasa-kilasha / Muhanta (Samb.), Mvepe (Swa.), Abelwinyo / Bel winyo / Kapanga (Ach.), Abelwinyo / Bel awele (Lan.), Kayuukiyuuki (Lug.), Musojore (Lugwe.), Kapanga (Luso.), Ehuuki / Omuhuuki (Runyan.), Omusekera (Ruto.), Itonaio (Madi)

Description and ecology
Small, scrambling, weak-stemmed herbaceous shrub usually 1–1.5m tall, occasionally up to 3m. Stems with bristle-like hairs rather than prickles, branches 4-angled. Leaves aromatic, stalked, with 3 leaflets, ovate to lanceolate to ovate-oblong, margins serrate. Flowers purplish pink, in round terminal or axillary heads clustered on long stalks. Fruits small globose drupes 2–3mm long, shiny green, turning mauve to purple when ripe. Grows at upland forest edges and in bush margins, grasslands and bushland at elevations of 900–2,300m.

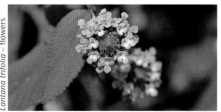

Lantana trifolia – flowers

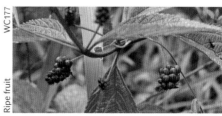

WC177

Ripe fruit

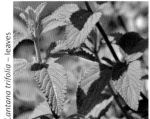
Lantana trifolia – leaves

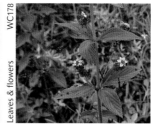
WC178 / Leaves & flowers

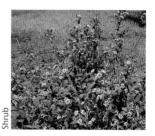
Shrub

USAGE AND TREATMENT

PARTS USED Root, leaves, stems and seeds.
TRADITIONAL MEDICINAL USES Decoctions of leaves are taken for liver diseases and indigestion.[M4] Pounded leaves are used to treat sore eyes[M4, M70] and convulsions in children with malaria.[M32] Leaves are used to treat coughs,[M39] colds,[M54, M91, M112] respiratory ailments, chest pain and gonorrhoea, and in external applications for ringworm[M54, M91, M112] and leprosy.[M53] Stems can function as toothbrushes.[M26] Leaves are crushed and mixed in hot water, the liquid then drunk to treat rheumatism, general body pain and indigestion.[M91, M112] Roots are a remedy for rheumatism.[M4]

PREPARATION AND DOSAGE
SORE EYES Apply 3g of pounded fresh leaves in hot water. Wash the eyes with the warm solution, taking care that it is the right temperature for the eyes.
COUGHS AND COLDS Boil 3g of crushed fresh leaves or a tablespoon of leaf powder in a cup of water. Drink 2 or 3 cups a day, freshly prepared.
RHEUMATISM, GENERAL BODY PAIN AND INDIGESTION Boil 2–3g of crushed fresh roots, or root powder or fresh crushed or dry leaf powder, in a cup of water. Drink 2 or 3 cups a day, preparing afresh every time.

PHARMACOLOGY AND CHEMISTRY

PHARMACOLOGICAL PROPERTIES
Essential oil from aerial parts of *Lantana camara* shows antibacterial and antifungal activities.[P328] The bark and leaves show smooth muscle stimulant activities.[P329] Aerial parts of *L. trifolia* produce anti-asthmatic activity.[P330]

COMPOUNDS REPORTED
Compounds isolated from *Lantana* species include sesquiterpenes (e.g. α-acorenol),[P331] triterpenes (e.g. α-amyrin),[P332] phenylpropanoids (e.g. calceolarioside A)[P333] and an antimicrobial flavonoid, umuhengerin.[P334] The triterpene oleanonic acid, isolated from *L. camara*, showed anti-inflammatory and anticancer activities.[P335]

α-Amyrin

Umuhengerin

a. *Leonotis nepetifolia*   Indigenous

Common names Leonotis, Christmas Candlestick, Lion's Ear • **Local names** Mucii (Kik.), Chemosibit (Kip.), Nyanyodhi (Luo), Ol-bibi (Maa.), Kachichin / Ilkesheni (Pok.), Ewat (Tur.), Lisanzauki (Hehe), Mfyomfyo (Nyam.), Achukia (Ate.), Ejuju (Ate.T.), Ocuru (Lan.), Ekifumufumu (Lug.), Olususuni (Lugw.), Susunu (Luso.), Lolemwo (Ngaka.), Ekicumucumu (Ruki., Runyan., Runy., Ruto.)

Description and ecology

Tall, woody, annual or short-lived plant 0.8–3m tall. **Leaves** ovate, base wedge-shaped, apex pointed, very soft, dark green, hairy or non-hairy, drooping, 2–9 × 1–6cm, margin dentate, stalk up to 4cm long. **Flowers** striking, lipped, commonly orange but can be red or cream, grouped in 1–4 dense spherical masses at intervals up the stem, 3–6cm across, petals covered with hairs, calyx funnel-shaped and with 8 spines, very prickly when dry. **Fruits** smooth, long, thin nutlets. Common along forest margins, roadsides, in abandoned cultivated and overgrazed areas, flood plains and in wetlands, growing almost as a weed, at 900–2,300m.

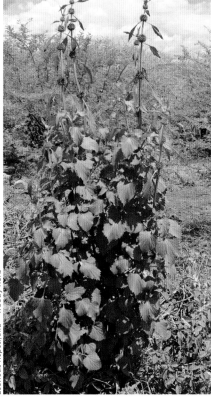

Leonotis nepetifolia – woody herb

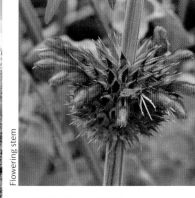

Flowering stem

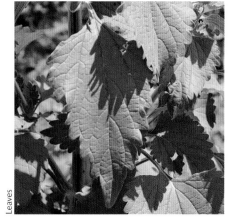

Leaves

PARTS USED All parts of the plant.
TRADITIONAL MEDICINAL USES Infusions of *Leonotis* roots are taken to treat dysentery, intestinal worms and digestive disorders.[M112] Fresh leaves are used as a remedy for stomach cramps. Young leaves are used to treat conjunctivitis.[M70] Brewed leaves are used as a tea for fever, coughs, womb prolapse and malaria. A decoction of the whole plant is taken for diarrhoea and heavy cramps, as a diuretic and as a tonic to strengthen the back.[M112] Leaf and root decoctions are also used to treat wounds, boils, eczema, itching and muscular pain.[M1]

PREPARATION AND DOSAGE
SKIN AILMENTS (BOILS, ECZEMA, FUNGAL DISEASES) Boil a handful of fresh leaves or roots in half a litre of water for 5–10 minutes. Apply the warm decoction to the affected areas.
DYSENTERY AND INTESTINAL WORMS Steep a handful of pounded fresh roots in a litre of cold boiled water. Leave for 30 minutes. Filter and then drink a cup of the infusion 3 times daily before meals.
STOMACH CRAMPS AND DIURETIC Wash 2 or 3 fresh leaves in cold boiled water before chewing them and swallowing the juice.

b. *Leonotis ocymifolia* (*Leonotis mollissima*)   Indigenous

Common names Leonotis, Rock Lion's Paw • **Local names** Ezewe (Kam.), Nyantodhi (Luo), Mosibit (Kik.), Ol-bibi (Maa.), Kipserere (Mar.)

Description and ecology
Erect, woody, roughly hairy herb or shrub 1–3m high, branching from a thick woody base, branches with widely spaced internodes along the stems, all parts with a strong smell. **Leaves** woolly, stalked, ovate to almost round, 5–15 × 2–7cm, apex pointed, base subcordate, margin toothed, slightly sandpapery and finely hairy above, silvery densely white-hairy below. **Flowers** bright orange, spherical, grouped in 1–3 terminal masses (well-spaced, ball-shaped whorls). Very common along upland forest margins, on rocky slopes and in montane forest as well as on hills and mountains, at 1,500–2,600m.

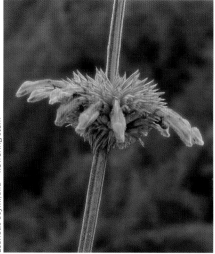
Leonotis ocymifolia – flowering stem

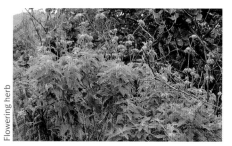
Flowering herb

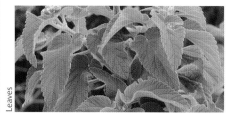
Leaves

USAGE AND TREATMENT

PARTS USED Roots, leaves and stems.

TRADITIONAL MEDICINAL USES A root decoction is used against stomach ache and to treat diarrhoea.[M33] Leaves are used for eczema and other skin irritations.[M112] A decoction of leaves and flowering stems is taken as an emmenagogue and purgative and is also used in the treatment of diabetes, hypertension and anaemia.[M112]

PREPARATION AND DOSAGE

SKIN IRRITATION AND ECZEMA Boil a handful of fresh leaves in half a litre of water for 5–10 minutes. Apply the warm decoction to the affected areas.

PHARMACOLOGY AND CHEMISTRY

PHARMACOLOGICAL PROPERTIES

In the β-carotene bleaching test, high antioxidant activities have been reported for both leaf and stem extracts of *Leonotis* species.[P336]

COMPOUNDS REPORTED

Species of *Leonotis* contain both essential oils and several diterpenoid lactones, such as marrubiin, which has been isolated from *L. leonurus* (not described here).[P337] Two labdane terpenoids have also been isolated from *L. leonurus*.[P337, P338] Examination of the different parts of *L. nepetifolia* showed that the plant has antimicrobial and antileishmanial activities and these are associated with flavonoids apigenin, cirsiliol apigenin-7-O-glucoside, luteolin, luteolin-4'-O-glucoside, luteolin-4'-O-glucuronide and luteolin-7-O-glucoside identified from the plant.[P339] The presence of diterpenes such as leonitin has been reported from leaves of *L. ocymifolia* var. *raineriana*.[P340]

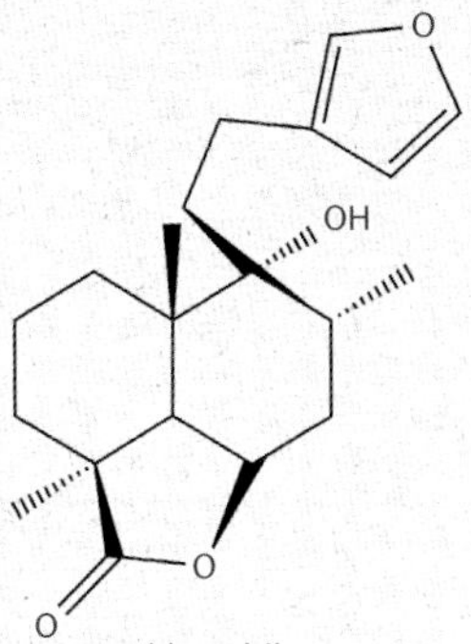

Marrubiin

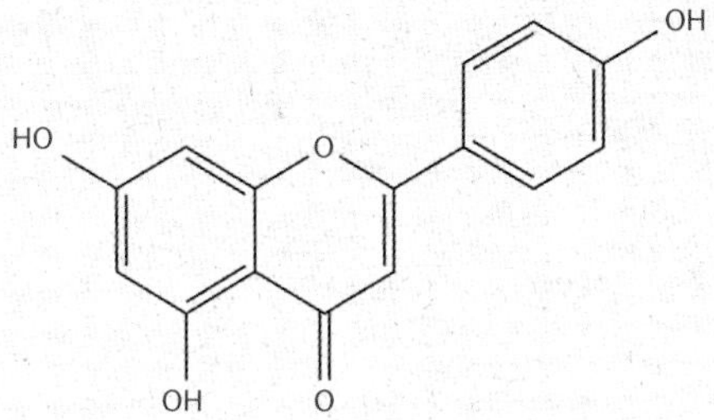

Apigenin

a. *Lippia javanica*   Indigenous

Common names Lippia Bush, Fever Tea • **Local names** Kyulu / Mutithi (Kam.), Muthoroti (Kik.),
Mwokyot (Kip.), Onyinkwa (Kis.), Ang'we-rao / Mweny (Luo), Sulasula (Luh.), Ol-sinoni (Maa.),
Mwokio (Mar.), Chepngosoriet (Nan.), Sunoni (Sam.), Karnet (Sebei), Arwo (Ach.)

Description and ecology
Erect, multi-stemmed, woody shrub 1–2.5m high,
with branched, hairy, reddish-purplish stems.
Leaves 2–4(–6)cm long, ovate to elliptic, base
wedge-shaped, apex acute, margin dentate,
veins prominent, hairy on both sides, sandpapery
above, emitting a lemon-like smell when crushed.
Flowers white or creamy white, on short stalks,
in dense, rounded heads at apex of stem. **Fruits**
dry, hairy mericarps. Abundant in disturbed areas
and in rocky soils in dry woodland, secondary
bushland or grassland, at 1,100–2,300m.

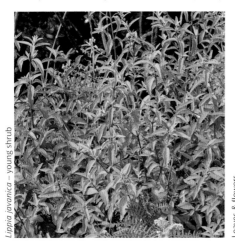

Lippia javanica – young shrub

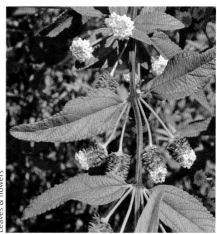

Leaves & flowers

USAGE AND TREATMENT

PARTS USED Leaves, twigs and flowers.
TRADITIONAL MEDICINAL USES Strong leaf and twig infusions are taken for coughs, colds,
influenza, bronchitis and fever.[M2, M70, M116] Leaves and flowers are sniffed to clear a stuffy,
blocked nose.[M1] Leaf decoctions are used to treat fever, especially in cases of malaria,
influenza,[M2, M116] stomach ailments and headache.[M2] A leaf paste is applied to wounds.[M70]
Leaf juice is swallowed for relief from tapeworm or to overcome indigestion.[M2, M70]

PREPARATION AND DOSAGE
COUGHS, COLDS, INFLUENZA, FEVER AND BRONCHITIS Steep a handful of fresh leaves in half
a litre of hot water. Drink 2 or 3 times daily, preparing afresh every time.
NASAL CONGESTION Rub some fresh leaves and flowers between the palms until a strong
scent is emitted. Sniff deeply to clear the nostrils, sneezing as it takes effect. Inhaling the steam
from crushed fresh leaves immersed in boiling water 3 times a day will also help to clear the
nasal passages.
WOUNDS, CUTS AND BRUISES Apply some pounded fresh leaves to affected areas of the skin.

b. *Lippia kituiensis*

Indigenous

Common names Lippia Bush, Wild Tea • **Local names** Muthiiti / Muthiethi (Kam.), Muthiriti / Muthoroti (Kik.), Mwokiot (Kip.), Osinoni / Olsinoni (Maa.), Muthirith / Muthiritii (Mer.), Mosonyon / Mojonyon (Pok.), Sinoni / Kaziti-wanda / Mvuti (Samb.), Mvudi (Tai.), Efurie (Chag.), Luhongole (Hehe), Mpugambu (Nyam.), Mvuti (Swa.Tan., Zig.)

Description and ecology

Much-branched, aromatic herb or shrub 1–3.5(–6)m tall, with hairy stems. **Leaves** opposite, ovate to elliptic, dark green, broad at base, pointed at apex, margin finely toothed, veins prominent, sandpapery on both sides, softly hairy below, aromatic when crushed.

Flowers small, white to cream with a yellow throat, in rounded or globose heads 0.5–2.0cm across, on stalks 2–3.5cm long. **Fruits** densely hairy mericarps, the two dry fruiting sections each with 1 seed. Found in bushland, woodland, grassland, often on rocky ground, volcanic soil or lava rocks, at 900–2,500m.

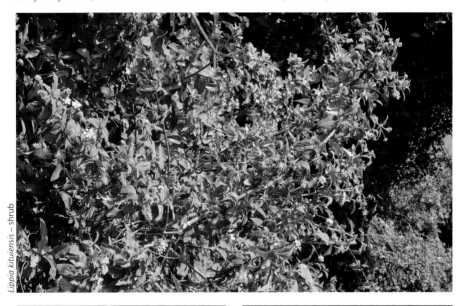

Lippia kituiensis – shrub

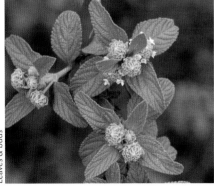

Leaves & buds

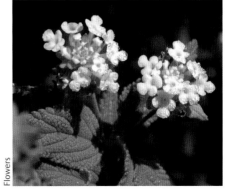

Flowers

PARTS USED Leaves only.

TRADITIONAL MEDICINAL USES Fresh leaves are used to treat coughs, colds and both nasal and chest congestion.[M3, M91] Pounded fresh leaves are applied to fresh wounds and cuts.[M70] Leaves are also used to treat malaria and chronic joint pains caused by osteoarthritis and/or rheumatoid arthritis.[M117]

PREPARATION AND DOSAGE

NASAL CONGESTION, COUGHS AND COLDS Add some crushed fresh leaves to boiling water and inhale the vapour 3 times a day. A herbal tea can be made by adding a few fresh leaves to half a litre of hot water. Drink the resulting infusion 3 times a day.

 WARNING! Internal treatments should be taken with great care, as species of *Lippia* contain some toxic compounds. Do not exceed the stated dosages.

PHARMACOLOGY AND CHEMISTRY

PHARMACOLOGICAL PROPERTIES

Hydrodistilled oil from the leaves of *Lippia multiflora* (not described here), commonly known as lippia oil, produces fungicidal and bactericidal activities.[P341] Volatile oil obtained from *L. javanica* shows antimicrobial activity against both *Escherichia coli* and *Staphylococcus aureus*, and antiplasmodial activity against *Plasmodium falciparum*.[P342]

COMPOUNDS REPORTED

From the extract of *L. rubella* (not described here), two new phenylpropanoid glycosides, lippiarubelloside A and lippiarubelloside B, with antifungal activity have been isolated.[P343] *L. javanica* contains monoterpenoids such as myrcene, linalool, caryophyllene and p-cymene.[P344, P345] From *L. javanica* triterpenoids, iridoid glycosides and phenylethanoid glycosides (verbascoside and isoverbascoside) have been identified.[P346]

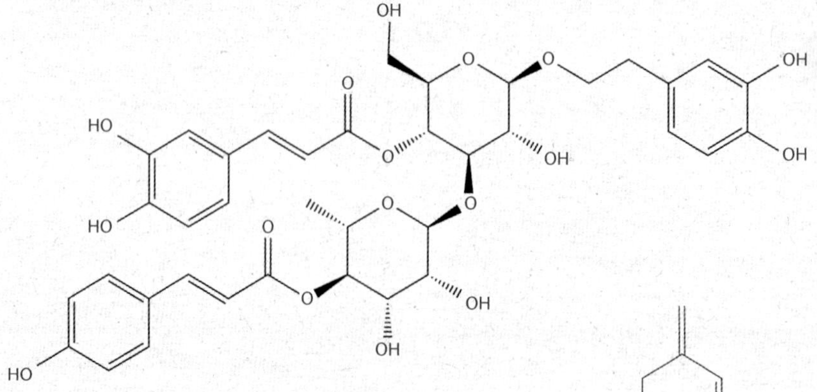

Lippiarubelloside B

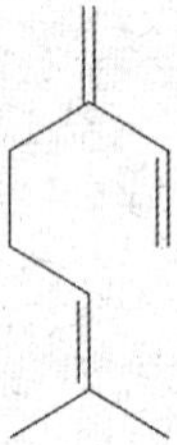

Myrcene

Indigenous

Common names Macaranga, Forest Macaranga • **Local names** Mukuhakuha (Kik.), Mukalati (Kam.), Mukaho (Luh.), Kibgetouoa (Mar.), Mukarati (Mer.), Sebesebet (Nan.), Kaptebema (Sebei), Logomaita (Kip.), Mudwess / Luwessu (Lugi.), Muburashasha / Murara / Mushasha (Ruki.), Muhunga (Ruko.), Muhoti (Ruto.), Kaptebema (Sebei-Ug.)

Description and ecology
Evergreen or semi-deciduous, fast-growing tree 6–20m tall but sometimes up to 24m, with a straight or fluted trunk and a dense much-branched, spreading crown of shiny leaves. In thickets sometimes a low, multi-stemmed shrub. **Bark** green at first, later becoming pale red-brown or dark grey, young branches hairy. **Leaves** heart-shaped, 5–15 × 3–10cm, densely hairy, tip long and pointed, base usually rounded, veins prominent, margin entire, stalk 7–8cm long. **Flowers** tiny, yellow-green, in panicles 2–10cm long. **Fruits** small, dull green capsules, subglobose or 2-lobed, about 6mm long, 1-seeded. An abundant, fast-growing species in East Africa's wetter montane forests, riverine forests and often regenerating profusely along forest edges, at 1,500–3,000m.

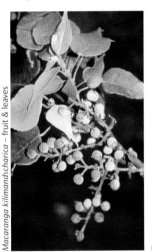

Macaranga kilimandscharica – fruit & leaves

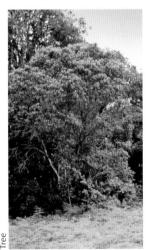

Tree

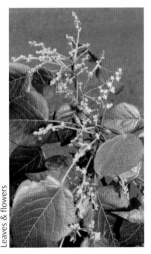

Leaves & flowers

USAGE AND TREATMENT

PARTS USED Roots and leaves.
TRADITIONAL MEDICINAL USES Leaves are used to treat stomach ailments.[M1, M111] Roots are included in remedies for coughs and are also used in the treatment of schistosomiasis.[M111, M112]

PREPARATION AND DOSAGE
SCHISTOSOMIASIS (BILHARZIA) Steep a handful of fresh roots or 3g of dry root powder in a litre of cold boiled water. Stir and filter after 30 minutes. Drink 3 cups daily for 2 or 3 days.
STOMACH AILMENTS Boil a handful of fresh leaves in a litre of water for 10 minutes. Leave to cool, then drink 3 cups of the decoction daily for 2 or 3 days.

PHARMACOLOGICAL PROPERTIES

The entire dried plant has a uterine stimulant effect[P347] and shows antibacterial and antifungal activities against some organisms.[P348] Dried leaves show immunomodulator[P104] and weak skeletal muscle stimulant activities.[P349] The plant as a whole has a toxic effect, but shows no antitumour activity.[P350] An extract from the leaves showed anti-measles activity by blocking the viral replication.[P257] The quercetin derivatives, 3,3',4',7-tetramethylquercetin and 3,7-dimethylquercetin, isolated from leaves of *Macaranga triloba*, show potent quinone reductase (QR) activities (QR is a phase II detoxifying enzyme whose induction is considered an important cancer chemopreventive mechanism at the initiation stage).[P349] Extracts of leaves, stems and roots of *M. capensis* (not described here), *M. kilimandscharica* and *M. conglomerata* (not described here) showed antibacterial activity towards 13 micro-organisms, including drug-sensitive and multidrug-resistant strains.[P351]

COMPOUNDS REPORTED

No phytochemical work has yet been done on *M. kilimandscharica*. However, from *M. triloba* (not described here), a new rotenoid, 4,5-dihydro-5'α-hydroxy-4'α-methoxy-6a,12a-dehydro-α-toxicarol, has been isolated, together with other known compounds such as (+)-clovan-2β,9α-diol, ferulic acid and quercetin derivatives (e.g. 3,3',4',7-tetramethylquercetin).[P349]

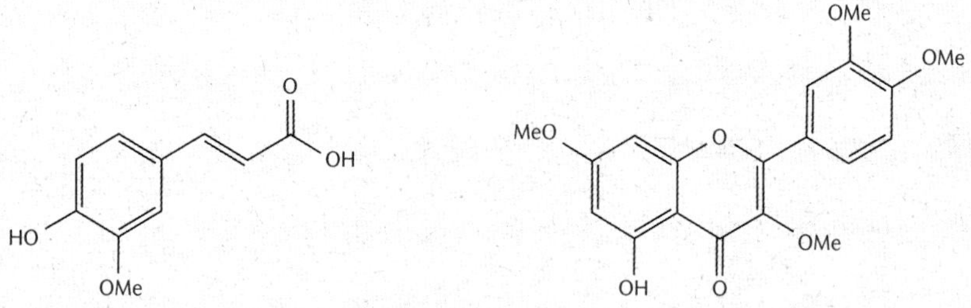

Ferulic acid

3,3',4',7-Tetramethylquercetin

Indigenous

Common name Maesa • **Local names** Mundume / Mundonge (Kik.), Omoterere (Kis.), Mushebeshebe (Luh.), Kalatera (Luo), Ol-reteti (Maa.), Mborio / Ribotio (Mar.), Mwenyuka (Mer.), Kibabustanient (Nan., Tug.), Likoi (Hehe), Lisebesebe (Luny.), Kiwondowondo (Lug.), Naporo / Kisangulu (Lugi.), Kusekseke (Luso.), Muhanga (Ruki.), Mahanga-honga (Ruko.), Muhangabagenzi (Runyan., Ruto.), Gogorwo (Sebei-Ug.)

Description and ecology
Straggling, evergreen shrub 2–4m high or small, much-branched, single-stemmed tree 6–8m tall. **Bark** grey-brown, rough, branches dotted with pale breathing pores, hairy or non-hairy, with orange or red resin. **Leaves** simple, oval, wide, up to 10cm long, with wavy margin and pointed tip, thick and leathery, shiny green above, pale below, stalk 2–3cm long. **Flowers** tiny, creamy white, scented, in branched axillary panicles up to 10cm long. **Fruit** small, fleshy, 3–4mm in diameter, round, greenish to pale pink, in clusters. **Seeds** numerous, small, blackish, embedded in the fruit flesh. Common in woodland, along dry evergreen forest margins, on mountain slopes and beside upland streams, often in secondary forest, at 1,200–2,800m.

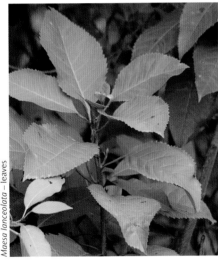

Maesa lanceolata – leaves

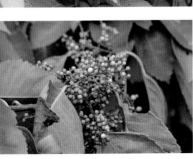

Ripe fruit

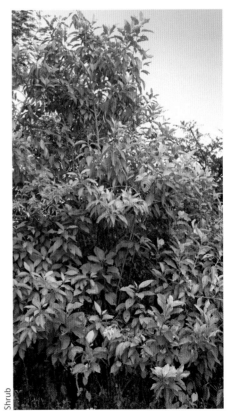

Shrub

PARTS USED Roots, bark, leaves and fruits.
TRADITIONAL MEDICINAL USES Fruits are used as a purgative, for treating a sore throat, and as remedy for tapeworm.[M58, M70] An infusion of dried fruits may be used to prevent cholera.[M59] Root or bark decoctions are taken to relieve lower abdominal pain during pregnancy and can soothe stomach ailments in children. A decoction of roots is used to expel tapeworms.[M58] Leaves serve as an anthelmintic.[M57] A fresh bark infusion acts as a body stimulant.[M115]

PREPARATION AND DOSAGE
SORE THROAT Eating five mature, ripe fruits will help to bring relief.
PURGATIVE AND ANTHELMINTIC Eating 10–12 mature, ripe fruits will have a purgative effect and will help to eliminate tapeworm. For anthelmintic use, steep a handful of dried roots, chopped into small pieces, in half a litre of hot boiled water for 30 minutes and drink a cup of the resulting mixture 3 times daily before meals.
LOWER ABDOMINAL PAIN Boil a handful of dried roots or bark in a litre of water and drink warm in small quantities 3 times daily for 3 days.

 WARNING! The fruits and leaves may prove toxic if consumed in excess.

PHARMACOLOGICAL PROPERTIES
Powdered fruits have shown taenicide activity when taken orally by adult humans.[P312] Maesaquinone, a benzoquinone present in all parts of *Maesa lanceolata*, has lowered testosterone levels in male New Zealand rabbits that were given intramuscular injections.[P352]

COMPOUNDS REPORTED
Benzoquinones (e.g. maesanin),[P353] flavonoids (e.g. quercetin),[P354] and triterpenes (e.g. maesasaponin I)[P355] have all been isolated from different parts of *M. lanceolata*. Quercitrin, a quercetin glycoside, has been identified from seeds of *M. lanceolata* as producing antitumour activity against HCT116 human colon cancer cells.[P356]

Maesanin R = Me
Maesaquinone R = H

Quercetin

a. *Melia azedarach*

Native to Asia and the Himalayas

Common names Indian Lilac, Persian Lilac, Bead Tree • **Local names** Dwele (Luo), Mmelia / Mwarubaini nusu (Swa.), Lira (Lug., Lugb.), Bakam-limbo (Guj.), Bakain / Dek / Drek / Mallan-nim (Hind., Urd.)

Description and ecology

Deciduous tree 10–12m tall, with spreading crown and bumpy lenticels on its branches. **Bark** smooth, greenish brown when young, turning grey, rough and fissured with age. **Leaves** borne in terminal bunches, alternate, 20–40cm long, bipinnately compound, with up to 6 pairs of pinnae, each with 3–9 pairs of leaflets, narrow, pale green at first, becoming dark and shiny, margins wavy, tips pointed, with pungent smell when crushed. **Flowers** small, fragrant, showy, in axillary panicles 20–25cm long, pale lilac, turning white, with a dark purple staminal tube. **Fruit** a fleshy, green to yellow drupe, nearly round, up to 1.5cm in diameter, in clusters that persist on the tree. **Seed** oblong, smooth, brown, surrounded by pulp. Termite resistant and fast growing at higher altitudes, therefore suitable for forestry and reforestation schemes. Grows in moist soils, at 0–2,000m.

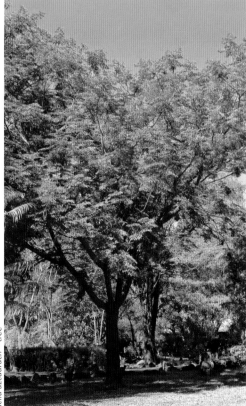

Melia azedarach – tree

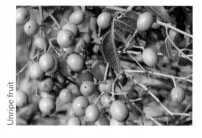

Unripe fruit

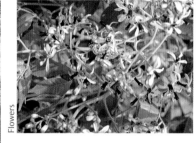

Flowers

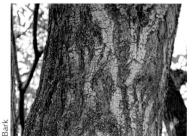

Bark

PARTS USED Leaves, roots, bark, fruit and seeds.
TRADITIONAL MEDICINAL USES Leaves, roots and stem bark are used to treat malaria and are also anthelmintic agents.[M4, M6, M7, M111] Seed oil is used to treat skin rashes and itching.[M7, M111] Leaves are used to heal infected wounds, scabies and skin itching.[M112] Bark decoctions are a remedy for fever[M7] and for body pain.[M1] The fruit kernels are applied externally for treating haemorrhoids.[M7] The leaf juice serves as anthelmintic, diuretic and emmenagogue, and a leaf decoction is used to treat diarrhoea and stomach pain.[M112] Dried or fresh stem bark can be used as anthelmintic, astringent and bitter tonic. Ripe fruit pulp is used as a vermifuge.[M112]

PREPARATION AND DOSAGE

MALARIA, BODY PAIN, INTESTINAL WORMS Steep 4g of dry leaf or bark powder or 20 fresh leaves in a litre of boiling water. Drink at intervals over 3 days.
SKIN INFECTIONS Apply seed oil directly to affected areas of the skin.
WOUNDS, SCABIES AND RASHES Steep a handful of crushed fresh leaves in half a litre of boiling water for 10 minutes. Wash and bathe wounds with this decoction.

b. *Melia volkensii*   Indigenous

Common name Melia • **Local names** Bamba (Bor., Orm.), Mukau (Kam., Kik.), Maramarui (Sam.), Baba (Som.), Mkowe (Tav.), Kirumbutu / Mukumbutu (Tai.).

Description and ecology

Deciduous tree 6–20m tall, with a rounded, open crown of drooping branches. **Bark** grey, smooth in young trees, becoming brown, rough and flaking with age. **Leaves** compound, light to bright green, with subopposite, oval to lance-shaped leaflets 2–5 × 05–2.5cm, non-hairy, apices tapering, margins entire or sometimes toothed. **Flowers** small, white, scented, in dense axillary panicles up to 12cm long. **Fruit** a drupe, oval, up to 4cm long, green turning yellow, in clusters that persist on bare trees. Common in association with *Acacia–Commiphora* in dry bushland, drier wooded grassland and bush or woodland, at 400–1,700m.

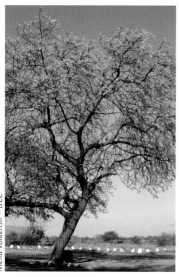

Melia volkensii – tree

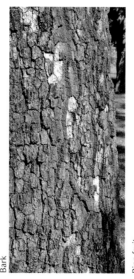

Bark

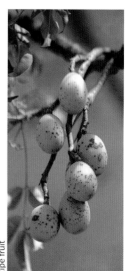

Ripe fruit

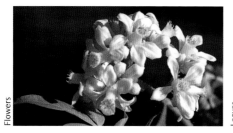
Flowers

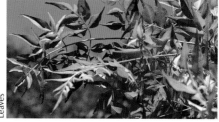
Leaves

USAGE AND TREATMENT

PARTS USED Leaves, roots and bark.
TRADITIONAL MEDICINAL USES A root infusion is taken as an emetic. Bark is used to relieve body ache and pain.[M1, M70] Leaves are used to treat skin rashes and eczema.[M70]

PREPARATION AND DOSAGE
SKIN INFECTIONS Apply some pounded fresh leaves directly to affected areas, or rub with a paste made from crushed seeds.
BODY ACHES Boil a teaspoon of dried bark powder in a litre of water for 10 minutes. Leave to cool, then filter and drink a cup 3 times a day.

 WARNING! Internal use of *Melia* is not recommended for pregnant women and patients with a heart condition. Overdosing can be harmful.

PHARMACOLOGY AND CHEMISTRY

PHARMACOLOGICAL PROPERTIES
Bark of *Melia* species produces an anthelmintic effect,[P357] while entire plants show an antiviral effect.[P358] Antifungal[P359] activities are reported for dried kernels and seed oil, especially of *M. azedarach*. Kulactone and other triterpenes in seeds of *M. volkensii* have shown activity against *Mycobacterium tuberculosis*.[P360]

COMPOUNDS REPORTED
Species of *Melia* contain triterpenoids (e.g. amoorastatone).[P361] Limonoids (e.g. volkensinin) are present in *M. volkensii* root bark,[P362] quinoids (e.g. 1,8-dihydroxy-2-methylanthraquinone) in stem bark,[P363] and flavones (e.g. apigenin-5-O-β-D-galactoside) in roots[P364] of *M. azedarach*. Seeds of *M. volkensii* elaborate a triterpene called kulactone.[P360] Different metabolites (e.g. melianin, meliavolkensin A and B), isolated from *M. volkensii*, showed cytotoxicity against different human tumour cell lines.[P365]

Volkensinin

Kulactone

Native to Central and South America

Common names Marvel of Peru, Four O'Clock Plant, Four O'Clock Flower • **Local names** Gul-abbas (Hind.), Gul-e-Abbas (Urd.), Abasi (Punj., Guj.)

Description and ecology

Herbaceous perennial of bushy habit growing 0.6–1m high, rarely up to 2m. **Leaves** opposite, oval, soft, shiny green, with pointed apex and prominent veins. **Flowers** clustered in groups of 3–7, more or less stalkless, tubular, scented, in a variety of colours including red, yellow, white, pink or streaked, opening at about four o'clock in the afternoon (hence some of its common names), remaining open all night. **Fruit** a small, 1-seeded capsule. **Seeds** black and wrinkled. In East Africa, it grows as a naturalised weed along roadsides and on waste ground, flowering continuously where there is sufficient water, at 200–2,200m.

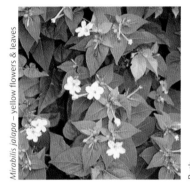

Mirabilis jalapa – yellow flowers & leaves

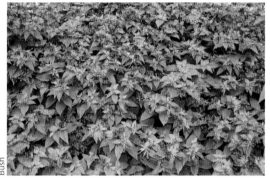

Bush

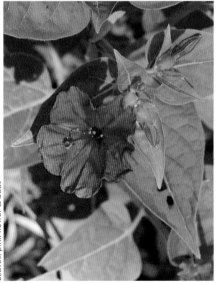

Leaves, pink flower & buds

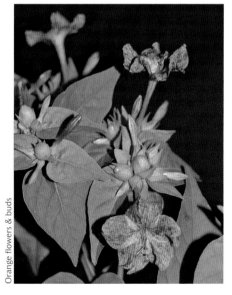

Orange flowers & buds

USAGE AND TREATMENT

PARTS USED Leaves, roots and flowers.
TRADITIONAL MEDICINAL USES Medicinal solutions of the roots are taken as a purgative and diuretic.[M9] Leaves and roots are used together to heal body swellings, wounds, abscesses and boils.[M7, M70, M112] Flowers can be used in treatments for haemorrhoids.[M70] A root decoction is used for treating gonorrhoea and scabies, and is also taken as an aphrodisiac.[M7, M112] Root infusions are used to treat tuberculosis. Cooked leaves are eaten in cases of jaundice.[M7] Juice of the roots is used in the treatment of diarrhoea, indigestion and fever.[M112]

PREPARATION AND DOSAGE
PURGATIVE AND DIURETIC Add 2g of root powder to half a litre of hot water, sweeten with a spoonful of brown sugar or honey, stir and drink early in the morning before breakfast.
GONORRHOEA Boil a tablespoon of root powder in a litre of water for 10 minutes. Leave to cool, then strain and drink a cup 3 times daily for 2 or 3 days.
HAEMORRHOIDS (PILES) Swallow a teaspoon of powdered dry flowers with water twice daily for 3 or 4 days.
BODY SWELLINGS, SCABIES, WOUNDS, ABSCESSES The paste or juice of fresh roots or leaves is applied as a poultice on affected areas.

 WARNING! No part of this plant should be ingested during pregnancy or given to people with intestinal ulcers or colitis. Overdosage can be harmful.

PHARMACOLOGY AND CHEMISTRY

PHARMACOLOGICAL PROPERTIES
Roots of *Mirabilis jalapa* have produced both antispasmodic effects[P366] and antibacterial activity against various organisms, including *Salmonella typhosa*, *Shigella flexneri* and *Vibrio cholera*.[P367] Dried roots have shown reverse transcriptase inhibition against HIV-1.[P368] Extracts of leaves show antibacterial and antifungal activities.[P369] Leaves and stems have produced an antinociceptive activity in mice, supporting the folkloric use of *M. jalapa* as an analgesic agent.[P370] In addition, extracts of the plant have showed anti-inflammatory, anthelmintic, analgesic, muscle relaxant and anti-asthmatic activities as well as protection against hepatotoxicity induced by antitubercular drugs.[P369]

COMPOUNDS REPORTED
Some isoflavonoids, such as boeravinone C and mirabijalone C, have been isolated from the roots of *M. jalapa*.[P368] Betaxanthins, such as betanin, occur in the flowers.[P371] The strong purgative properties of the roots are probably due to the presence of isoflavonoids and jalapine.

Boeravinone C

Betanin

a. *Moringa oleifera*   Native to the western Himalayas and India

Common names Moringa, Drumstick Tree, Horseradish Tree, Ben Oil Tree. • **Local names** Muzungwi (Chon.), Muzungi / Muzumbwi / Muzungwi (Gir.), Mzunze / Mronge (Swa.Ken.), Muguunda (Tha.), Mlongo (Swa.Tan.), Mlonge / Mlonje (Lugu.), Saragwuu (Guj.), Singhii (Urd.)

Description and ecology

Small to medium-sized, deciduous tree with sparse, feathery foliage, reaching 6–8(–10)m, usually much shorter, bole crooked, often forked from the base. **Bark** grey, thick, corky, peeling in patches, branches drooping and fragile, young twigs and shoots covered in dense hairs. **Leaves** alternate, 30–40cm long, tripinnately compound, leaflets 1–2cm long, dark green, elliptical to obovate. **Flowers** creamy white fading to yellow, in long sprays or panicles 10–20cm long, sweetly scented. **Fruits** hanging, stick-like capsules up to 45cm long, bluntly triangular in cross section, green when young, turning brown at maturity, splitting when dry to release dark brown, 3-winged seeds. In East Africa, widely grown by Indian families in their gardens and backyards, today planted in well-drained soils throughout the tropics. Has become naturalised in coastal areas of East Africa, at 0–1,000m.

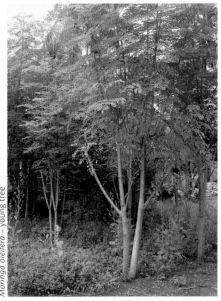

Moringa oleifera – young tree

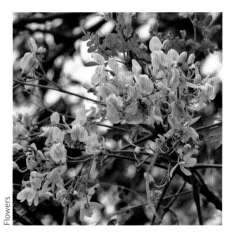

Flowers

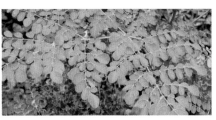

Leaves

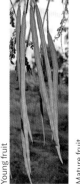

Young fruit

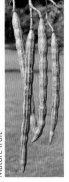

Mature fruit

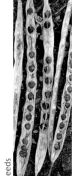

Seeds

PARTS USED Roots, leaves, flowers, fruits, seed oil and gum.
TRADITIONAL MEDICINAL USES A root infusion is used for impotence[M3] and stomach ache. Roots are diuretic and are used as a laxative and for purifying the blood as well as in remedies for inflammation, bronchitis and haemorrhoids.[M6, M7] Leaves are also used to treat diarrhoea, anaemia, ulcers, diabetes[M1] and scurvy. Leaf decoctions and squeezed leaf juice are used as an anthelmintic. Leaves and pods are administered for malnutrition. The seed oil, known as ben oil, is used in poultices to relieve painful body swellings and skin infections.[M6, M14, M111] The oil also helps to relieve rheumatism, gout and stomach ailments. The bark serves as an appetiser and digestive.[M111] Root and bark decoctions are taken as a remedy for arthritis, rheumatism, fever and leprosy.[M4, M70] Roots and bark are also used as an antiscorbutic and are applied externally as anti-irritants.[M114] A decoction of flowers is used as a cold remedy. Infusions of flowers are taken orally as a stimulant and aphrodisiac. Decoctions of dried fruit and leaves are taken for dysentery and diarrhoea.[M10, M70] Gum from the tree is used for fungal infections.[M4, M70] The gum is diuretic, astringent and abortifacient and is also used against asthma.

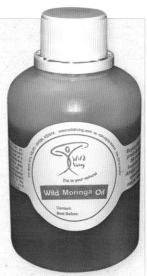

Moringa oleifera seed oil, also known as ben oil, is used for a range of ailments.

PREPARATION AND DOSAGE

SKIN AND FUNGAL INFECTIONS Dissolve some gum in water. Apply to affected areas of the skin. A paste made from the seed oil can be applied to treat eczema, itching, boils and scabies.
DIABETES Steep 5g of dried leaf powder in a litre of hot water for 15–20 minutes, stirring intermittently. Strain and drink 3 times a day for a few days, making a fresh infusion every time.
IMPOTENCE Boil a tablespoon of crushed dry bark or roots in a litre of water for 15 minutes. Drink the decoction at intervals during the day.
MALNUTRITION Leaves can be eaten fresh. Alternatively, they can be dried in the shade and crushed to make a powder for adding to rice, sauces, chutneys and other dishes. A spoonful of dried leaf powder can be given to malnourished children 3 times a day.
ARTHRITIS Add a teaspoon of dried bark powder to half a litre of hot water. Leave for 20 minutes. Drink twice daily for a few days.

b. *Moringa stenopetala* Indigenous

Common names African Moringa, African Drumstick Tree, African Horseradish Tree • **Local names** Safara (Bon.), Lorsanjo (Sam.), Mau / Mawali / Mawe (Som.), Muguunda (Tha.), Etebusoit (Tur.)

Description and ecology
Deciduous medium-sized tree 10–12(–14)m tall, with a dense, heavily branched crown, young shoots densely hairy, bole swollen, bottle-shaped and up to 1m in diameter. **Bark** conspicuous silvery white to pale grey, smooth. **Leaves** alternate, 45–55cm long, bipinnate to tripinnate, leaflets oval or elliptic, 3.2–6.0 × 1.8–3.2cm, rounded at the bases and pointed at the apices. **Flowers** abundant, creamish white, sweetly scented, in many-flowered panicles 10–60cm long. **Fruit** a long, 3-angled capsule 20–50 × 2–4cm, with many thin-winged seeds. Found along rivers and lakes in dry areas, often on rocky ground, at 400–1,050m.

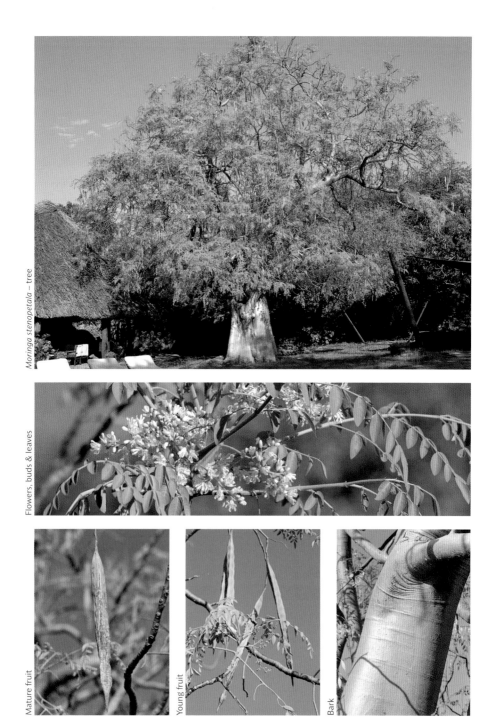

Moringa stenopetala – tree

Flowers, buds & leaves

Mature fruit

Young fruit

Bark

USAGE AND TREATMENT

PARTS USED Bark, leaves and seeds.
TRADITIONAL MEDICINAL USES A leaf infusion is taken as a remedy for leprosy and fever.[M115] Leaves are used to treat diabetes, hypertension, colds and asthma, also as an anthelmintic and to induce vomiting.[M115] Decoctions of bark are a remedy for arthritis and fresh bark is chewed as a treatment for coughs.[M115] Roots are used to treat stomach pain and infertility.[M3] Decoctions of leaves and roots are used as a remedy for malaria, stomach problems and diabetes.[M115] The seed oil is used in poultices to relieve painful body swellings and other skin ailments, including itching, eczema and fungal infections.[M4, M70]

PREPARATION AND DOSAGE
SKIN AND FUNGAL INFECTIONS Dissolve some gum in water. Apply to affected areas of the skin. Apply the seed oil to relieve eczema and itching.
DIABETES Steep 5g of dried leaf powder in a litre of hot water for 15–20 minutes, stirring intermittently. Strain and drink 3 times a day, preparing a fresh infusion every time.
ARTHRITIS Add a teaspoon of dried bark powder to half a litre of hot water. Leave for 20 minutes. Drink twice daily for a few days.

PHARMACOLOGY AND CHEMISTRY

PHARMACOLOGICAL PROPERTIES
Dried leaves of *Moringa stenopetala* have shown hypoglycaemic activity.[P372] Fresh leaves have weak antibacterial and smooth muscle relaxant activities.[P373] A fresh root wood ethanol extract and dried leaf acetone extract were found to be active against *Trypanosoma brucei*.[P374] Antibacterial and antihistamine activities have been reported for the roots. Dried seeds have produced anti-yeast, antispasmodic and hyperglycaemic activity and have wound-healing properties.[P79]

COMPOUNDS REPORTED
Compounds isolated from species of *Moringa* include sulfur compounds (e.g. glucoconringiin in seeds[P375]) and benzenoids such as 4-(α-L-4'-O-acetyloxyrhamnosyl)-benzaldehyde.[P376] Flavonoids (e.g. rutin) have been found in the leaves of *M. stenopetala*.[P376] Compounds reported for different parts of *M. oleifera* include amylase, 4-hydroxyphenylacetamide, benzenoids, ß-sitosterol, ß-carotene, rutin, and vitamins A, B-1 and B-2.[P79] *Moringa* isothiocyanates, including isothiocyanate-1, are responsible for anti-inflammatory activity of *M. oleifera*.[P377]

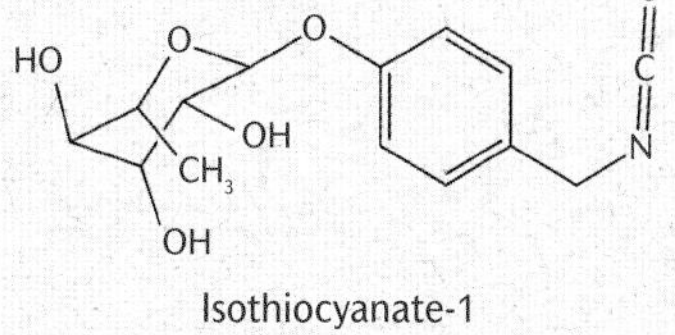

Isothiocyanate-1

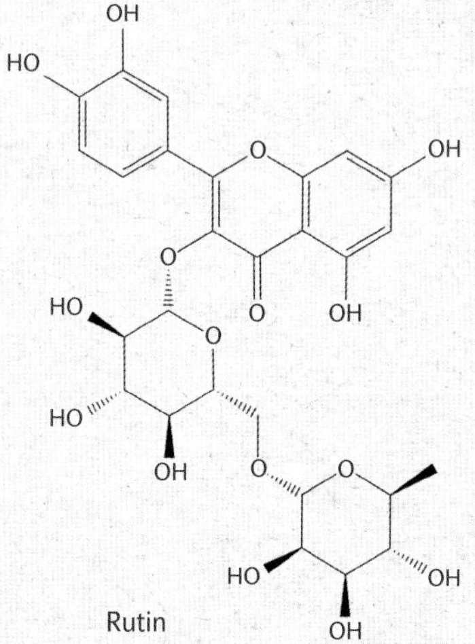

Rutin

64 *Ocimum* species

LAMIACEAE

a. *Ocimum gratissimum*

Indigenous

Common names African Basil, Wild Basil, Clove Basil • **Local names** Manjabbi / Anchabbi (Bor.), Vumba manga (Dig.), Vamba manga (Gir.), Mukandu (Kam.), Mugio (Kik.), Olururuecha (Luo), Ol-emoran (Maa.), Yoiyoiya / Jemasat / Chesimia (Mar.), Kirumbasi (Swa.), Lemurran (Sam.), Omujaaja (Lug.), Mujaaja (Luso.), Omwenyi (Runy.), Ekijaaja (Ruto.)

Description and ecology

Erect, much-branched herb or small, woody shrub 0.5–2(–3)m high, hairy and strongly but pleasantly aromatic. **Leaves** elliptical to ovate but variable in shape, 1.5–10 × 1–4(–5)cm, softly hairy below, with pointed tip and toothed margin, stalk 1–4mm long. **Flowers** small, white-purple, 2-lipped, crowded along a simple or branched 6–10-flowered terminal raceme 5–25cm long, softly hairy. **Fruit** consisting of 4 ovoid or subglobose, dry, rough, 1-seeded nutlets in a persistent calyx, 1.5mm long, brown. Common in coastal scrub, along lakeshores, on roadsides, in cleared lands, as a secondary shrub at forest edges, in thickets and bushland, occurring naturally at 0–2,400m.

USAGE AND TREATMENT

PARTS USED Leaves, stems and seeds.
TRADITIONAL MEDICINAL USES The strongly scented leaves are rubbed between the palms and snuffed as a treatment for headache, influenza and a blocked or runny nose.[M1, M111] Leaves are also used to treat diarrhoea,[M14] abdominal pain, eye sores, ear troubles and coughs. An infusion of leaves serves as a disinfectant and an insect repellent.[M14, M111] The seeds have laxative properties and are used against gonorrhoea; pounded leaves and young twigs are used for diarrhoea, stomach pain, ear and eye infections and for skin diseases.[M111]

PREPARATION AND DOSAGE
INFLUENZA, HEADACHE, COUGH AND BLOCKED NOSE Rub a few fresh leaves between the palms and snuff it 3 or 4 times a day.
INSECT REPELLENT (MOSQUITOES, TICKS ETC.) AND SKIN DISEASES Grind some fresh leaves and rub their juice directly on exposed skin. Alternatively, add some pounded leaves to a litre of hot water, leave the mixture for 20 minutes, then stir, sieve and use for bathing or as a body wash.

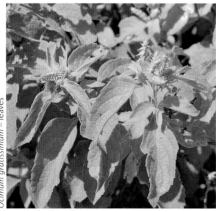

Ocimum gratissimum – leaves

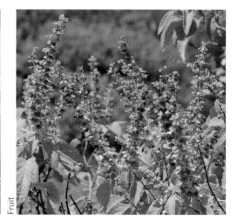

Fruit

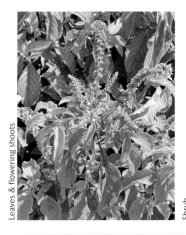

Leaves & flowering shoots

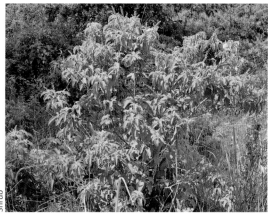

Shrub

b. *Ocimum kilimandscharicum*   Indigenous

Common names Camphor-scented Basil, African Basil, Fever Plant • **Local names** Makoli (Emb.), Mwenye / Wenye (Kam.), Okita / Bwar (Luo.), Mwonyi (Luh.), Makuru (Mer.), Supko (Pok.), Kameteber (Tur.), Esilokha (Luny.), Mzugwa (Samb.), Kirumbasi (Swa.)

Description and ecology
Erect, branching, perennial, hairy, woody herb or subshrub 0.5–1.5(–2)m tall, branchlets quadrangular, pubescent, purplish. **Leaves** opposite, 1.5–5.5 × 0.6–3cm, ovate-elliptic, pale green, hairy on both surfaces, with acute apex and broad base, margin slightly wavy, strongly aromatic when crushed. **Flowers** white with purple bracts, in clusters on elongated, terminal racemes 10–20cm long. Common on rocky ground in evergreen wooded upland vegetation and also in riverine grasslands, at 1,100–2,550m.

Ocimum kilimandscharicum – flowers

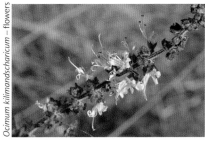

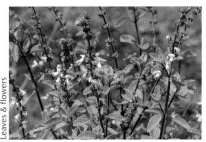

Leaves & flowers

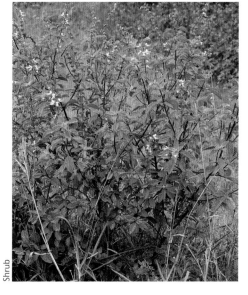

Shrub

PARTS USED Leaves and flowers.
TRADITIONAL MEDICINAL USES The plant is generally used to lower fever and deter mosquitoes.[M112] Leaves are used as a remedy for colds and coughs,[M33] as well as for malaria, stomach pain, sore eyes and measles in children.[M1, M70] Leaves are also applied to fungal and other skin infections, including wounds, boils, eczema, herpes and itching. Other very common indigenous species of *Ocimum* are *O. suave* (which is used to treat many of the same afflictions as *O. kilimandscharicum*) and *O. gratissimum* (whose leaves are used for treating diarrhoea, but which are also prized as an insect repellent).[M114]

PREPARATION AND DOSAGE
COUGHS AND COLDS Chew a few fresh leaves 2 or 3 times a day. Fresh leaves can also be added to bath water. Inhaling the steam vapour of boiled leaves can be effective, and fresh leaves, rubbed between the palms and taken as snuff, will help to clear a blocked nose.
MOSQUITO REPELLENT Grind some fresh leaves and rub their juice over exposed skin.
MALARIA AND FEVER Pour a litre of boiling water over 20g of fresh leaves and flowers. Leave for 5 minutes. Filter and drink a third of this mixture warm, 3 times daily after meals.
SKIN INFECTIONS Mix a tablespoon of powdered leaves with a teaspoon of lemon juice to form a paste. Apply directly to affected areas.
MEASLES Steep some pounded fresh leaves in warm water for a few minutes. Use the warm mixture to wash and bathe a baby suffering from measles.
SORE AND INFLAMED EYES Steep some pounded fresh leaves in hot water. Leave to cool, then wash the eyes with the warm infusion 3 times a day.

c. *Ocimum tenuiflorum* (*Ocimum sanctum*)
Native to the Indian subcontinent

Common names Holy Basil, Tulsi • **Local names** Chivumbani (Dig.), Bwar (Luo), Kurimbasi (Swa.), Jrumba yaza (Nyam.), Tulsi (Guj., Hind., Urd., Punj.)

Description and ecology
Erect, many-branched, perennial, woody herb or subshrub or small shrub, reaching 0.5–2m, with hairy stems. **Leaves** simple, 3–6 × 1–2.5cm, elliptic to oblong, green, softly hairy, with toothed margin and pointed tip, strongly aromatic when crushed, stalk 1–2.5cm long. **Flowers** small, pale pink or purplish, in terminal, elongated racemes or panicles 4–10cm long.

Fruits consisting of purple-green to brown nutlets, broadly ellipsoid, 0.8–1.2mm long, smooth to minutely pitted, swelling in water. Hindus consider tulsi as a sacred plant and worship it, planting it in temples and near entrances to dwellings. Widely grown in Africa and around the world as a garden herb. Tulsi grows best in full sun and moist, well-drained soils, at 0–2,800m.

PARTS USED Leaves and flowers.
TRADITIONAL MEDICINAL USES The leaf juice is used as eardrops to relieve earache.[M7, M45] Leaves are used to treat ringworm and itching of the skin.[M7] Infusions of fresh leaves are taken as a remedy for chronic fever and flatulence.[M6, M7, M45] Chewing the fresh leaves is a popular remedy for asthma, coughs and colds.[M45] Basil helps to ease migraine and digestive disorders. It also relieves stomach ache, bloating and belching and facilitates rapid digestion. It boosts milk production in breast-feeding mothers and eases menstrual spasms and pain. The herb is also recommended for relief from hypotension, fatigue and nervous exhaustion.[M9]

PREPARATION AND DOSAGE

DIGESTIVE DISORDERS, FEVER, FLATULENCE AND MENSTRUAL PAIN Steep 20g of fresh leaves and flowers in a litre of boiling water for 5 minutes. Filter and drink a cup after every meal.

ITCHING AND RINGWORM Apply a paste made from a tablespoon of leaves mixed with a teaspoon of lemon juice directly to affected areas.

COUGHS AND COLDS Chew a few fresh leaves 2 or 3 times a day. Fresh leaves can also be added to bath water. Inhaling the steam vapour of boiled leaves can also be effective. Fresh leaves, rubbed between the palms and inhaled as snuff, will help to clear a blocked nose.

STOMACH AILMENTS AND FLATULENCE Boil 15–20g of fresh leaves and twigs in a litre of water for 5 minutes. Leave to cool. Strain and drink in small quantities during the day.

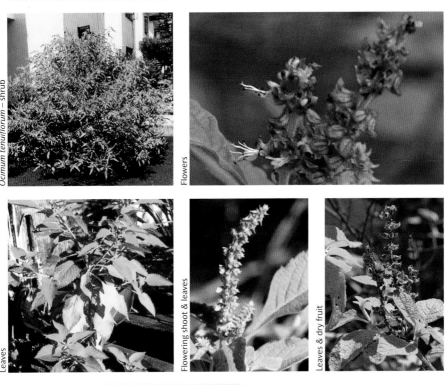

Ocimum tenuiflorum – shrub

Flowers

Leaves

Flowering shoot & leaves

Leaves & dry fruit

PHARMACOLOGY AND CHEMISTRY

PHARMACOLOGICAL PROPERTIES

Essential oils in species of *Ocimum* are responsible for a range of properties, including effects as an emmenagogue and antispasmodic, while also countering arterial hypotension, asthenia and nervous exhaustion.[P84] Leaf extracts are highly toxic to mosquito larvae and may also be useful in the management and control of the larvae of other vectors of disease.[P378] Essential oil from the aerial part has shown anthelmintic,[P379] antibacterial[P380] and antimicrobial activities against a variety of bacterial and fungal organisms.[P381] Spermicidal effects in humans have also been reported for the essential oil.[P382] Aerial parts of the plants have shown anti-ulcer,[P383] antioxidant,[P384] and strong acid neutralisation[P385] activities.

COMPOUNDS REPORTED

The essential oil of the whole plant is rich in estragol, eugenol and linalool.[P84] Other compounds isolated from species of *Ocimum* include sesquiterpenes (e.g. α-bisabolene[P385] and α-epicadinol[P386]), monoterpenes (e.g. camphor[P386]), benzenoids (e.g. benzaldehyde[P387]) and phenylpropanoids (e.g. rosmarinic acid).[P388] Camphor is the major component among 35 compounds identified from the essential oil of *O. kilimandscharicum*. [P386] Six major compounds (camphor, limonene, 4-terpeneol, 1,8-cineole, camphene and trans-caryophyllene) of the essential oil of *O. kilimandscharicum* were found to be largely responsible for the toxic action of its essential oil against post-harvest insect pests *Sitophilus zeamais* and *Rhyzopertha dominica*.[P389] In addition, there are several chemical constituents isolated in *O. tenuiflorum* (*O. sanctum*), including oleanolic acid, rosmarinic acid, ursolic acid, eugenol, linalool, carvacrol, β-elemene, β-caryophyllene and germacrene.[P390]

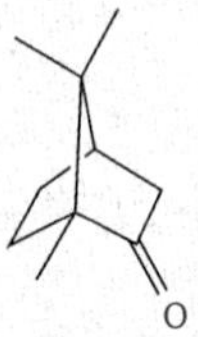

Camphor 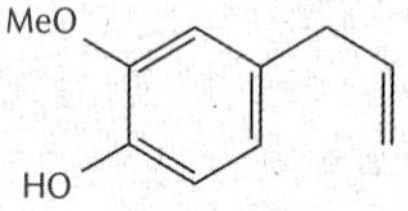   Eugenol 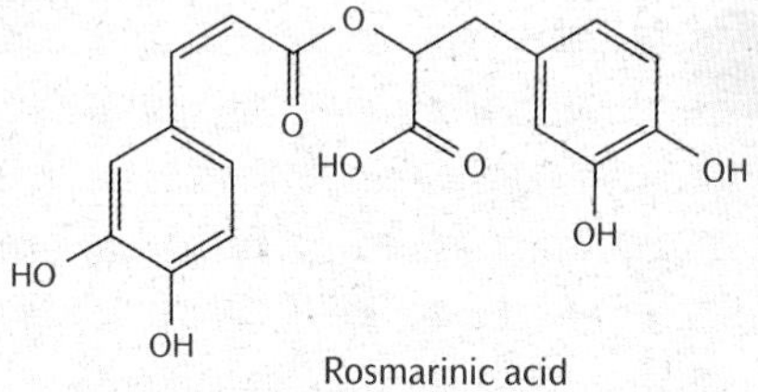   Rosmarinic acid

Indigenous

Common names Camphor Tree, East African Camphorwood • **Local names** Muthaiti (Kik.), Muura (Mer.), Muthura / Muzura (Emb.), Mkulo / Mukongo (Swa.), Mkongo / Mulongo / Munganga (Tai.), Mseri / Muwong / Mwawong (Chag.), Muheti (Hehe), Msibisibi (Nyak.), Maasi / Maase (Pare), Mkulo / Mtoa-mada / Mkenene (Samb.), Mwiha (Ruki.)

Description and ecology

Medium-sized to large, evergreen timber tree 15–30(–45)m tall, bole straight, 2–3m in diameter, with dense spreading crown, often slightly fluted, slightly buttressed at the base. **Bark** greyish brown to reddish brown, granular, scaly or flaky, inner bark white to pale pink, with sweet, camphor-like scent. **Leaves** alternate or subopposite, 4–10 × 3–5cm, broadly oval to rounded, dark green above, pale below, apex tapering, base rounded, margin entire and rolled under in mature leaves, camphor-scented when crushed, stalk 0.5–2cm long. **Flowers** greenish yellow or whitish, in axillary and terminal clusters, on short, branched hairy stalks. **Fruits** very small drupes up to 6 × 5mm, smooth, green, ellipsoid to nearly globose, 1-seeded. Once dominant in Kenya's wet and moist forests, but rare in these habitats today, having long since been felled for its excellent hardwood timber. Now considered an endangered forest species. Tanzania's natural camphor forests in the Usambara Mountains and on Kilimanjaro are under intensive management, however. It requires deep, fertile soils with good drainage and grows in wet montane forests, at 1,700–2,600m.

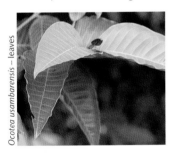

Ocotea usambarensis – leaves

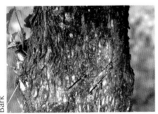

Bark

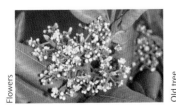

Flowers

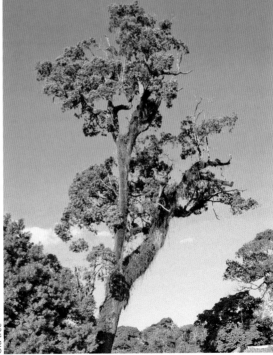

Old tree

PARTS USED Root bark and stem bark only.

TRADITIONAL MEDICINAL USES Stem bark is used for treating whooping cough, bronchitis, stomach pain and headache.[M70, M111] Powdered root bark is used to dress wounds and to heal abscesses. A poultice made of fresh or dried root or stem bark is applied to body swellings, including swollen glands and cancer-related tumours, wounds and boils.[M70, M115] A poultice may also be applied as a remedy for measles. A root infusion is taken for relief from backache and headache, and to treat malaria.[M1, M4, M70, M71, M112, M115]

PREPARATION AND DOSAGE

MALARIA AND BACKACHE Soak a handful of pounded fresh roots in a litre of cold boiled water for half an hour. Stir, strain and drink a cup of the infusion 3 times during the day.
HEADACHE Use some ground root or stem bark as snuff, or burn and inhale the smoke.
WHOOPING COUGH, BRONCHITIS AND STOMACH PAIN Boil a handful of fresh or dry stem bark in a litre of water for 10–15 minutes. Drink a cup of the decoction 3 times a day.
WOUNDS AND ABSCESSES Apply dry bark powder as a dressing over the affected areas.

PHARMACOLOGY AND CHEMISTRY

PHARMACOLOGICAL PROPERTIES

Dried bark of *Ocotea usambarensis* has not shown any antifungal activity.[P391] Methanol extract of stem bark of *O. usambarensis* showed antiplasmodial activity against the chloroquine-sensitive D6 (IC50 = 0.98µg/mL) and the chloroquine-resistant W2 (IC50 = 2.40µg/mL) strains of *Plasmodium falciparum*.[P392]

COMPOUNDS REPORTED

Bark of *O. usambarensis* contains several lignans, including (+)-sesamin.[P393] The bark is also rich in volatile compounds such as monoterpenoids (e.g. β-pinene)[P391] and sesquiterpenes (e.g. β-bisabolol).[P391]

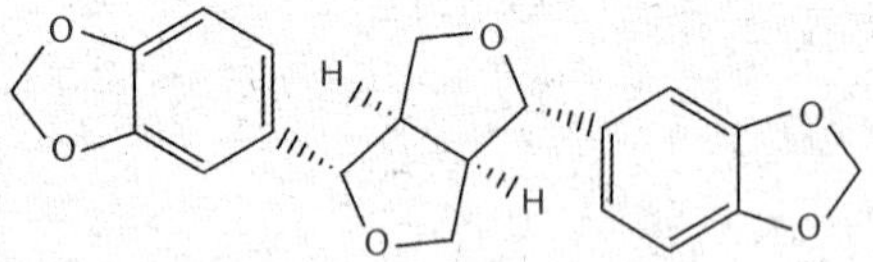

(+)-Sesamin

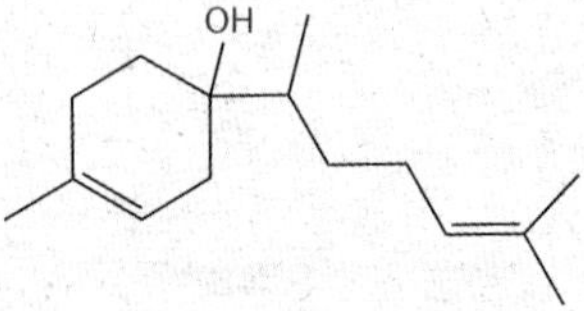

β-Bisabolol

Indigenous

Common names Wild African Olive, African Olive, Wild Olive • **Local names** Ejarse / Ejass (Bor.), Ejerssa (Gab.), Muthata (Kam., Mer.), Mutamaiyu (Kik.), Emitiot (Kip.), Kang'o (Luo), Yemit (Mar., Tug.), Ol'oirien / Olorien (Maa.Ken., Maa.Tan., Aru.), Emidit (Nan.), Ilnyirei / Lorien (Sam.), Wera (Som.), Mzeituni (Swa.), Mkumbi (Tai.), Euriepei (Tur.), Mlamuru / Msenefu / Mtamioi (Chag.), Mhagati / Muhagati (Hehe, Zig.), Muranganji (Pare), Mziaghembe / Mzilaghembe (Samb.), Murama (Runyan.), Yemit (Sebei, Sebei-Ug.)

Description and ecology

Much-branched, small to medium-sized, evergreen tree 5–10(–15)m tall, occasionally reaching 18–20m, with dense, rounded crown. Bark grey to brown, smooth when young, rough, dark brown and deeply fissured when old. **Leaves** opposite, 2–9 × 0.5–3cm, narrowly oval, stiff, grey-green and glossy above, greyish below with a dense covering of silvery, golden or brown scales, both ends sharply pointed, with prominent midrib and entire margin,

slender stalk up to 10mm long. **Flowers** small, greenish white or cream, sweetly scented, in terminal branched cymes 5–6cm long. **Fruit** a thinly fleshy drupe, green to purple or black when ripe, spherical to oval, 0.5–1cm long. Widespread in a variety of habitats such as woodland, on lava flows, on termite mounds, in dry rocky places, riverine habitats, often near water and also found in dry upland evergreen forest (often in association with *Juniperus procera*) and forest margins, at 900–3,000m.

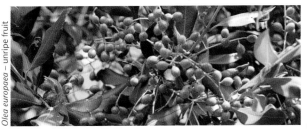

Olea europaea – unripe fruit

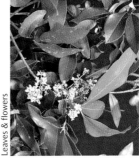

Leaves & Flowers

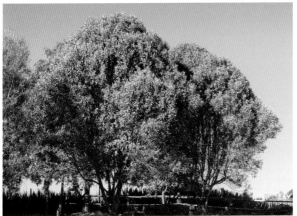

Trees

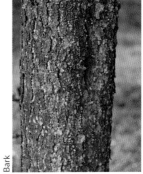

Bark

PARTS USED Roots, bark and leaves.

TRADITIONAL MEDICINAL USES Root, bark or leaf decoctions are used as a remedy for malaria and fever.[M33, M71, M111] A bark decoction is used for skin rashes and irritations, and also as a laxative and an anthelmintic, especially against tapeworm.[M4, M70, M71] Leaf decoctions are taken for the treatment of liver diseases.[M4, M70] Leaves are also taken as a remedy for hypertension, arteriosclerosis and as an aid in regulating proper renal function.[M2] In southern Africa, leaves or leaf extracts of subsp. *africana* are mainly used as an eye lotion, as a styptic to treat fresh wounds, and to treat a cold and sore throat.[M118] Roots and bark are commonly used for urinary ailments, colic, rheumatism and other afflictions.[M118]

PREPARATION AND DOSAGE

SKIN RASHES AND ITCHING Boil a handful of fresh bark in a litre of water. Steam-bath the affected areas of the skin.

INTESTINAL WORMS Steep a handful of pounded fresh bark or 4g of dry bark powder in a litre of hot water for 5–10 minutes. Drink a cup of the mixture 3 times daily before meals. Pounded fresh bark, left to soak in cold boiled water overnight, can also be used and taken in the same way.

MALARIA Boil 5g of powdered root or bark in a litre of water for 10 minutes. Leave to cool, then filter and drink a cup of the decoction 3 times daily for 3 days.

HIGH BLOOD PRESSURE AND BLOCKED ARTERIES Add a handful of pounded fresh leaves to half a litre of hot boiled water. Leave for 15 minutes. Drink a cup of the mixture 2 or 3 times a day.

PHARMACOLOGICAL PROPERTIES

The major compound of species of *Olea*, oleuropein, has characteristic antispasmodic and antioxidant activity;[P96] it also reduces blood pressure (hypertensive), constituting one of the most effective vegetal remedies against hypertension, while also enhancing coronary flow in cases of arteriosclerosis.[P84, P394] Oleacein, meanwhile, stops angiotension-converting enzymes (ACE).[P394] The two compounds work in combination.[P394] Oleanolic acid and ursonic acid, two triterpenes present in the leaves of *O. europaea*, have vasodepressor, cardiotonic and antidysrhythmic effects.[P395] Based on its potent antihypertensive, antihyperlipemic (anti-atherosclerotic), hypoglycaemic and antioxidant effects, this plant has been recommended as a highly effective, inexpensive and non-toxic treatment for salt-sensitive, insulin-resistant types of hypertension.[P396]

COMPOUNDS REPORTED

Olea leaves contain two major secoiridoids (oleuropein and oleacein[P84, P96]), together with other secoiridoids and both triterpenoids and flavonoids.[P96] Compounds isolated from *Olea* bark include lignans, africanol, olivil and 8-hydroxypinoresinol derivatives. The leaves contain two triterpenes, namely oleanolic acid and ursonic acid.[P395, P396]

Oleuropein

Oleanolic acid R = H, R' = Me
Ursonic acid R = Me, R' = H

67 *Plectranthus barbatus* LAMIACEAE

Indigenous

Common name Plectranthus • **Local names** Muvou / Moiya (Kam.), Muigoya / Maigoya (Kik.), Okita / Akita (Luo), Shilauha (Luh.), Mwaraka (Mer.), Irakwet (Nan.)

Description and ecology
Aromatic, woody, perennial herb forming a dense bush or shrub 0.5–3(–4)m high, with erect or ascending, square stems and hairy, softly wooded, brittle branches. **Leaves** 0.9–20 × 0.5–11cm, ovate to broadly ovate, fleshy, densely covered with soft greyish hairs, margin serrate, with short leaf stalk.

Flowers bright blue to blue-purple, clustered in erect, hairy spikes 10–20(–30)cm long. **Fruits** pale brown to black nutlets, smooth, broadly ovoid, slightly flattened, 1.5–2mm long. Quite popular as a fast-growing hedge plant. Grows wild in moist upland bush, along forest margins and in wooded grassland, at 600–2,800m.

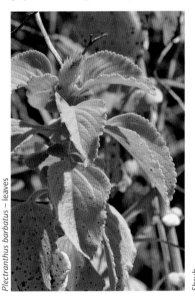

Plectranthus barbatus – leaves

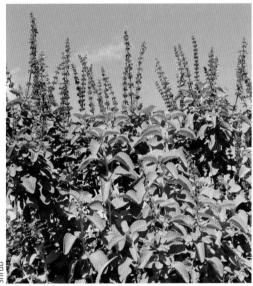

Shrub

USAGE AND TREATMENT

PARTS USED Leaves and soft stems and occasionally roots as well.
TRADITIONAL MEDICINAL USES Fresh leaf juice is a remedy for stomach ache and is also used as a purgative.[M70, M119] Leaves are used to treat measles in children.[M1, M70] Leaves and soft stems are recommended for a range of ailments, particularly intestinal disturbance and liver fatigue, respiratory problems, digestive disorders, heart diseases and certain nervous system conditions and skin infections.[M119]

PREPARATION AND DOSAGE
MEASLES IN CHILDREN Soak pounded fresh leaves in warm water used for bathing the child.
PURGATIVE AND STOMACH ACHE Steep a handful of crushed fresh leaves or roots in half a litre of warm water. Drink the infusion before breakfast in the morning.

PHARMACOLOGICAL PROPERTIES

Antibacterial,[P397] anti-inflammatory,[P397] antispasmodic[P398] and anti-allergic[P399] activities are reported for *Plectranthus barbatus*, whose relaxant and spasmolytic effects may be associated with α-pinene.[P398] Leaf extracts from *P. barbatus* stimulate gastric secretions, explaining the use of this plant for treating digestive disorders. The extracts stimulate the breakdown of fat as well; forskolin, a diterpene, is mainly responsible for this activity.[P400]

COMPOUNDS REPORTED

The volatile oil of *P. barbatus* contains monoterpenes (e.g. α-pinene)[P398] and diterpenes (e.g. forskolin).[P400] Forskolin is added to pharmaceutical preparations used for the treatment of several ailments. The water-soluble analogue of forskolin, 6-(3-dimethylaminopropionyl) forskolin hydrochloride (NKH477), is widely used in the treatment of a number of diseases, including cardiovascular disorders.[P401]

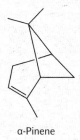

α-Pinene   Forskolin

a. *Plumbago auriculata*
Native to South Africa

Common names Blue Plumbago, Cape Plumbago, Cape Leadwort

Description and ecology
Evergreen, multi-stemmed, bushy, scrambling shrub 2–3m high, sometimes reaching 6m as a climber. **Leaves** simple, alternate, oblong, 2–5cm long, entire, sticky, glossy green above, greyish green below, thin in texture, leaf stalk winged at the base, clasping the stem. **Flowers** sticky, pale blue, blue or violet, rarely white, borne in terminal clusters (corymb-like racemes) at branch tips. A garden favourite, clambering over other shrubs, making striking hedges, and sprawling down banks and up walls. Grows at 1,600–2,200m.

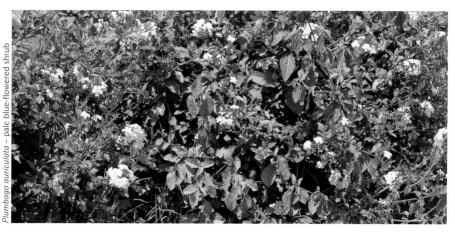

Plumbago auriculata – pale blue-flowered shrub

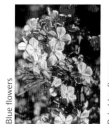

Blue flowers

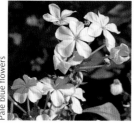

Pale blue flowers

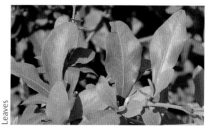

Leaves

USAGE AND TREATMENT

PARTS USED Roots and leaves.
TRADITIONAL MEDICINAL USES Roots and leaves are used to relieve headache.[M70, M116] Roots are also used for removing warts and for treating wounds and fractures.[M2, M4, M116]

PREPARATION AND DOSAGE
HEADACHE Use powdered roots or leaves as snuff.
WARTS Make a paste from powdered dry roots and apply locally.
FRACTURES Roast dry root powder, make a paste and rub on the affected areas.

b. *Plumbago zeylanica* — Indigenous

Common names Wild Plumbago, Wild White Leadwort, Wild Leadwort • **Local names** Wala (Kam.), Takale (Tai.), Lkimantus (Sam.)

Description and ecology

Evergreen, trailing or scrambling, multi-stemmed shrub 0.5–2m high. Stems and slender branches hairless, climbing, prostrate or erect, reaching lengths of 1.5m or even 2.5m. Leaves simple, alternate, ovate, entire, soft, pale green and shiny above, greyish below. Flowers white or rarely pale blue, star-shaped, very sticky, in small bunches on an elongated terminal raceme. Fruit an oblong capsule, 7.5–8.0mm long, 1-seeded. Seed oblong, 5–6mm long, brown to dark brown. Common in dry bushland in low-rainfall areas, in deciduous woodland, along roadsides, often near rivers and on lake margins or on termite mounds, at 0–2,000m.

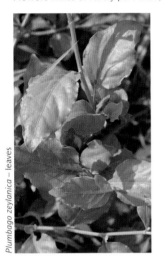

Plumbago zeylanica – leaves

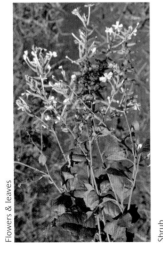

Flowers & leaves

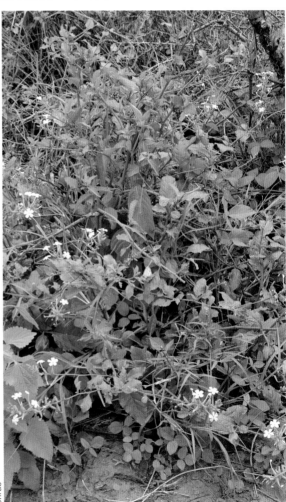

Shrub

USAGE AND TREATMENT

PARTS USED Roots, bark and aerial parts.

TRADITIONAL MEDICINAL USES The roots are widely used throughout Africa as a remedy for parasitic diseases of the skin, especially leprosy, and also to treat scabies, acne, sores, ringworm and ulcers.[M14, M115] A decoction of roots is taken to treat diarrhoea, for stomach ailments and as a remedy for hookworm.[M1, M70, M115] Such a decoction is also applied externally to swellings, fractures and blisters. A root decoction with boiled milk is swallowed to treat inflammation in the mouth, throat and chest.[M115] Pulped roots or aerial parts are inserted into the vagina as an abortifacient.[M115] Powdered bark, roots or leaves are used for gonorrhoea, syphilis, tuberculosis, rheumatic pain, swellings and wounds.[M115] Pounded roots are applied to swollen legs and to treat itchy skin.[M115]

PREPARATION AND DOSAGE

SKIN AFFLICTIONS Apply a paste made from powdered roots to the affected areas of the skin, or use a warm root decoction for this purpose.

DIARRHOEA AND STOMACH WORMS Steep a handful of crushed roots in half a litre of warm water. Drink the infusion before breakfast in the morning.

 WARNING! Plumbagin, one of the major compounds in the roots, is toxic in high doses.

PHARMACOLOGY AND CHEMISTRY

PHARMACOLOGICAL PROPERTIES

Both roots and leaves of species of *Plumbago* have shown some antibacterial and antifungal activities against certain organisms.[P183, P188] Roots also have anti-atherogenic, cardiotonic, hepatoprotective and neuroprotective properties.[P402] Aerial parts show weak antiviral activity against hepatitis B.[P403]

COMPOUNDS REPORTED

Compounds identified in *Plumbago* roots include some benzenoids (e.g. plumbagic acid),[P404] naphthoquinones (e.g. plumbagin)[P17] and quinoids (e.g. anthraquinone).[P405] Triterpenes (e.g. lupenone) have been isolated from the aerial parts.[P406] Tannins, anthocyanin pigments and phenolic acids have also been reported.[P17] Plumbagin exhibits a wide spectrum of biological activities, which include anticancer, antifungal, anti-inflammatory, antibacterial, contraceptive, antimalarial, antidiabetic and antioxidant properties.[P407]

Lupenone

Plumbagin

Plumbagic acid

Indigenous

Common names Red Stinkwood, African Cherry • **Local names** Mutimailu / Mumbaume (Kam.), Muiri (Kik.), Arareut (Kip.), Omoiri (Kis.), Mwiritsa / Kumuturu (Luh.), Kiburabura (Swa.), Kunukwa / Kunyukwa (Tug.), Olkoijuka / Olkoijuk (Maa.Ken.), Mweria (Mer.Ken.), Tendwet (Nan.), Tenduet (Mar.), Oromoti (Sebei), Lemalan (Sam.), Ol gujuk / Olkonjuku (Aru.), Mkonde-konde / Msendo (Chag.), Mwiluti (Hehe), Olkonjuku (Maa.Tan.), Kondekonde (Mer.Tan.), Mdundulu (Ngu.), Wami (Ran.), Mkomahoya (Samb.), Mufubia (Zin.), Ngwabuzito / Ntasesa (Lug.), Chiramat / Charamandi (Lugi.), Musuba (Ruki.)

Description and ecology

Tall, evergreen forest tree reaching 25m or more, in forests or plantations with high, open foliage and pendulous branches, but trees in grassland shorter, 8–12m high and with a more rounded crown. **Bark** rough, dark brown or black, scaling irregularly, sometimes into squares, branches brown and corky, branchlets dotted with breathing pores. **Leaves** simple, alternate, 6–14 × 1.5–6cm, elliptic or broadly oval, non-hairy, glossy dark green above, apex pointed,

base rounded, margin mildly serrate, leaf stalk typically pink or red and up to 2cm long. **Flowers** sweetly scented, small, greenish white or cream, borne singly or in short, axillary, 7–15-flowered sprays or racemes 2–5(–8)cm long. **Fruit** an ellipsoid, non-hairy drupe, 5–8 × 8–12mm, red to purplish brown when ripe, extremely bitter, often 2-lobed, with a seed in each lobe. Occurs in high-rainfall areas, in moist upland evergreen forest and in riverine forest, often in remnants or along margins, at 1,100–3,150m.

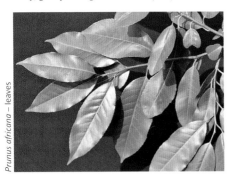

Prunus africana – leaves

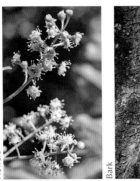

Flowers

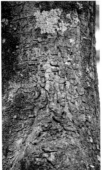

Bark

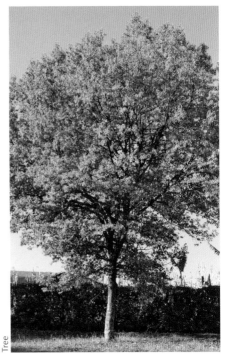

Tree

USAGE AND TREATMENT

PARTS USED Stem bark and leaves.
TRADITIONAL MEDICINAL USES Bark is used as
a purgative and to treat stomach ache,[M4] but is
best known throughout Africa as well as in Europe
and America as a remedy for benign prostate gland
hypertrophy[M2, M4, M60] and benign prostatic hyperplasia
(BPH).[M112] A leaf infusion is taken to stimulate the
appetite. Leaves are also used as an inhalant for relief from
fever.[M1, M70, M112] Bark is used for numerous ailments: as
a wound dressing, a purgative, and an appetite stimulant,
and to treat fever, malaria, arrow-poisoning, stomach pain,
kidney disease and gonorrhoea.[M120]

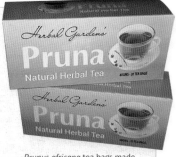

Prunus africana tea bags made
from dried powdered bark

PREPARATION AND DOSAGE
PROSTATITIS, MALARIA AND STOMACH PAIN Boil a handful of dried or fresh bark in a litre of
water for 10 minutes. Filter and drink the decoction in portions during the day for 5–7 days.

PHARMACOLOGY AND CHEMISTRY

PHARMACOLOGICAL PROPERTIES
ß-Sitosterol, found in the bark of *Prunus africana*, is said to show activity against prostatic
adenoma;[P96] the same compound is found in other plants that have traditionally been used
for this purpose.[P26, P96]

COMPOUNDS REPORTED
Stem bark extracts contain phytosterols, including β-sitosterol and campesterol.[P96] A
cyanogenic glycoside, amygdalin, has been reported.[P17, P26] The bark also contains pentacyclic
triterpenoid esters and ferulic acid esters.[P96] Several triterpenes (e.g. 2α-hydroxyoleanolic
acid) have been isolated from the stem bark.[P408] In addition to the phytosterol β-sitosterol,
which is the major compound of *P. africana*, other phytochemicals present in the bark of this
plant, namely triterpenes (e.g. oleanolic acid), phenolics (e.g. atraric acid), the sulfonamide
N-butylbenzene-sulfonamide and the fatty acid lauric acid, also contribute to the use of the
plant to treat prostate cancer.[P409, P410]

ß-Sitosterol

2α-Hydroxyoleanolic acid

Native to the Caribbean, South and Central America

Common name Guava • **Local names** Kivela (Kam.), Mubera (Kik.), Lipera (Luh.), Mapera (Luo), Mpera (Swa.), Zeitun (Som.), Mupeera (Lug.), Amrood (Hind., Urd.)

Description and ecology

Shrub or small, evergreen tree 2–6(–10)m tall and with irregular branches. **Bark** smooth, light reddish brown, later peeling and flaking showing greenish-brown inner bark, younger stems greenish, hairy and 4-angled. **Leaves** simple, opposite, large, 7–15cm long, ovate or oblong-elliptic, dull green, with pointed tip, rounded base and entire margin, stalk 4–10mm long. **Flowers** white, usually borne singly in the upper leaf axils, 2.5cm across, on hairy stalk 1–2.5cm long. **Fruits** rounded, egg-shaped or pear-shaped berries 2.5–8cm long, tipped by the remains of the calyx, green at first, turning yellow when ripe, with edible variably coloured pulp (pink, green, white or yellow) containing many seeds. **Seeds** yellowish and kidney-shaped. Widely cultivated in Africa as a fruit tree and has become naturalised and invasive in East Africa. Flourishes in moist conditions. Commonly found in agricultural areas, forest edges, natural forests, riparian zones and disturbed scrub or shrublands in higher-rainfall areas, at 0–2,200m.

AS214

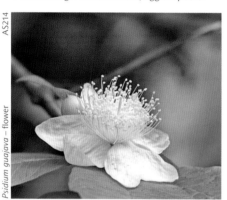

Psidium guajava – flower

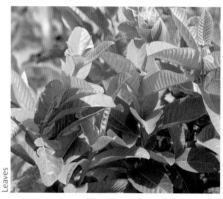

Leaves

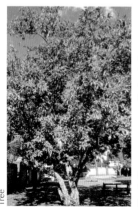

Tree

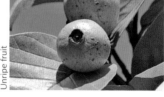

Unripe fruit

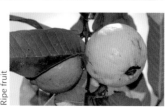

Ripe fruit

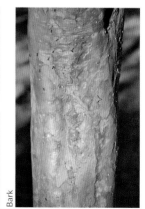

Bark

PARTS USED Root bark, stem bark, young leaves, buds, flowers and fruits.
TRADITIONAL MEDICINAL USES Leaves and root bark are a remedy for diarrhoea, amoebic dysentery and gastritis.[M6, M10, M70, M121] Leaves are also used for treating diabetes, fever, ulcers, coughs, boils, abscesses[M2, M121] and wounds, as well as in a vaginal wash after childbirth.[M6, M9] Fresh fruits are eaten to allay malnutrition and exhaustion or weakness, while also having a mild laxative effect.[M9, M70] Squeezed juice from buds and flowers is taken orally as an anthelmintic. A dried bark decoction is a remedy for stomach ache. A dried leaf decoction acts as an anti-emetic and treatment for diarrhoea,[M7, M10] and is also used to treat malaria.[M63] Hot-water extracts of flowers and fruits are taken as an emmenagogue.[M4, M70] Green (unripe) fruits are recommended as a remedy for dysentery, while leaves and fruits are used for diarrhoea.[M111] A warm decoction of leaves or bark is used externally as a lotion for skin complaints, ringworm, wounds and ulcers.[M111]

PREPARATION AND DOSAGE

GASTRITIS Boil a handful of fresh leaves in a litre of water for 10 minutes in a covered pot. Filter and add water to restore the volume to a litre. Drink in portions during the day.
DIARRHOEA Boil a handful of leaves in a litre of water for 10 minutes in a covered pot. Filter and add water to restore the volume to a litre. Add a teaspoon of salt and 4 tablespoons of honey or 2 or 3 tablespoons of sugar. Drink at intervals. Children should be given half of this dose.
DYSENTERY In mild cases, follow the procedure for diarrhoea (above). In severe cases, mix a handful each of paw-paw leaves, mango leaves and guava leaves and boil in a litre of water for 15 minutes. Filter and drink at intervals during the day.
DIABETES Steep a handful of pounded fresh leaves in a litre of boiled water. Sip this mixture at regular intervals.
COLDS Chew a young leaf 5 times daily, or drink a guava leaf tea made as for diarrhoea (above).
WOUNDS Boil 2 handfuls of fresh leaves in a litre of water until the volume reduces to 500ml. Strain and wash affected areas with the warm decoction.
ABSCESSES Apply a warm poultice made by adding a teaspoon each of salt and sugar to a handful of pounded fresh leaves in a saucepan and then heating the mixture (without adding water) until it turns brownish (but does not burn).
MALNUTRITION, PHYSICAL WEAKNESS, SCURVY (VITAMIN C DEFICIENCY) Eat plenty of ripe fruits or drink at least a glassful of fresh fruit juice every day.

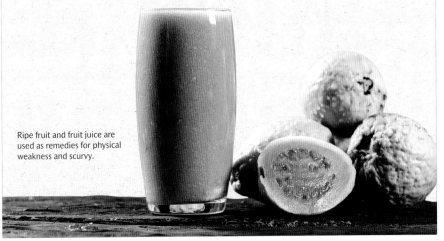

Ripe fruit and fruit juice are used as remedies for physical weakness and scurvy.

AS215

PHARMACOLOGICAL PROPERTIES

The volatile oils of *Psidium guajava* show antibacterial and antifungal activity, effective in the treatment of both internal and external infections.[P96] Different parts of the plant show analgesic, anti-oedema, antidiarrhoeal, anti-inflammatory, antimalarial, antispasmodic, antipyretic and antihyperglycaemic activity.[P79] Spasmolytic activity of the leaf extract is due mainly to the presence of aglycone quercetin, the glycosides of which are hydrolysed by gastrointestinal fluids.[P323] Leaves contain tannins and ellagic acid (with a protective effect on mucous membranes), explaining the enduring use of this plant for treating diarrhoea and dysentery.[P84] Quercetin and its glycosides are antioxidants with antibiotic, anti-HIV and anti-carcinogenic activities. The antiscorbutic, re-mineralising and invigorating properties of the fruits are helpful in addressing physical exhaustion and malnutrition.[P84]

COMPOUNDS REPORTED

The *P. guajava* fruit contains mucilage, pectin, small amounts of protein and fat, minerals (e.g. potassium, calcium, iron and phosphorus), and vitamins A and B. It is furthermore one of the richest of all fruits in vitamin C.[P84] The leaves contain numerous tannins, volatile oils and other phenolic compounds such as amritoside (a glycoside of ellagic acid)[P159] and quercetin and its glycosides.[P411] Various triterpenoids (including guavanoic acid) have also been isolated from the leaves.[P411] Antioxidant, antibacterial, antidiabetic and antihyperlipemic, antimutagenic and anticancer activities as well as cardioprotective effects of the leaves of *P. guajava* are associated with the phytochemicals quercetin and its glycosides, pentacyclic triterpenoids and polyphenolics isolated from this plant.[P411]

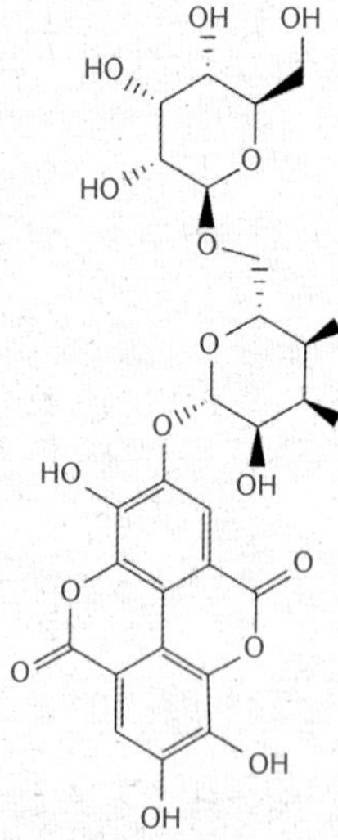

Amritoside

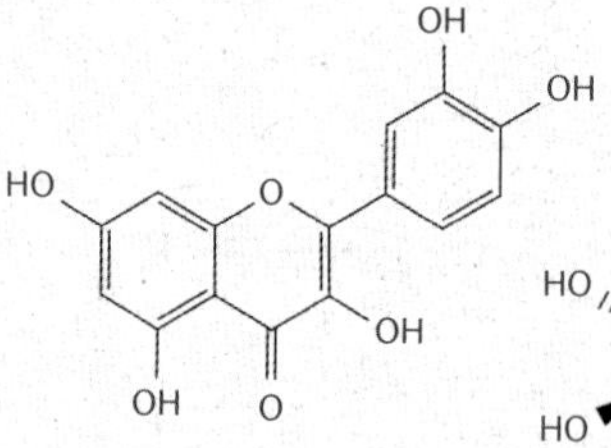

Quercetin

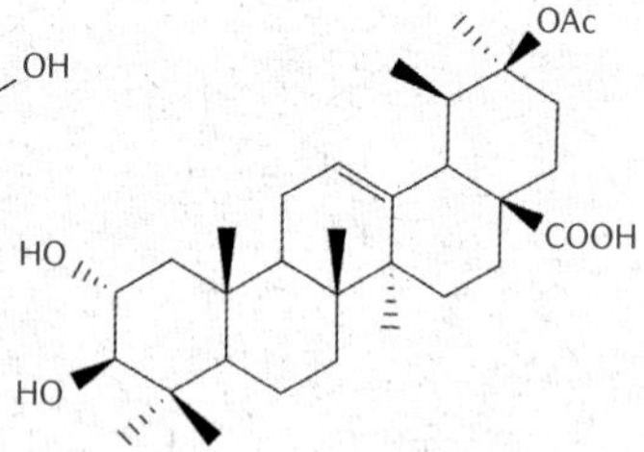

Guavanoic acid

Native to Iran and northern India

Common name Pomegranate • **Local names** Nkomawawanga (Lug.), Daram / Dadam (Guj.), Anar (Hind., Urd., Punj.)

Description and ecology

Multi-stemmed, semi-deciduous shrub or small tree 5–6(–8)m tall. Stem woody and spiny. **Bark** light brown or dark grey and smooth. **Leaves** simple, opposite, smooth and non-hairy, oval, coppery red when young, later shiny green. **Flowers** brilliant orange-red, about 3cm across, with wrinkly petals and 5–7 fleshy red calyx lobes, borne solitarily or in terminal clusters. **Fruit** a large, orange-sized berry with a tough, leathery rind. **Seeds** numerous, edible. Cultivated as a fruit and ornamental tree and has become naturalised in East Africa, occurring at 0–1,500m. Requires well-drained soil and plenty of sunshine.

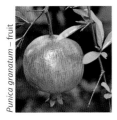

Punica granatum – fruit

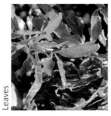

Leaves

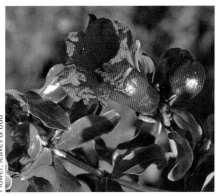

Flower, leaves & bud

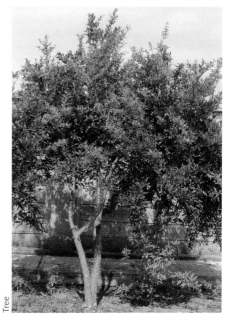

Tree

PARTS USED Root bark, stem bark, leaves, fruit rind and flowers.
TRADITIONAL MEDICINAL USES A decoction of fruit peel is taken to control excessive bleeding during menstruation. An extract of dried fruit is used for treating skin lesions. Root bark is used as an abortifacient and emmenagogue.[M10] Root and stem bark, mixed with some leaves, make a strong vermifuge against tapeworm.[M111] A mixture of fruit rind and flowers is taken for stomach ache, dysentery[M7, M45] and diarrhoea. Leaf decoctions are applied to sore eyes to relieve pain and redness. A decoction of fruit rind and flowers is used to heal inflamed and damaged gums,[M7] vaginal irritations (white vaginal flow), tonsillitis and pharyngitis.[M9] Unripe fruit and flowers are significant emetics and ripe fruits serve as a laxative.[M111]

PREPARATION AND DOSAGE

VERMIFUGE Steep 30–40g of dried root bark in a litre of water for 24 hours. Then boil until the liquid has reduced by half. Sweeten with honey and drink every morning on an empty stomach for 3 days. For children, use only 10–20g of root bark.

DIARRHOEA, DYSENTERY AND STOMACH ACHE Steep 20–30g of the flowers in a litre of water. Take a teaspoon of this mixture every hour until symptoms abate.

INFLAMED GUMS AND VAGINAL IRRITATION Add 30g of the flowers and 5g of the fruit rind to a litre of hot boiled water. Rinse the mouth and gargle with the warm decoction or use for vaginal cleansing.

 WARNING! Root bark of *Punica granatum* must never be given to infants on a milk diet, to pregnant women or to people with wasting conditions or nervous disorders. Stated doses should not be exceeded.

PHARMACOLOGY AND CHEMISTRY

PHARMACOLOGICAL PROPERTIES

Pelletierine and other alkaloids in *Punica granatum* root bark are active against tapeworm. [P156] The presence of tannins in the fruit rind explains its efficacy in treating diarrhoea and dysentery.[P412] Water extracts of dried fruit peel have shown anthelmintic, antibacterial, antidiarrhoeal, antioxidant, anti-yeast, uterine stimulant and weak anti-inflammatory effects on different organisms.[P79] Aerial parts of *P. granatum* have been found to have hypothermic and diuretic properties. Hypoglycaemic activities have been reported for the flowers.[P79]

COMPOUNDS REPORTED

Root bark of *P. granatum* contains several piperidine alkaloids, notably pelletierine[P17, P79] and isopelleterine.[P17, P79] Alkaloids are also present in stem and branch bark, but in lower concentrations. Root bark contains tannins and glycosides with astringent properties. Two gallotannins, punicalin and punicalagin,[P79] have been isolated from fruit. The heartwood contains ellagitannins[P17] such as diellagic acid rhamnosyl-(1-4) glucopyranoside.[P412] Other compounds isolated include ß-sitosterol (from bark), cynadin-3-glucoside (fruit), ellagic acid (bark), methyl pelletierine (root bark), mucilage (fruit rind) and p-coumarinic acid.[P79] Phytochemicals, anthocyanins, flavonoids, tannins and phenolic acids are associated with the health benefits of pomegranate peels.[P413]

Pelletierine

Diellagic acid rhamnosyl -(1-4) glucopyranoside

Indigenous

Common names Castor Oil Plant, Castor Bean • **Local names** Kobor (Bor.), Mwono (Dig.), Mwacariki (Emb.), M'bono (Gir.), Kivunu / Kyaiki / Mwaiki (Kam.), Mwariki (Kik.), Menuet / Imanek (Kip.), Omobono (Kis.), Mubonebone / Libono / Kumubono (Luh.), Odagwa / Obala ndagwa (Luo), Oldule / Orpaliki (Maa.), Manwa (Mar.), Mwariki (Mer.), Koboo (Orm.), Pondon (Pok.), Fololo (Ren.), Laibelelhi / Lampalegi (Sam.), Gitkalat (Som.), Mbono (Tai.), Ebune (Tur.), Mnyemba (Gogo, Hehe, Lugu.), Mhale (Nyam.), Mbono (Pare), Mzono (Samb.), Mbarika / Mbono / Nyonyo (Swa.), Nsogasoga (Lug.), Kasyoga / Kaisaja (Runyan.), Diveli / Arando (Guj.), Endi (Hind., Urd.), Arand (Punj.)

Description and ecology

Evergreen, softly woody, monoecious shrub or small tree 1–5m tall, with hollow stems and prominent leaf scars, shoots light bluish green or green or red. **Leaves** spirally arranged, very large, up to 50cm across, palmately compound, on long, stout, hollow leaf stalk, leaflets 5–9(–11), deeply lobed, with serrate margins. **Flowers** unisexual, borne on spikes 10–25cm long, male flowers with creamy yellow stamens, female flowers with showy red stigmas and clustered above male flowers. **Fruit** a spiny, green-brown, round capsule, 25mm across, 3-lobed and 3-seeded. **Seeds** oval, shiny, mottled silver, brown and black. Grows in various habitats from bushed grassland to upland forest but common on disturbed ground, at 0–2,100m.

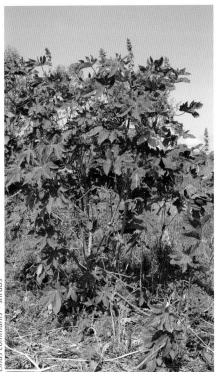

Ricinus communis – shrubs

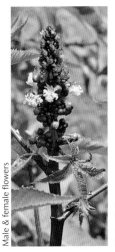

Male & female flowers

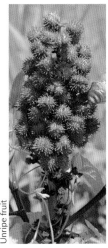

Unripe fruit

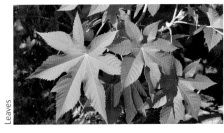

Leaves

PARTS USED Roots, stems, leaves and seeds.

TRADITIONAL MEDICINAL USES Castor oil is well known as a purgative and laxative.[M7, M9, M4, M122] A root decoction is taken to stimulate the appetite and for abdominal ailments.[M4] Infusions of leaves can relieve stomach ache.[M122] Seed, root and leaf poultices are applied to wounds, fungal infections, skin lesions, sores and boils.[M2, M6, M70] Leaves are used to reduce rheumatic pain and swellings,[M7, M122] as an antidote against snake venom, and as an emetic. The pure oil extract can be used for ear problems.[M7] Dried leaves are taken as a remedy for chronic headache.[M7, M64] Dried root infusions are used to treat intestinal worms, especially hookworm.[M64] A decoction of fresh roots may facilitate expulsion of the placenta or speed up a baby's delivery or labour.[M26] Shade-dried seeds are used as a contraceptive and for birth control in women.[M65] Seed kernels are used to treat paralysis, coughs and asthma and to reduce testicular swelling.[M7] Hot-water extracts from the entire fresh plant are taken orally to treat venereal diseases, ulcers and diarrhoea, and are applied as a fungicide or as eardrops.[M48, M70]

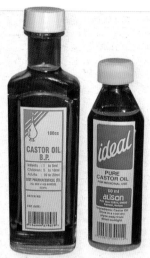

Seed oil of *Ricinus communis*, sold as castor oil, is a recognised purgative and laxative.

PREPARATION AND DOSAGE

INTESTINAL PARASITES, CONSTIPATION, STOMACH ACHE
Take a tablespoon of castor oil (available from chemists and most supermarkets) and half a teaspoon of honey an hour before breakfast daily until diarrhoea begins. Children should be given half this dose. A handful of pounded fresh leaves, steeped in a litre of cold water for 10 minutes and stirred intermittently, can be administered orally or as an enema to treat stomach ache. Alternatively, boil 20g of pounded fresh or crushed dry roots in a cup of water for 10 minutes and drink half a cup twice daily for 3 days.

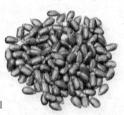

Dry seeds

SKIN AILMENTS Poultices made from powdered seeds, roots or crushed fresh leaves can be applied to the affected area on the body.

SNAKEBITE Orally administer a tablespoon of juice from pounded fresh leaves. This will cause vomiting and diarrhoea but will counter the effects of the venom. At the same time, juice from a crushed leaf shoot can be applied to the bite itself.

CHRONIC HEADACHE Add a handful of crushed dried leaves to a cup of olive oil. Massage the head with the mixture, placing a drop in each nostril.

 WARNING! Castor oil seeds contain ricin, one of the most toxic of all compounds. Intake of just two seeds can kill a child and 10–15 seeds may kill an adult.

PHARMACOLOGICAL PROPERTIES

The roots of *Ricinus communis* have shown anti-inflammatory activity[P414] and the leaves produce weak antiviral activity.[P366] The purgative action of the oil is ascribed to free ricinoleic acid and its stereoisomer, produced through hydrolysis in the duodenum.[P17] The highly toxic substance ricin is present in the seeds. Symptoms of ingestion may include (within 12 hours) nausea, vomiting, diarrhoea and abdominal pain, leading to hypotension, liver failure, renal dysfunction and death from multi-organ failure or cardiovascular collapse. Inhalation of ricin may lead (within 8 hours) to coughing, dyspnoea, arthralgia and fever.[P415]

COMPOUNDS REPORTED

Seeds of *R. communis* contain about 50% oil, ricinine (an alkaloid) and ricin, a highly toxic glycoprotein.[P416] Castor oil contains glycerides of ricinoleic, isoricinoleic, stearic and dihydroxystearic acids;[P17] aerial parts elaborate some flavonoids (e.g. quercitrin[P417]), while roots contain alkaloids (e.g. indole-3-acetic acid).[P418] Antibacterial and antifungal activities against 30 micro-organisms, including the genera *Bacillus* and *Aspergillus*, and *Escherichia coli* and *Candida albicans*, have been reported for extracts obtained from various plants of *R. communis*.[P419] Alkaloid and enriched extracts of the leaf, stem, root, capsule and seeds showed significant antioxidant activity.[P419] These activities are linked to the presence of alkaloids, flavonoids, coumarins, terpenoids and cardiac glycosides.

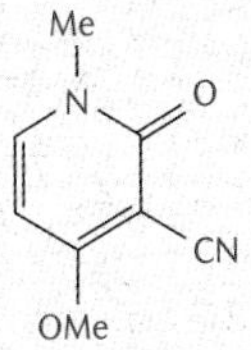

Ricinine

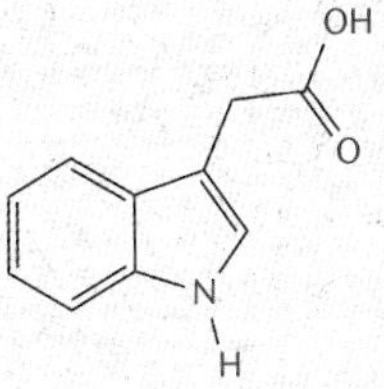

Indole-3-acetic acid

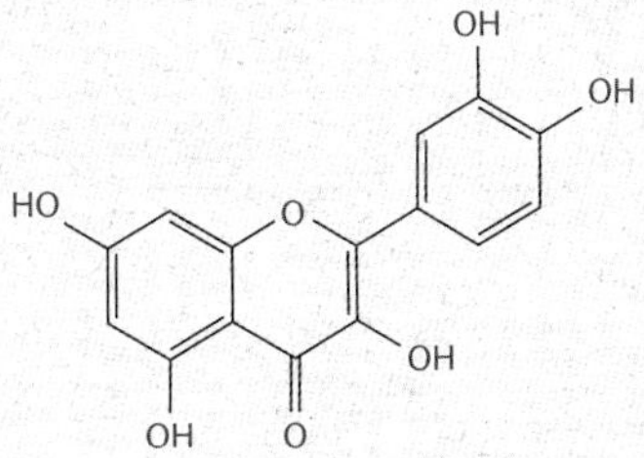

Quercitrin

Indigenous

Common names Butterfly Flower, Blue Butterfly Bush • **Local names** Mara-sisa (Bor.), Kiteangwai / Muvweia (Kam.), Munjugu (Kik.), Chesamisiet (Kip.), Shisilangokho (Luh.), Kurgweno / Okwero / Okwergweno (Luo), Ol-magotogot / Ol-makutukut (Maa.), Chesagon / Chebobet (Mar.), Makutukuti (Sam.), Gobetie (Tug.), Okwero (Ach.)

Description and ecology

Small, untidy, evergreen shrub or subshrub 1–3(–4)m tall, with many branches from the base. **Leaves** simple, opposite or in whorls, narrowly elliptic to ovate or obovate, 1.5–12cm long, often smaller, soft, apex pointed, base wedge-shaped, margin conspicuously wavy, stalk 0–25mm long. **Flowers** with 4 dark blue or purple petals spread like butterfly wings, fifth petal darker and more rounded. **Fruits** small berries, 5–6 × 8–10mm, green turning black, edible when ripe. In dry or semi-evergreen bushland and bushed or wooded grassland at forest margins, often on rocky sites, at 150–2,400m.

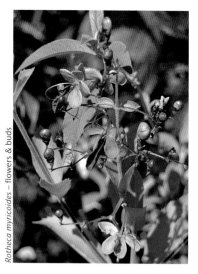

Rotheca myricoides – flowers & buds

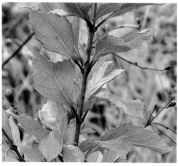

Leafy branch

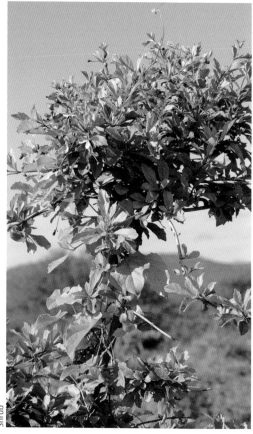

Shrub

PARTS USED Roots and leaves.

TRADITIONAL MEDICINAL USES A root decoction can be used to treat chest pain, malaria, tonsillitis, a sore throat and rheumatism. A root decoction can be used for sexually transmitted infections.[M88] Roots may also be used as an emetic, as a purgative and for the treatment of gonorrhoea.[M1, M70] Root infusions are taken as a remedy for a cold and to stop bleeding from the gums. A leaf poultice can be used for dressing wounds and treating fungal infections.[M70]

PREPARATION AND DOSAGE

CHEST PAIN, RHEUMATISM AND SORE THROAT Boil a handful of pounded roots in a litre of water. Drink the mixture at intervals during the day. Alternatively, wash some fresh roots in cold boiled water. Chew, swallowing the juice.

EMETIC OR PURGATIVE Boil 5g of dry root powder in a litre of water for 10 minutes. Drink all of the warm mixture before breakfast in the mornings.

GONORRHOEA Boil a handful of fresh roots or 5g of dry root powder in a litre of water for 10–15 minutes. Cool, filter and drink the mixture at intervals during the day.

> ⚠ **WARNING!** Fresh parts of *Rotheca myricoides* may be toxic if taken in high doses. Adverse symptoms of overdose include stomach ache, vomiting, diarrhoea, headache and weakness.

PHARMACOLOGICAL PROPERTIES

The leaves have produced antifungal and antibacterial activities, but no antiviral activity.[P254] Leaves and stems have a smooth muscle stimulant effect,[P347] while stems have also exhibited hypotensive (skeletal muscle relaxant) activity.[P347] An organic solvent extract of roots of *Rotheca myricoides* showed high activity against methicillin-resistant *Staphylococcus aureus* (MRSA), *Escherichia coli*, *Shigella sonnei*, *Candida albicans* and *Mycobacterium tuberculosis*, which are currently posing great public health challenges due to the development of drug resistance and as major sources for community and hospital-based infections.[P420]

COMPOUNDS REPORTED

A number of alkaloids (e.g. myricoidine) have been isolated from the whole plant,[P421] and a cyclohexapeptide, cleromyrine I, also from the whole plant.[P422] The genus *Clerodendrum* (under which *R. myricoides* was once classified) is known to contain iridoids and abietane diterpenoids (e.g. taxodione), and some of the abietane diterpenoids showed antiplasmodial and antileishmanial activities.[P423]

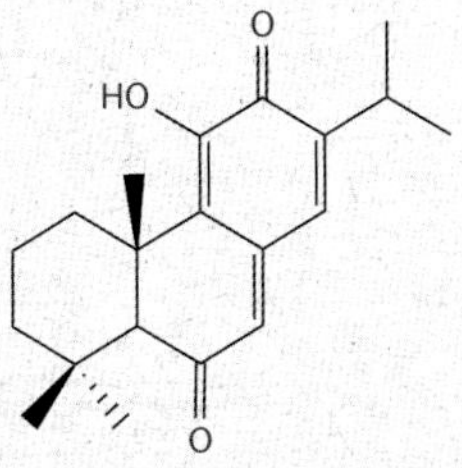

Taxodione

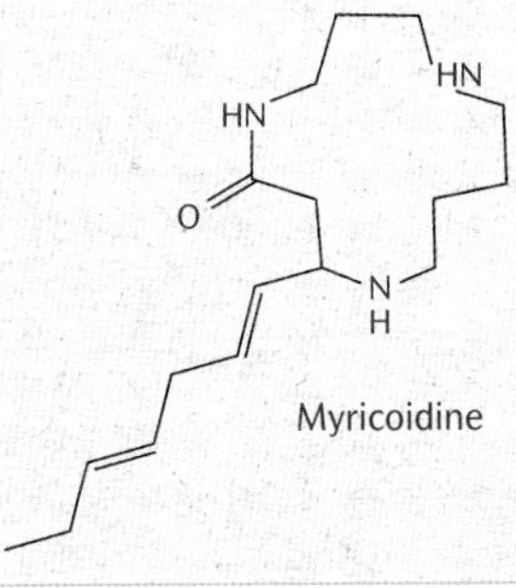

Myricoidine

Indigenous

Common names Rumex, Sorrel • **Local names** Kinyonywe (Kam.), Mugagatio (Kik.), Mindeiywet (Kip.), Bule / Msheshere (Tai.), Enkaiswishoi / Enkaisijoi (Maa.), Linyimbili (Hehe), Kchambo (Pare), Gentamana / Nywanywa (Samb.), Mchachu / Mchumvichumvi (Swa.), Nywanywa (Zig.), Omufumbwa (Ruki.), Omuka (Runyan.).

Description and ecology
Scrambling shrub 1–2m tall or weak, straggly climber reaching 3m or more. Stems very soft, juicy, brown-tinged, glabrous. **Leaves** narrowly to broadly elliptic, 2–11 × 0.5–4cm, non-hairy, with a pointed tip, 2 short lobes towards the base, a smooth margin and 3 distinct veins from the centre, stalk 1–4cm long. **Flowers** inconspicuous, up to 7mm long, brick-red, in much-branched panicles up to 30cm long and carried above the leaves. **Fruit** an oval, shiny, red-brown nutlet 2–2.5mm long, 3-angled. Common in upland or montane bush and grassland, also on roadsides, at forest edges, in rocky areas and near swamps in lowlands, at 900–2,400m.

USAGE AND TREATMENT

PARTS USED Roots, leaves and young stems.
TRADITIONAL MEDICINAL USES Roots are used for treating scabies.[M3] Leaves and young stems are used for coughs and pneumonia. A leaf infusion can be used to treat coughs, rheumatism, stomach ache and gastritis.[M112] Decoctions of roots or leaves are taken as a remedy for intestinal worms (tapeworm and roundworm) and stomach pain, and are also applied externally to heal wounds, boils and abscesses.[M1, M70, M112] Leaves of several species of *Rumex* are used in poultices on skin afflictions, including acne.[M25] Fresh leaves and roots are used as a diuretic and laxative.[M4, M70] *R. abyssinicus*, common at lower altitudes in East Africa, is put to similar medicinal uses.

PREPARATION AND DOSAGE
INTESTINAL WORMS AND AS A LAXATIVE Boil a handful of pounded fresh roots or leaves in half a litre of water. Drink the entire decoction before breakfast in the mornings for a few days.
WOUNDS, BOILS AND ABSCESSES Apply a warm poultice of powdered roots to the affected areas. A warm decoction of the whole plant can be used to wash wounds up to 3 times a day.
COUGHS, STOMACH ACHE AND GASTRITIS Pound and then soak a handful of fresh leaves in half a litre of cold water for an hour, then stir. Take half a cup of the infusion 2 or 3 times a day before meals.

 WARNING! Owing to high concentrations of oxalic acid, internal use is not recommended for people with gout or arthritis.

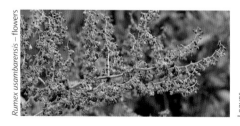

Rumex usambarensis – flowers

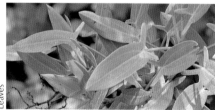

Leaves

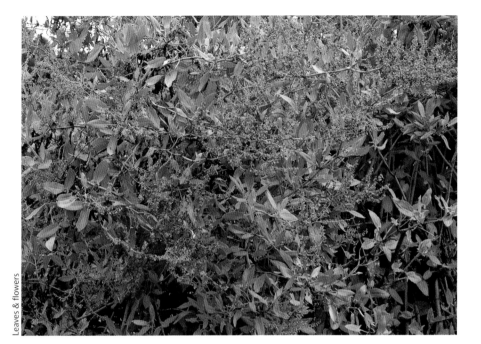

PHARMACOLOGY AND CHEMISTRY

PHARMACOLOGICAL PROPERTIES

Species of *Rumex* show antibacterial and antiviral activities, notably against coxsackie virus B3 and the influenza-A virus.[P243] None of the species produce any antifungal activity,[P243] however. Anti-inflammatory activity has been reported for *R. abyssinicus*.[P243] Water extract of *R. dentatus* shows molluscicidal activities, ascribed to anthraquinones.[P424] The laxative properties of anthraquinones such as chrysophanol and related anthraquinone glycosides are well documented.[P84]

COMPOUNDS REPORTED

All sorrels are acidic and sour tasting owing to the presence of tartaric acid, vitamin C and both oxalic acids and oxalic salts (mostly potassium hydrogen oxalate).[P84, P156] Roots of *Rumex* species contain anthraquinones, such as chrysophanol, and chromones, such as 7-hydroxy-2,5-dimethylchromone.[P243, P424] It was further shown that the anthraquinones chrysophanol, physcion and emodin are found in the roots, seeds, stem and leaves of five species of *Rumex*, including *R. usambarensis*.[P352]

Chrysophanol

7-Hydroxy-2,5-dimethylchromone

Oxalic acid

a. *Searsia natalensis (Rhus natalensis)*

Indigenous

Common names Rhus Bush, Giraffe Bush, Currant Rhus • **Local names** Dabobiss (Bor.), Mbwananyahi / Mgwanyahi (Dig.), Dabobbessa (Gab.), Ntheu / Mutheu (Kam.), Muthigio (Kik.), Suriet (Kip.), Busangura nabili / Kumusangura nabili / Obusangura (Luh.), Osangla / Sangla (Luo), Muthanguta / Mutheru / Muthiigi (Mbe.), Mirikitha (Mer.), Monjororioyot (Nan.), Siriewo / Siria (Pok.), Ilmisingiyot / Lmisigiyoi (Sam.), Ilka adeis (Som.), Mtishangwe / Mkono-chuma (Swa.Ken.), Siriande (Tug.), Ekadetewa (Tur.), Kitarika (Tai.), Ormisigiyoi (Aru.), Mpungulu (Chag.), Msagara (Haya), Mtunumbi (Hehe), Ol mesigie / Ol misigiyoi / Ilmisigiyo (Maa.), Msakasaka (Ran.), Mhunguru (Samb., Suk.), Mkumba / Mkono-chuma (Swa.Tan.), Msense (Zin.), Ewayo (Ate.), Karagba (Lugb.), Keregwe (Madi), Omusheeshe (Runyan.)

Description and ecology

Much-branched, evergreen, bushy and woody shrub up to 3m high, occasionally a small tree reaching 6–8m. **Bark** grey-brown, rough, dotted with breathing pores. **Leaves** 3-foliolately compound, the 3 leaflets elliptic or obovate, central one the largest, dark olive-green above and light green below, leathery, hairless, margins toothed or entire, wider towards tips, narrowed towards bases, leaf stalk 2–4cm long, young leaves shiny red, smelling of apples when crushed. **Flowers** small, greenish cream, in groups on loose panicles up to 12cm long. **Fruits** oblong to kidney-shaped berries, 5–6mm across, flattened, smooth and shiny, green, turning reddish brown on ripening. Widespread in wooded grassland, along dry forest edges, beside rivers and in bushland and thickets, at 0–2,700m.

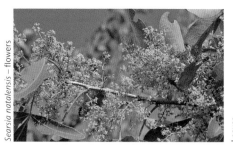

Searsia natalensis – flowers

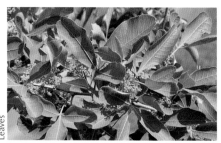

Leaves

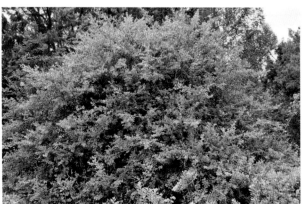

Shrub

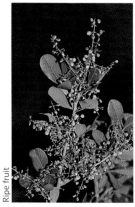

Ripe fruit

PARTS USED Leaves, branches and roots.

TRADITIONAL MEDICINAL USES Leaves are used for heartburn and stomach ache[M3] and as a hot-water inhalant for coughs and colds.[M4, M70] Branches are used to treat stomach complaints.[M3] Root decoctions are taken for gastrointestinal ailments,[M4, M28, M91, M112] influenza, headache, constipation, neck pain,[M35] diarrhoea,[M3, M112] gonorrhoea[M4, M48, M91] and as an anthelmintic against hookworm.[M1, M91, M112] A root decoction is also given to a woman who has suffered an abortion or stillbirth.[M112] Fresh stems are used for toothache, while the twigs are useful chewing sticks.[M26]

PREPARATION AND DOSAGE

HEARTBURN, COUGHS AND COLDS Steep a handful of pounded fresh leaves in a litre of hot water. Drink a cup of the infusion 3 times daily after meals. Inhale steam vapour from boiled leaves or chew some fresh leaves for relief from a cold and headache.

ABDOMINAL PAIN Boil 3g of pounded fresh leaves and branches in half a litre of water. Drink warm 2 or 3 times daily until symptoms abate.

GONORRHOEA AND HOOKWORM Steep a handful of pounded fresh roots or 5g of dry root powder in half a litre of hot or cold water. Drink a cup of the mixture 2 or 3 times a day. For hookworm, a cup daily before breakfast for 2 or 3 days is sufficient.

b. *Searsia pyroides* (*Rhus vulgaris*)   Indigenous

Common names Rhus, Currant Rhus, Common Wild Currant • **Local names** Mbwanyahi (Dig.), Kitheu / Mutheu (Kam.), Muthigiu / Muthigio (Emb., Kik.), Siriat / Suriet (Kip.), Busangura-busecha / Kumusangura-kamusecha / Obusangura / Omusangura (Luh.), Awayo / Sangla-madhako / Sangla-madoung (Luo), Ol-misigiyioi / Ol-munyushi / Ilmisigiyioi / Ormisigiyioi (Maa.Ken., Maa.Tan.), Muthanguta / Mutheru / Muthigiyo (Mbe.), Mirimuthu / Muthigiu (Mer.), Monjororioyat (Nan.), Siriewo kaptamu (Pok.), Sioloran / Lejoro (Sam.), Njowaruwa (Sebei), Mlishangwe / Mlama mwitu / Mkono chuma (Swa.), Mkungu / Seria (Tai.), Nyungu / Mpungulu (Chag.), Datlaii (Goro.), Umusagara / Msagara (Haya), Muhehefu (Hehe), Muizi / Msakasaka / Mwiizi (Ran.), Mtuntano (Samb.), Awaca (Ach.), Awaya / Awaca (Lan.), Kakwansokwanso / Eakansokanso (Lug.), Owayo (Lugw.), Busojole (Luso.), Obukaanja (Runyan.), Obukanjakanja (Runy.)

Description and ecology

Hairy, much-branched, multi-stemmed, deciduous shrub or small tree 1.5–5(–9)m tall. **Bark** smooth, dark brown and rough in older trees, branches thickly covered with soft hair. **Leaves** 3-foliolately compound, 4–11 × 2–6cm, central leaflet larger than lateral leaflets, smooth and velvety above and hairy below, leaf stalk about 3mm long. **Flowers** small, inconspicuous, greenish cream, borne in bunches in leaf axils on terminal, branched panicles 5–20cm long. **Fruit** a round, flat drupe, 3–4mm in diameter, reddish brown when ripe. Found in wooded or bushed grassland, thickets, rocky areas and dry forest margins, at 1,200–2,700m.

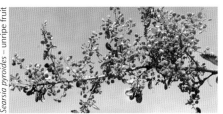

Searsia pyroides – unripe fruit

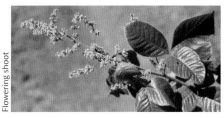

Flowering shoot

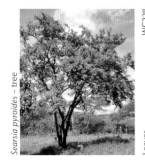

Searsia pyroides – tree

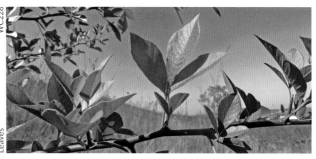

WC228

Leaves

PARTS USED Stems, leaves, roots and fruits.

TRADITIONAL MEDICINAL USES The entire dried plant can be used to treat colic.[M40] Liquid from boiled stem bark can be used on wounds.[M1, M70, M91] A fruit decoction is taken as a remedy for diarrhoea.[M4, M33, M91] Leaves are used for haemorrhoids and sores.[M40, M91] Decoctions of powdered roots or fruits are administered for gonorrhoea.[M1, M91] Hot-water root extracts are taken to ease childbirth and for treating infertility.

PREPARATION AND DOSAGE

DIARRHOEA Boil a handful of ripe fruits in a litre of water for 5–10 minutes. Leave to cool, then filter and drink at intervals during the day.

WOUNDS Boil some fresh or dry stems in water. Apply warm directly to affected areas.

GONORRHOEA, COLIC AND ABDOMINAL PAIN Steep a handful of pounded fresh roots or 5g of dry root powder in a litre of hot or cold water. Drink 3 or 4 times daily, preparing afresh every time.

PHARMACOLOGICAL PROPERTIES

Root extracts from *Searsia natalensis* (*Rhus natalensis*) have shown strong antigiardiasis activity,[P211] while dried fruit extracts of *S. pyroides* (*R. vulgaris*) show smooth muscle stimulant activity[P347] and a weak uterine stimulant effect.[P347] Dried leaves of *Searsia* (*Rhus*) species produce some antifungal activity.[P254]

COMPOUNDS REPORTED

The benzenoid 2-hydroxy-4-methoxybenzaldehyde, which is a potent tyrosinase inhibitor, has been isolated from roots of *S. pyroides* (*R. vulgaris*).[P425] Some species contain flavonoids; the flavonol fisetin, present in *Toxicodendron vernicifluum* (*R. vernciflua*),[P425] has potential therapeutic use in the treatment of angiogenesis-related diseases.[P426] Three bioflavonoids, including rhuschromone, have been isolated from root bark of *S. natalensis* (*R. natalensis*). An extract of roots of this plant showed cytotoxicity to HeLa cancer cells, and from this extract a new compound, 3-((Z)-heptadec-14-enyl) benzene-1-ol, was isolated and showed weak cytotoxicity.[P427]

2-Hydroxy-4-methoxybenzaldehyde

Fisetin

a. *Solanum incanum* Indigenous

Common names Sodom Apple, Bitter Apple • **Local names** Idi-gaga (Bor.), Mtunguza-koma (Dig.), Iddi-loonni (Gab.), Mtonda (Gir.), Muhidi (Ilw.), Mukondu (Kam.), Mutongu (Kik., Mer.), Omotobo (Kis.), Lobotwet (Kip.), Indulandula (Luh.), Ochok (Luo), Endulelei (Maa.), Jemokimnerkeny (Mar.), Hidi (Orm.), Yohola (Ren.), Ltulelei (Sam.), Mutunguja-mwilu (Swa.), Karir (Som.), Mtunguja mwitu (Swa.), Etulelo (Tur.), Ndula (Hehe), Etengoeddene (Lug.)

Description and ecology

Erect, multi-stemmed herb or softly woody shrub 0.5–1.8m high, sometimes up to 3m, often with prickles on stem, branches and leaves. **Leaves** simple, alternate, entire, oval to lance-shaped, 4–18 × 2–8cm, densely softly and velvety hairy, stalked. **Flowers** blue, purple or violet, rarely white, solitary or in few-flowered axillary racemes. **Fruit** a round berry, yellow, becoming blackish brown when ripe, 18–40mm in diameter. **Seeds** numerous, 3.5 × 3mm, lentil-shaped, pale yellow-brown. Common throughout East Africa as an invasive weed in disturbed and overgrazed grasslands, on waste ground, along margins of riverine and evergreen forest and in eroded soil along roadsides, at 0–2,300m.

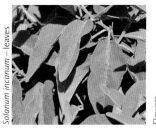

Solanum incanum – leaves

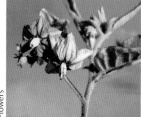

Flowers

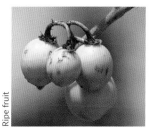

Ripe fruit

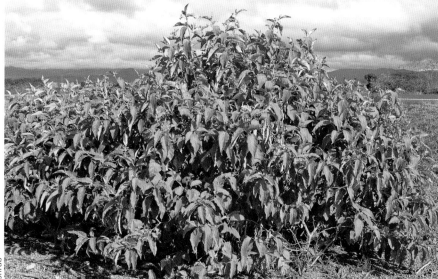

Shrub

PARTS USED Roots, leaves and fruits.

TRADITIONAL MEDICINAL USES Roots are used to alleviate toothache. A decoction of roots is taken for fever, dyspepsia, stomach ache, colic and indigestion.[M1] Infusions of leaves are administered as a remedy for earache[M4] and as a topical application for snakebite.[M1] Fruit pulp is applied to warts, rashes, burns, benign tumours, ulcers, bleeding wounds, fresh cuts and for toothache,[M112, M115] as well as to fungal afflictions, ringworm and other skin ailments.[M4, M70, M112, M115] Though poisonous, fruits are sometimes given to children as an emetic. A leaf infusion can be used as an eye bath to treat ophthalmia.[M115] To treat snakebite, a decoction of roots is drunk, the roots are chewed and the sap is swallowed, and chewed young leaves or pulped fresh roots are applied externally to the bite wound.[M115] Infusions of leaves or flowers are used as eardrops to soothe inflammation.[M112, M115]

PREPARATION AND DOSAGE

WARTS, BLEEDING WOUNDS, RASHES AND RINGWORM Apply fresh fruit pulp directly to affected areas of the skin.

EARACHE Crush a few fresh leaves and steep in half a cup of warm water for 20–30 minutes. Drain the mixture and apply as eardrops.

ABDOMINAL PAIN, FEVER AND INDIGESTION Boil 5g of pounded fresh roots in a litre of water for 10 minutes. Cool and filter the decoction. Drink a cup 3 times a day.

b. *Solanum nigrum* Indigenous

Common names Black Nightshade, Blackberry Nightshade • **Local names** Managu (Emb.), Munavu (Gir.), Kitulu / Ndulu (Kam.), Manangu (Kik., Mer.), Isoiyot (Kip.), Rinagu (Kis.), Namasaka / Litsusa / Yimboka (Luh.), Osuga (Luo), Ormomoi (Maa.), Ksoya (Pok.), Gengalat (Ren.), Imomoi (Sam.), Mnavu / Mnafu (Swa.), Ndunda (Tai.), Kisuchot (Tug.), Esuja / Abune (Tur.), Ocuga (Ach.), Piludi (Guj.), Mako (Hind.), Kachmach (Punj.)

Description and ecology

Erect, herbaceous, short-lived herb or perennial shrub 0.4–1m high or more. Stems sparsely hairy or sometimes hairless, rough, green or purplish green when young. **Leaves** simple, alternate, soft, slightly hairy or hairless, oval to heart-shaped, margin toothed, stalk 1–3cm long. **Flowers** small, star-shaped, greenish white or white, borne in several-flowered terminal clusters in leaf axils. **Fruit** a round berry 5–8mm in diameter, dull green, maturing to dull black or purplish black. **Seeds** numerous, yellowish, kidney-shaped, 1.5mm × 1mm. Widespread in East Africa, growing with other weeds on cultivated lands, disturbed lands, in waste areas, under shade trees and along fences, at 0–2,600m.

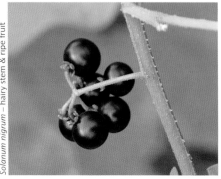

Solanum nigrum – hairy stem & ripe fruit

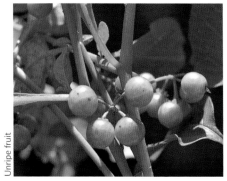

Unripe fruit

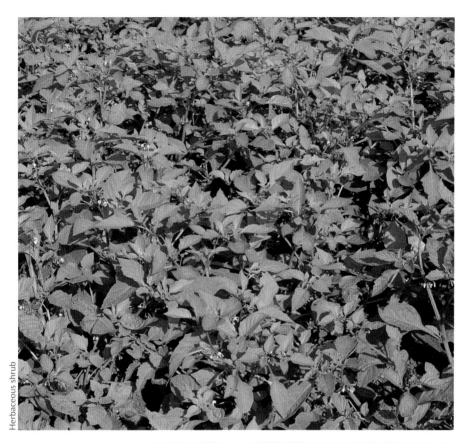

Herbaceous shrub

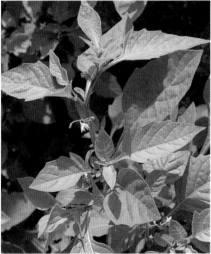

Leaves

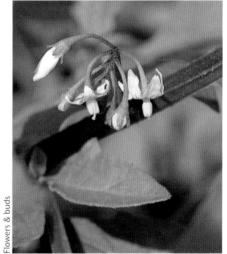

Flowers & buds

PARTS USED Roots, leaves and fruits.

TRADITIONAL MEDICINAL USES Leaves are a remedy for stomach ache.[M3, M70] Fresh leaf juice is a remedy for oedema of the liver (usually in cases of jaundice), the gall bladder, stomach, intestines or the uterus.[M7] Leaf and fruit extracts are taken for tonsillitis. Fresh leaves, stems and roots are used externally as a poultice and wash in the treatment of cancerous sores, boils, leucoderma and wounds.[M112] Fruit or leaf juice is applied to infected skin ulcers, wounds and eczema. Fruits are used to treat dysentery, stomach ulcers and abdominal pain.[M70] Ripe fruit serves as an aphrodisiac, a diuretic and a laxative; a paste of unripe fruit is applied as a poultice to treat headache and ringworm.[M112] Unripe fruits are used to relieve toothache and are also applied to ease a baby's teething pains.[M3, M70] Roots boiled in milk are given to children as a tonic.

PREPARATION AND DOSAGE

TOOTHACHE AND PAINFUL GUMS Squeeze some juice from unripe fruits onto an aching tooth or rub it onto the painful gums of a teething baby. Do not use internally.
SKIN ULCERS, WOUNDS AND ECZEMA Squeeze some juice from fresh fruits or leaves and apply directly to the affected areas, or use pounded fresh leaves, stems and roots externally as a poultice.

> ⚠ **WARNING!** Fruits and aerial parts of all species of *Solanum* can have strong toxic effects if ingested in high doses. Internal use is not recommended for pregnant women or for people with heart or respiratory conditions.

PHARMACOLOGICAL PROPERTIES

Antihyperglycaemic,[P428] antitumour,[P429] antimalarial[P147] and anti-ulcer[P381] activities are ascribed to some species of *Solanum*. Symptoms of high doses of aerial parts of these plants might include stupefaction, staggering, dilation of the pupils, convulsions and paralysis of both body and respiratory muscles.[P430]

COMPOUNDS REPORTED

Compounds isolated from species of *Solanum* include sapogenins (e.g. diosgenin[P431] and neochlorogenin[P432]) from fruits, phenylpropanoids (e.g. caffeic acid[P433] and chlorogenic acid) from leaves, and flavonoids (e.g. astragalin[P433]) and proteids (e.g. 2-aminoadipic acid) [P434] from aerial parts. The seeds contain triterpenoids, including daturaolone.[P435] Steroidal alkaloids such as solasodine occur in *S. incanum*.[P17] Saponins were identified as the active principles conferring antimicrobial effects of extracts of roots of *S. nigrum*. The plant has also been described as an anticancer, anticonvulsant, hepatoprotective and anti-inflammatory agent.[P436]

Diosgenin

Chlorogenic acid

a. *Syzygium cordatum* — Indigenous

Common names Waterberry Tree, Cordate Syzygium, Waterwood • **Local names** Muziahi / Muzihae (Dig.), Muriru / Mukoe / Ngoe (Kik.), Muvuena / Kivueni (Kam.), Lemeyet (Kip.), Omosambarao (Kis.), Kumusemwa / Musioma / Omusemwa / Tsisirnya (Luh.), Mukutan achak (Luo), Oloiragai / Ololobironi (Maa.), Muriru / Mukui (Mbe.), Reper / Reperwo (Pok.), Lamulii / Lairakai / Ngilenyai (Sam.), Mkarafuu / Msambarau / Mzambarau wa mwitu / Myamayu (Swa.), Musu (Tai.), Muhulo / Muhuu (Gogo), Mugege (Haya), Muvengi / Lulenga (Hehe), Mshihwi / Msungudi (Samb.), Kasyamongo (Nyam.), Mpegele (Nyak.), Mondoyanjoghu (Nyat.), Msungunde (Ngu.), Mlama (Pare), Msuharu (Ran.), Mzeze (Zin.), Kanzironziro / Muziti (Lug.), Anigo / Kuzu (Lugb.), Chiemo / Sizanzass / Wandiviri (Lugi.), Mutuli (Lugw.), Kano (Luo-Ug.), Mufumba / Mukondo (Ruki.), Munyabarika / Musimangwa (Runyan.), Lemaiyua / Reberwo (Sebei-Ug.)

Description and ecology

Evergreen, medium-sized tree 8–15(–20)m tall and with a rounded or spreading crown on a short, thick trunk, sometimes a flowering shrub. **Bark** dark brown, rough and fissured. **Leaves** numerous near ends of branches, simple, opposite, oblong to circular, 4–12 × 2–6cm, leathery, blue-green above, paler green below, leaf base heart-shaped, margin entire, young leaves reddish. **Flowers** in dense, many-flowered, terminal clusters, pink-white with conspicuous fluffy stamens, fragrant. **Fruit** fleshy, oval berries, 1.3–1.8cm long, green, turning deep purple-black when ripe, 1-seeded. Seed whitish. Growing near water, along streams, in swampy areas, in riverine thickets and in forest margins, at 300–1,800(–2,400)m.

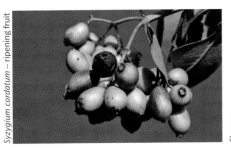

Syzygium cordatum – ripening fruit

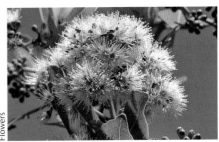

Flowers

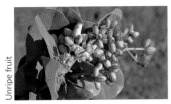

Unripe fruit

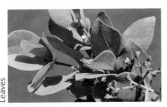

Leaves

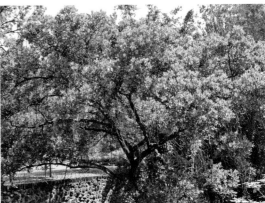

Tree

PARTS USED Roots, bark and leaves.
TRADITIONAL MEDICINAL USES Various parts of the plant are often used in traditional medicine. A decoction of roots is drunk as a treatment for amenorrhoea.M115 Infusions of roots or bark are used for stomach ache, indigestion and diarrhoea.M1, M2, M3, M91, M116 Leaf infusions also serve as a purgative and are used to treat diarrhoea, stomach problems and coughs.M91 Decoctions of root bark and stem bark are taken for the treatment of malaria.M115 Fresh or dried ground leaves, bark and roots are steeped in water and then applied externally as a poultice.M112, M115 Bark is emetic and can be used for diarrhoea, stomach problems, headache and amenorrhoea, and also for wounds and respiratory problems.M112, M115

PREPARATION AND DOSAGE
STOMACH ACHE AND INDIGESTION Steep a handful of pounded fresh bark or roots in a litre of cold water. Stir, filter and drink a cup of the mixture 3 times a day after meals.
DIARRHOEA Steep 3g of pounded fresh young leaves in a cup of cold water for 15 minutes. Strain the mixture and take a third of it 3 times a day.

b. *Syzygium cuminii*

Native to India, Pakistan, Myanmar, Sri Lanka, Philippines

Common names Java Plum, Jambolan, Indian Blackberry • **Local names** Mzambarau / Zambarau (Dig., Gir., Swa.), Jamna (Luo), Lushanaku (Haya), Jambura / Jambu (Guj.), Jamun / Jaman (Hind., Punj., Urd.)

Description and ecology

Evergreen, compact, fast-growing tree 10–15m tall but can reach 30m, with bole straight, short, usually 0.6–1m in diameter, with low, leafy branches and dense foliage. **Bark** brown and rough, cracking and flaking with age. **Leaves** simple, opposite, large and oval, smooth and shiny, tip pointed, aromatic when crushed, older leaves glossy dark green above, lighter green below, young leaves pinkish or reddish. **Flowers** small, scented, in clusters, white at first, becoming rose-pink, rapidly shed,

remains with many stamens. **Fruits** round or oblong berries, 1.3–4cm long, green at first, becoming deep purple or nearly black when ripe, with thin, smooth, glossy skin and purple or purplish-white pulp, very juicy, edible, 1-seeded. **Seed** up to 4cm long, oblong, green or brown. In India and Pakistan, medicinal use of this tree goes back over more than a century. Considered a naturalised fruit tree in East Africa, cultivated for its fruits and grown in garden compounds and backyards, also along avenues, at 0–1,800m.

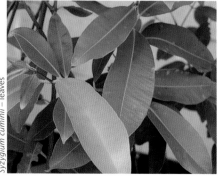

Syzygium cuminii – leaves

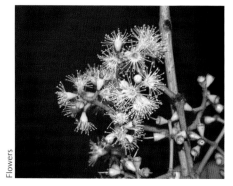

Flowers

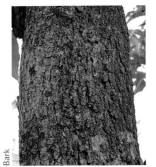

Bark

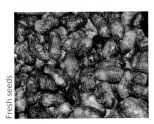

Fresh seeds

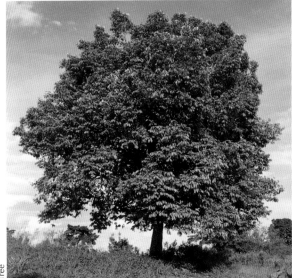

Tree

PARTS USED All parts except flowers.

TRADITIONAL MEDICINAL USES Fruit kernels are used as a remedy for colic, diarrhoea, dysentery, diabetes[M7, M111, M123] and high blood pressure.[M66] Young leaf shoots are also used for diarrhoea. Fresh leaves are taken to treat leucorrhoea.[M10] Stem bark can be used as an astringent, possibly helping to heal bleeding gums and treat mouth ulcers[M111] and fresh wounds.[M7] Ripe fruit may be used as a treatment for diabetes[M111] and is also eaten as a tonic and for treating stomach, liver or spleen ailments. Dry seeds help to stop nosebleeds. Fresh root and bark decoctions are taken as a purgative.[M4, M123] Fresh or dried aerial parts are used for treating diabetes and diarrhoea.[M112, M123] A dried or fresh bark infusion is taken orally as a remedy for dysentery, irregular menstruation and diarrhoea.[M111]

PREPARATION AND DOSAGE

DIABETES AND DIARRHOEA Take a teaspoon of powdered dry fruit kernels in the morning and evening. A mixture of half a teaspoon of kernel powder with half a teaspoon of mango kernel powder can be taken twice a day. To stop diarrhoea, steep 5g of pounded fresh leaf shoots in half a litre of water, strain and take 2 or 3 times daily.

WEAK OR BLEEDING GUMS Boil a handful of fresh bark in half a litre of water for 10–15 minutes. Use the warm decoction as a mouthwash to strengthen the teeth and gums.

WOUNDS AND NOSEBLEEDS Use finely ground seeds as snuff powder to stop nosebleeds or as a dusting powder to stop bleeding from wounds.

DYSENTERY Mix 3g of dry bark powder in half a cup of plain yogurt and take 3 times daily for 2 days. Alternatively, prepare and drink a decoction of bark boiled in water.

LEUCORRHOEA Chew two fresh young leaves with cold water for 3 or 4 days.

WARNING! Ripe *Syzygium cuminii* fruits have nutritional attributes but can cause abdominal pain when eaten in large quantities on an empty stomach. They are best eaten after meals and with a little added salt.

c. *Syzygium guineense* Indigenous

Common names Woodland Waterberry, Water Pear, Waterberry • **Local names** Kada (Bor.), Muziahi / Mugiaki (Dig.), Muvueni / Kivuena (Kam.), Mukoe / Ngoe (Kik.), Lamaiyat (Kip.), Kumusitole / Busitole / Obusitole / Omusitole (Luh.), Oleragai / Olairagai (Maa.), Lamayuet / Lemaiyua (Mar., Nan.), Lamaiwa / Lamaiyua (Pok.), Lairakai / Lamulii (Sam.), Mzuari / Mzambarau (Swa.Ken.), Musu / Mkongo (Tai.), Mase (Tav.), Lomoiwo / Lamack / Lamaywet (Tug.), Msadi / Mmasai (Chag.), Muhulo / Muhuu (Gogo), Mchwezi (Haya), Muvengi (Hehe), Msalazi (Lugu.), Msengele (Nyak.), Kasyammongo / Mzambalawe (Nyam.), Mlama (Pare), Mkamati / Mkomati (Ran.), Mshiwi / Mschichui / Muhula (Samb.), Mzuari (Swa.Ken.), Mzambarau mwitu / Mzuari (Swa.Tan.), Muvenge / Muwenge (Zig.), Msangura / Mgege (Zin.), Kalunginsavu / Muziti (Lug.), Anigo / Amigo (Lugb.), Chiemo / Wandiviri / Garaviri (Lugi.), Kano (Luo-A), Ozu / Ologua (Madi), Mugote / Mufumba (Ruki.) Musimangwa (Runyan.).

Description and ecology
Medium-sized to large, evergreen forest tree 15–20m tall but can reach 25m, with a broad trunk, dense, heavy, rounded crown and drooping branches. **Bark** smooth when young, turning black, dark brown, rough and flaking with age. **Leaves** simple, opposite, 4–12 × 2–6cm, lance-shaped to slightly oval, mature leaves glossy dark green, shiny and smooth on both surfaces, stalk 0.2–2.0cm long, slightly fragrant when crushed, young leaves purple-red. **Flowers** creamy white, borne in heads up to 10 × 10cm, in dense clusters of terminal panicles, sweetly scented. **Fruits** oval drupes 1.3–3cm long, borne in bunches, shiny, purple-black, juicy, edible, 1-seeded. **Seeds** round, 1.3–1.4cm in diameter, yellowish to brownish. Prefers moist soils on a high water table in riverine forest, lowland rain forest and wooded grassland, at 0–2,100m.

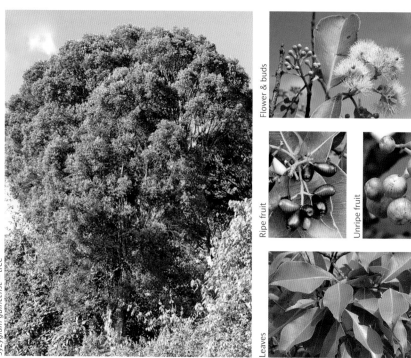

Syzygium guineense – tree

Flower & buds

Ripe fruit

Unripe fruit

Leaves

PARTS USED Roots, stem bark, leaves, twigs and fruit.
TRADITIONAL MEDICINAL USES A decoction of twigs and leaves can be used as an enema and drunk for its purgative properties and against colic, diarrhoea and abdominal pain;[M91, M115] it is also taken orally for amenorrhoea and cerebral malaria.[M115] Root and stem bark infusions are drunk for stomach ache and also as a laxative, anthelmintic and purgative.[M4, M70, M91, M112] Bark infusions are taken for infertility.[M70] A root infusion may be taken by drinking and bathing to treat epilepsy.[M115] A bark decoction or infusion can be a remedy for stomach ache, diarrhoea, malaria, intestinal worms, a cough, asthma and throat problems.[M91, M115] Fruits are eaten as a treatment for dysentery.[M91, M115]

PREPARATION AND DOSAGE
STOMACH ACHE AND AS AN ANTHELMINTIC Mix 5g of pounded fresh bark and 5g of pounded fresh roots in a litre of cold water. Stir, filter and drink a cup of the infusion 3 times a day.

PHARMACOLOGICAL PROPERTIES
Seeds of *Syzygium cuminii* produce antibacterial activities,[P437] while leaves show antifungal activity against *Cryptococcus neoformans*.[P438] Experiments with seeds, bark and fruit have shown that *S. cuminii* reduces glycaemia in different animal models.[P439] Clinical human trials, though, have not shown any significant antiglycaemic activity.[P439] Fruit skin of *S. cuminii* shows significant antioxidant activity.[P440] Leaves of *S. guineense* produce antibacterial activity against some organisms.[P441] A short-term hypoglycaemic effect in rats of orally administered *S. cordatum* leaf extract has been reported. Findings suggest the leaf extract might be effective in treating mild diabetes mellitus or glucose tolerance impairment, but less effective in cases of severe hyperglycaemia.[P442] Triterpenes, including 6-hydroxyasiatic acid, oleanolic acid and ursolic acid, account for the antibacterial activity of leaves of some species of *Syzygium*.[P441, P442] C-methylated chalcones such as 2',4'-dihydroxy-3',5'-dimethyl-6'-methoxychalcone, isolated from *S. samarangense*, have produced cytotoxic activity against the SW-480 human colon cancer cell line. Quercetin and its glycosides account for the plant's antioxidant activities.[P443]

COMPOUNDS REPORTED
Constituents isolated from *S. cuminii* fruits include vitamin C, gallic acid, tannins and anthocyanins (cyanidin, petunidin and malvidin-glucoside).[P440, P445] Pulp and seed extracts from *S. samarangense* fruits elaborate C-methylated chalcones (including 2',4'-dihydroxy-3',5'-dimethyl-6'-methoxychalcone), quercetin and its glycosides (e.g. reynoutrin), a flavanone, (S)-pinocembrin, and two phenolic acids (gallic and ellagic acid).[P443, P445] Leaves of *Syzygium* species contain polyphenols and triterpenes such as arjunolic acid, asiatic acid, terminolic acid, 6-hydroxyasiatic acid,[P441] oleanolic acid and ursolic acid,[P442] all compounds triggering antibacterial activity.[P441, P442] The isocoumarin bergenin and its derivatives have shown antinociceptive, anti-arrhythmic, anti-oxidative, antimicrobial, hepatoprotective, gastric-ulcer-protective, anti-inflammatory, insulin-enhancing, lypolytic and wound-healing activities.[P444, P445]

Gallic acid

2',4'-Dihydroxy-3',5'-dimethyl-6'-methoxychalcone

Ursolic acid

Indigenous

Common names Tamarind, Tamarind Tree, Indian Sour Date • **Local names** Mukai (Bon.), Roka (Bor.), Mkwaju / Kwaju (Dig., Gir., Nyat., Ran.), Muthithi, Muthithu (Emb., Mer.), Kithumula / Kikwasu / Nzumula / Ngwasu (Kam.), Lamaiyat (Kip.), Kumukhuwa (Luh.), Ochwa / Chwaa (Luo), Oloisijoi (Maa.Ken.), Aron / Oron (Mar., Pok.), Muthithi (Mbe., Tha.), Limaiyua / Lamayuet (Nan.), Roqa (Orm.), Rogei (Sam.), Hamar / Raqee / Roghe (Som.), Mkwaju / Msisi / Ukwaju (Swa.), Mkwachu (Tai.), Mase / Muzumura (Tav.), Aryek / Arwe (Tug.), Epeduru (Tur.), Olmasambrai (Aru.), Moya / Mkakyi (Chag.), Msisi (Gogo, Nyam.), Mnyali / Munyali (Hehe), Mdai (Lugu.), Olmasambrai / Oloisijoi / Masamburai (Maa.Tan.), Nshishi / Mkwazu (Samb.), Bushishi / Nshishi (Suk.), Msisa (Zin.), Cwa (Ach.), Epeduru (Ate.), Cwao (Lan.), Mukoge (Lug.), Iti (Lugb., Madi), Mokoge / Nkoge (Luso.), Mukoge (Lugwe.), Epedura (Ngaka.), Mukoge / Munondo (Runy.), Nondwa (Ruto.), Imli (Hind., Punj., Urd.), Ambli (Guj.)

Description and ecology

Medium-sized, long-lived, slow-growing tree 12–18m tall, sometimes reaching 25–30m, with a dense, extensive, low-spreading crown, evergreen or deciduous in arid areas, bole up to 1m in diameter. **Bark** rough, dark grey-brown, strongly fissured. **Leaves** alternate, compound, feathery, with 10–20 pairs of small opposite leaflets, dull green, oblong, up to 3cm long, tips and bases rounded, with prominent veins, young leaves red. **Flowers** elongated, red and yellow with streaks of yellow, orange or red, borne in small, few-flowered racemes, buds red. **Fruit** a straight or curved legume pod, 10–12 × 2–3cm, indehiscent, green, maturing to rusty brown, shell brittle. **Seeds** 3–10 per pod, brownish black, shiny, smooth, hard-textured. Adaptable, drought resistant and hardy, it is widespread in semi-arid areas and wooded grassland, often along rivers and streams in dry areas, at 0–1,600m.

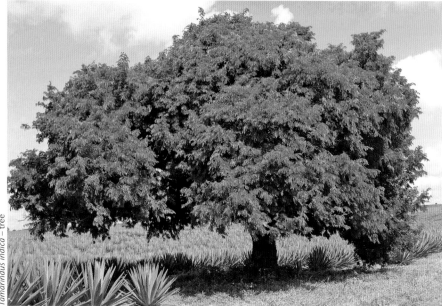

Tamarindus indica – tree

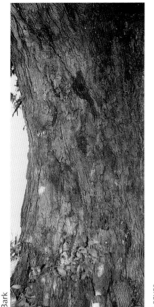
Bark

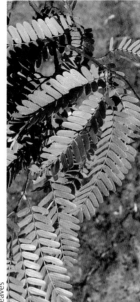
Leaves

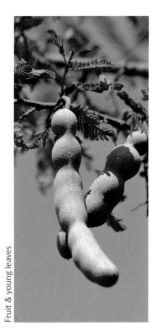
Fruit & young leaves

USAGE AND TREATMENT

PARTS USED All parts.

TRADITIONAL MEDICINAL USES A root decoction is taken for coughs and fever.[M1, M4, M112] Leaves and fruits are used as a laxative. Fruit pulp may also be used as a mild laxative and to treat scurvy.[M111, M112] Decoctions of dried fruit peel are also beneficial as laxatives.[M10] A leaf infusion is taken for stomach ache[M3] and for expelling intestinal worms.[M9, M70] Leaves are applied as an astringent to skin infections[M6] and to inflamed eyes.[M3] Leaves and fruits are taken as mild laxatives[M4] and are eaten to remedy constipation,[M3, M70] to reduce fever, for relief from nausea, to avoid vomiting during pregnancy,[M7] to reduce blood sugar levels, for relief from heart palpitations and to treat heart complaints.[M6] Fresh or raw fruits are eaten as an appetiser, as a digestive aid and as a tonic to boost energy.[M7] Seed kernels are used to treat spermatorrhoea and premature ejaculation as well as dysentery and diarrhoea.[M7] A leaf decoction is taken for malaria[M4, M70] and to treat throat infection, coughs, fever and intestinal worms.[M111] Leaf juice is taken for diarrhoea. A hot-water extract of trunk bark is taken for amenorrhoea. Poultices of dried bark powder can relieve sores, ulcers, boils and rashes.[M111]

PREPARATION AND DOSAGE

SPERMATORRHOEA AND PREMATURE EJACULATION Roast some seeds in the oven. Shell and then grind them to a powder. Take a tablespoon of powder with a cup of milk every morning before breakfast.

DYSENTERY AND DIARRHOEA Take a tablespoon of powdered seed kernels with a cup of water 3 times a day.

INDIGESTION, AS AN ENERGISER, AS AN APPETISER, FOR FEVER, NAUSEA AND VOMITING Peel some ripe fruit and remove the seeds from the pith. Steep 10g of pith in a litre of hot water for 15 minutes. Filter, sweeten with sugar, jaggery or honey and drink twice a day.

STOMACH ACHE AND INTESTINAL WORMS Steep 30g of crushed fresh young leaves in a litre of water. Drink a cup of the mixture after meals 3 times daily for 2 days.

PHARMACOLOGICAL PROPERTIES

Methanolic extracts of pericarps and seeds of *Tamarindus indica* have shown a significant antioxidant capacity.[P446] Leaves show anthelmintic and vermifugal properties and astringent effects.[P84, P221] Fruits show mild choleretic and cholagogic effects and are recommended for liver and gall bladder disorders, also for helping to empty the gall bladder.[P84] Dried fruits, dried stem bark and leaves produce antimalarial activity against *Plasmodium falciparum*.[P79, P303] Antiviral,[P447] antifungal[P448] and antibacterial[P449] activities have been reported for bark and dried fruits.

COMPOUNDS REPORTED

Seeds of *T. indica* are a rich source of catechin, a flavonoid, and its monomeric, dimeric and trimeric derivatives.[P446] Fruits are rich in vitamin C,[P84, P221] sugar (60–65%) and organic acids such as citric, malic and tartaric acid, and also contain pectin.[P79, P84] Other compounds isolated from species of *Tamarindus* include benzenoids (e.g. 3,4-dihydroxybenzoic acid) from seeds,[P450] sesquiterpenes (e.g. aromadendrene) from fruit pulp,[P451] and oxygen heterocycles (including 2-acetylfuran) from fruits.[P452] Fixed oil from seeds contains a mixture of glycerides of saturated and unsaturated (oleic, linoleic) acids.[P79, P446] Seeds of *T. indica* appear to be important sources of potential cancer chemopreventive natural products, including the procyanidins and flavonoids.[P446]

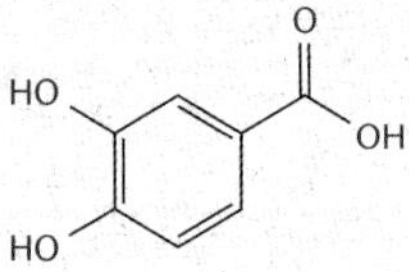

3,4-Dihydroxybenzoic acid 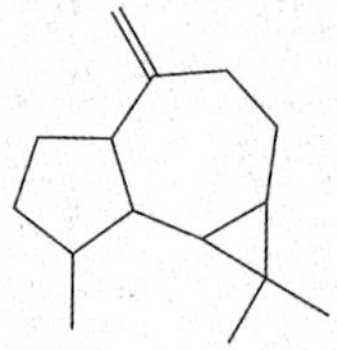   Aromadendrene 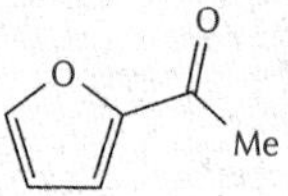   2-Acetylfuran

Indigenous

Common names Leleshwa Bush, Camphor Bush • **Local names** Kileleshwa / Mururicua (Kik.), Lelechuet (Kip., Tug.), Ol'leleshwa (Maa.), Mkalambati (Swa.), Elewa (Tug.)

Description and ecology
Medium-sized, much-branched, evergreen, bushy dioecious shrub or sometimes small tree 4–6(–8)m tall. **Bark** rough, greyish, fissured. **Leaves** narrowly elliptic, 1.5–4 × 1–3cm, green above, silvery white and covered with dense white hairs below, base rounded, apex pointed, margin entire or finely toothed, camphor-scented when crushed. **Flowers** unisexual, small, creamy white, bell-shaped, in heads 4–5mm across and clustered in large, leafy, terminal panicles 6–20cm long at ends of branches. **Fruits** small, with tiny seeds covered with dense, fluffy, cotton wool-like white hairs, strongly scented. Common in evergreen or semi-deciduous bushland, bushed grassland, woodland, wooded grassland, often on poorer, stony soils, at 1,200–2,300m.

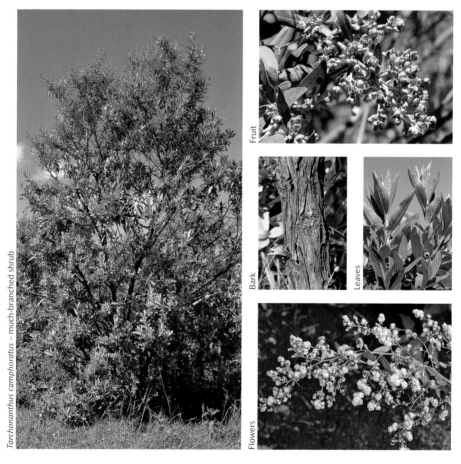

Tarchonanthus camphoratus – much-branched shrub

Fruit

Bark

Leaves

Flowers

PARTS USED Leaves and young twigs.

TRADITIONAL MEDICINAL USES Decoctions or mixtures of leaves and twigs are used for treating asthma, bronchitis, headache, abdominal disorders and toothache.[M4, M70, M116] Fresh leaves are applied to fresh cuts, wounds, bruises and fungal infections. Problems such as blocked sinuses and headache can be treated by inhaling the smoke from burning green leaves.[M116] Leaves contain essential oils found to be excellent cosmetic and dermatological remedies with soothing and anti-irritation effects on conditions such as sensitive skin, dermatitis, sunburn and bedsores.[M111]

PREPARATION AND DOSAGE

ASTHMA, BRONCHITIS AND HEADACHE Inhale smoke or fumes from fresh or dried aerial parts 3 times a day. Make a hot poultice from dry powdered leaves and twigs and apply over the chest, under a covering blanket. Steep 5g of crushed fresh leaves and branches in half a litre of cold water for 15 minutes. Filter and drink the infusion twice a day.

TOOTHACHE AND STOMACH AILMENTS Chew 2 or 3 fresh leaves twice daily. Steep 5g of crushed fresh leaves and branches in half a litre of cold water for 15 minutes. Filter and drink a third of the infusion 3 times a day after meals to relieve abdominal pain. For toothache, gargle the warm infusion.

CUTS, WOUNDS, BRUISES AND FUNGAL INFECTION Squeeze the juice from some fresh young leaves and apply directly to the affected areas.

PHARMACOLOGICAL PROPERTIES

Aerial parts of *Tarchonanthus camphoratus* show antispasmodic, decongestant and analgesic effects, ascribed to the volatile oil and to flavonoids.[P96] The essential oil shows antimicrobial activity against both Gram-positive and Gram-negative bacteria and against the pathogenic fungus *Candida albicans*. The monoterpenes 1,8-cineole, terpinen-4-ol and another minor monoterpene alcohol, linalool, have been linked with the antibacterial and antifungal activities of the essential oil.[P453]

COMPOUNDS REPORTED

Aerial parts of *T. camphoratus* contain the flavanone pinocembrin.[P454] The volatile oil contains very small concentrations of camphor.[P455] The monoterpenes fenchol, 1,8-cineole and α-terpineol are the main components of the essential oil.[P453] The presence of sesquiterpenes such as β-eudesmol has also been reported in the essential oil.[P453] Two sesquiterpenes were identified as antitrypanosomal principles in the aerial parts of *T. camphoratus*.[P456]

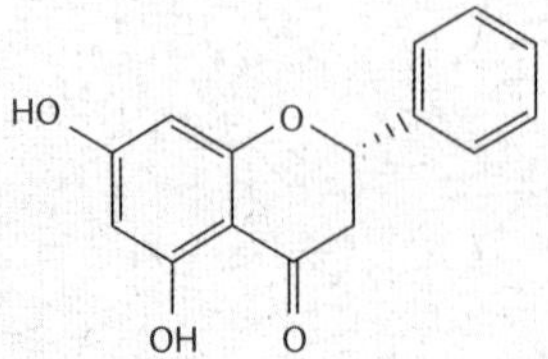

Pinocembrin

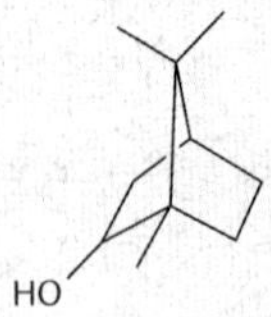

Fenchol

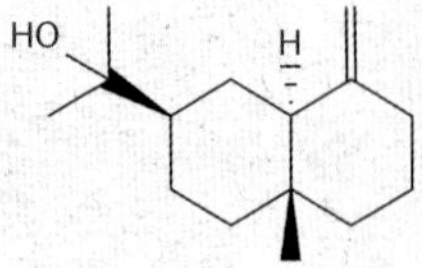

β-Eudesmol

Indigenous

Common names Toddalia, Orange Climber • **Local names** Chikombe za chui (Dig.), Mururue (Kik.), Maluia (Kam.), Luabare (Luh.), Ajua (Luo), Ole-barmonyo (Maa.), Kipkeres (Mar.), Mukongura (Mer.), Ketemwe (Tug.), Usuet (Nan.), Etokebengu (Tur.), Llaramunyo (Sam.)

Description and Ecology

Woody, climbing shrub or liana up to 10m in forests using other trees for support. Stems corky, stems, branches, twigs and underside of leaves covered with hooked prickles. **Leaves** shiny, dark green, 3-foliolately compound, leaflets oval, 3–8 × 1–3cm, hairless, strongly citrus-scented when crushed. **Flowers** greenish yellow, borne in axillary and terminal clusters. **Fruits** round, fleshy, orange-yellow berries 5–8mm in diameter, tasting like orange peel. **Seeds** dark brown, hard, smooth, up to 4mm long. Grows in coastal lowland areas, along forest margins, in riverine forest and grassland thickets, at 0–450m and 1,200–3,000m.

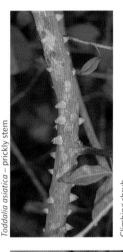

Toddalia asiatica – prickly stem

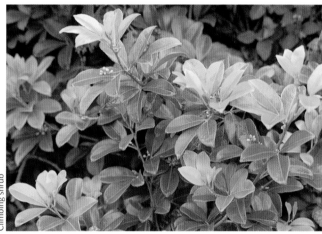

Climbing shrub

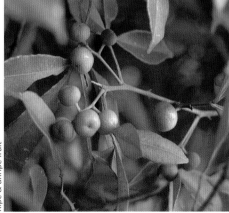

Ripe & unripe fruit

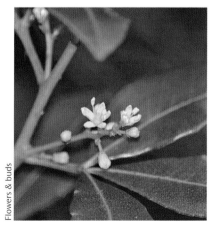

Flowers & buds

PARTS USED Roots, leaves, branches and fruit.

TRADITIONAL MEDICINAL USES Leaf infusions are used to treat malaria[M67, M44] and toothache,[M23] while also serving as an appetite restorer. Root decoctions are taken for gastrointestinal ailments,[M28] malaria,[M124] rheumatism, coughs and stomach ache[M124] and also as an anthelmintic,[M44] emetic and purgative. Infusions of dried root bark are used for fever.[M70, M124] Juice from roots is taken orally as an emetic and is also a remedy for paralysis caused by snakebite.[M1] Juice of a chewed fruit is a remedy for coughs and colds. Leaves and branches relieve nasal and bronchial pain,[M1, M70] diarrhoea, syphilis, cholera, lung diseases, toothache, pneumonia and fever.[M44]

PREPARATION AND DOSAGE

BRONCHITIS AND NASAL CONGESTION Boil some fresh leaves and branches in water and inhale the steam vapour.

EMETIC, PURGATIVE OR ANTHELMINTIC AND FOR STOMACH AILMENTS Boil a teaspoon or 5g of dry root powder in a cup of water for 10 minutes. Cool and filter. Drink a cup of the mixture twice a day.

MALARIA AND FEVER Boil a teaspoon of root or leaf powder in a cup of water for 10 minutes. Cool and filter. Drink a cup of the mixture twice daily.

PHARMACOLOGY AND CHEMISTRY

PHARMACOLOGICAL PROPERTIES

Antibacterial,[P118, P457] antifungal,[P457] vasorelaxation,[P458] antimalarial,[P459] antigiardiasis[P211] and diuretic[P460] properties have all been identified in different parts of *Toddalia* species. The alkaloid nitidine, isolated from *T. asiatica*, has shown potent antiplasmodial activity.[P461] The methanol extract of wood of *T. asiatica* has shown strong anti-platelet-aggregation activity, with chelerythrine identified as one of the active principles.[P462]

COMPOUNDS REPORTED

Underground parts of *T. asiatica* contain a number of triterpenes (e.g. β-amyrin),[P463] alkaloids (e.g. dihydroavicine)[P464] and coumarins (e.g. toddalenol).[P465] The coumarin flindersine, isolated from the leaves of *T. asiatica*, showed antibacterial and antifungal activity.[P466]

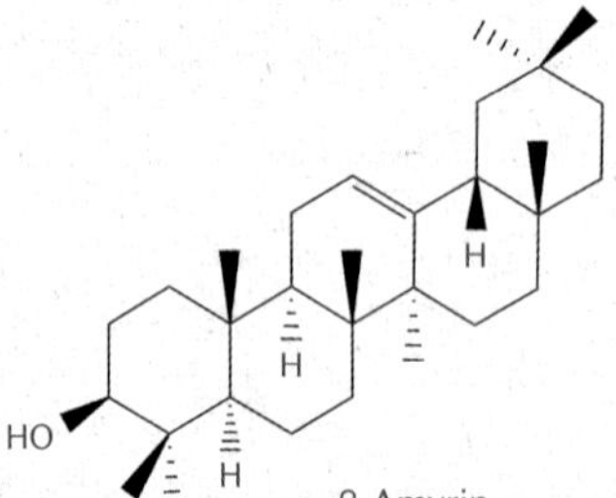

β-Amyrin

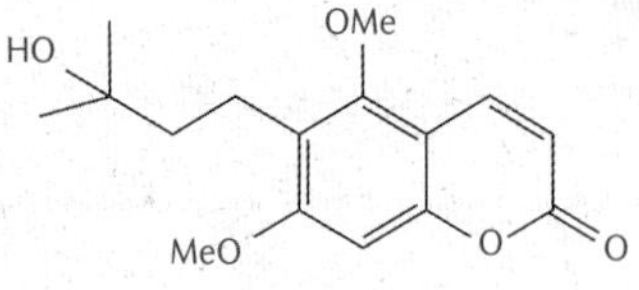

Toddalenol

81 *Trichilia emetica* MELIACEAE

Indigenous

Common names Trichilia, Cape Mahogany • **Local names** Anona (Bor.), Munwa-madzi (Dig., Gir.), Mururi (Kik.), Musambo / Mutuluku (Kam.), Ochond rateng' / Ohcond athuth (Luo), Munyama / Musinzi / Irojo (Luh.), Kurteswa (Mar.), Mutuati (Mer., Tha.), Muwamaji (Swa.Ken., Gir.), Soke (Orm.), Ilberi (Sam.), Ekuyen (Tur.), Korteswa (Pok.), Mchengo / Mututu / Mkongoni (Chag.), Nyembe mwitu (Gogo), Mtengotengo (Lugu.), Mgolimazi (Ngu., Samb., Zig.), Msanguti (Nyak.), Sungute (Suk.), Mkungwina / Mtimaji / Mtimai (Swa.Tan.), Sekoba (Lug.)

Description and ecology

Striking, medium-sized to large evergreen tree 15–21(–25)m tall, with dense, spreading crown and cylindrical bole up to 80cm in diameter, the trunk swollen at the base and fluted with age. **Bark** grey-brown or red-brown, corky and scaling with age. **Leaves** large, opposite or alternate, crowded near ends of branches and twigs, compound, with 3–5 pairs of leaflets plus a terminal one, 4–15 × 2.5–5cm, dark glossy green above, sparsely hairy below, tips pointed or rounded, margins smooth. **Flowers** creamy white to pale yellow-green, sweetly scented, in axillary cymes up to 10cm long. **Fruits** round, furry, grey-brown or red-brown capsules, 2.5–3cm in diameter, splitting into 3 or 4 parts, with 3–6 shiny black seeds, a fleshy orange-red aril covering the seeds. Common along riparian forests, swamp forests, rivers and in areas with a high water table. Prefers rich, well-drained soils. Found throughout East Africa at 0–1,850m.

USAGE AND TREATMENT

PARTS USED Stem bark, roots, leaves and seeds.

TRADITIONAL MEDICINAL USES A root decoction is taken for a cold, as a diuretic and to induce labour in pregnant women.[M1, M70] An infusion of pounded or unpounded bark can be used for pneumonia.[M1, M40, M70, M111] Decoctions of roots and bark combined are taken as a remedy for a cold, pneumonia and fever or as a purgative and for intestinal disorders.[M71, M112, M115] Bark, roots and leaves are used to treat intestinal complaints, including indigestion, dysentery and infestation with parasites.[M2] An infusion of bark, roots and leaves may help in the treatment of malaria.[M71] Leaf and seed poultices are applied to bruises, cuts and eczema.[M4, M70] Seed oil is applied to relieve rheumatism.[M111] An infusion of roots acts as an emetic.[M1, M33] Leaves are used for malaria. A decoction of powdered bark is a remedy for stomach and intestinal ailments.[M116] Oil obtained from grounded seeds is applied externally to treat leprosy, sores, ringworm and other skin diseases.[M111]

PREPARATION AND DOSAGE

SKIN AILMENTS (ECZEMA, BRUISING AND CUTS) Mix some pounded fresh leaves or seeds in water to form a paste. Apply directly to affected areas of the skin.

RHEUMATISM Rub seed oil onto affected areas.

PURGATIVE Boil 5g of dry root or leaf powder in a litre of water for 10 minutes. Cool, strain and drink a cup an hour before breakfast.

MALARIA AND FEVER Steep a handful of pounded fresh leaves, bark or roots in a litre of hot water for 15 minutes. Filter and drink a cup 2 or 3 times a day.

 WARNING! Roots may be lethal if consumed in excessive doses.

PHARMACOLOGY AND CHEMISTRY

PHARMACOLOGICAL PROPERTIES

The limonoids of *Trichilia* species are known for their insect antifeedant activities.[P467] Anti-inflammatory and antimicrobial activities against some organisms have also been reported.[P96] Leaves of *T. emetica* show antiplasmodial activity against both chloroquine-sensitive (Dd2) and chloroquine-resistant (3D7) strains of *Plasmodium falciparum*.[P303] The complement activating effect reported for the leaf water extract may accelerate the healing of burns and wounds.[P468] Antipyretic activity has been confirmed, vindicating traditional use of this plant as an antipyretic agent.[P469]

COMPOUNDS REPORTED

Several limonoids such as trichilin A and dregeanin have been isolated from the seed oil of *Trichilia* species.[P467, P470, P471] Root bark of *T. emetica* also contains trichilin A.[P467] Limonoids isolated from *T. emetica* are responsible for the anticancer, hepatoprotective activity. The plant also shows antioxidant, antitrypanosomal, anticonvulsant, antiplasmodial, antischistosomal, anti-inflammatory and antimicrobial activities.[P472]

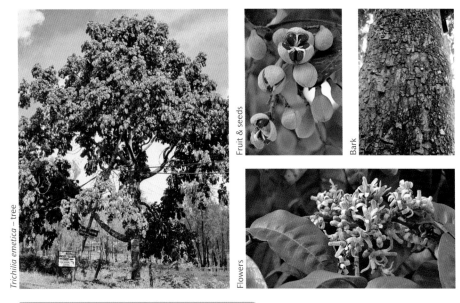

Trichilin A   Dregeanin

Native to southern Europe and Mediterranean region

Common name Fenugreek • **Local name** Methi (Guj., Hind., Punj., Urd.)

Description and ecology

Smooth, erect annual herb 40–80cm tall, all parts infused with strong aroma. **Leaves** alternate, 3-foliolately compound, leaflets oval, 2–3.5cm long, hairy below. **Flowers** whitish or yellow, irregular, butterfly-like, either solitary or in axillary pairs. **Fruits** straight or sickle-shaped pods 2–6(–8)cm long, thin, narrow, pointed, green to brown. **Seeds** 10–20 per pod, oblong or square, yellow to amber or brownish, with strong spicy odour when pounded. Grows optimally in full sun, in well-drained soils in areas with annual temperature ranges of 10–27°C and annual rainfall of 400–1,500mm. Cultivated as an annual herb and sold at most vegetable markets in East African cities. A long-standing favourite herb among Arabs and widely used in Indian cooking as well, the leaves as a vegetable and the seeds in curries and pickles.

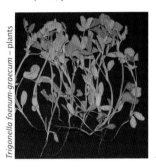

Trigonella foenum-graecum – plants

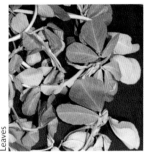

Leaves

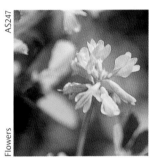

AS247

Flowers

USAGE AND TREATMENT

PARTS USED Fresh leaves and seeds.

TRADITIONAL MEDICINAL USES Leaves are used for colds, coughs, asthma and rheumatism as well as for relieving constipation and haemorrhoids.[M7, M70] Seeds are a remedy for constipation, indigestion,[M25] coughs and asthma.[M7] Seeds are also a prized remedy for anaemia, lack of appetite, weight gain and stomach ailments.[M7, M9, M25, M70] Seed powder is applied locally to reduce haemorrhoid inflammation, for pain relief in cases of inflamed or aching joints, in arthritis or rheumatism, and for healing wounds, skin ulcers, cracked lips or nipples, abscesses, furuncles and infected sores.[M9, M70]

PREPARATION AND DOSAGE

COUGHS, COLDS, ASTHMA AND RHEUMATISM Boil a tablespoon of seed powder in a cup of water for 10 minutes. Strain, sweeten with honey or brown sugar and drink a cup of the mixture 3 times a day. Alternatively, cook 250g of leaves and young twigs for 5 minutes with a little oil and a pinch of salt and eat as a vegetable with meals. Another option is to mix 1g of seed powder with half a teaspoon of honey and take it 3 times a day after meals.

ARTHRITIS, RHEUMATISM, WOUNDS, SKIN ULCERS, CRACKED LIPS OR NIPPLES, ABSCESSES, FURUNCLES AND INFECTED SORES Grind some seeds into a fine powder. Add hot water to make a paste and apply as a warm poultice over the affected areas.

HAEMORRHOIDS Apply the previous preparation of powdered seeds as a cold poultice directly to the anus.

PHARMACOLOGICAL PROPERTIES

Mucilage in fenugreek seeds has a mild laxative and emollient effect that aids the digestive process;[P84] seeds also have a carminative effect that is helpful for dyspepsia.[P156] Seeds contain significant amounts of protein, minerals and vitamins, and are recommended for promoting weight gain in cases of anaemia.[P84]

COMPOUNDS REPORTED

Major constituents found in fenugreek seeds include trigonelline, choline, flavone pigments, lecithin and phytosterols.[P156] Seeds are very rich in assimilated protein (27% by mass) and mucilage (30% by mass) as well as in minerals (iron, phosphorus, sulfur) and vitamins.[P84] Seeds contain steroidal sapogenins, most notably diosgenin. Two furostanol glycosides have also been recorded.[P17] Phenolic acids (e.g. 3-coumaric acid) and flavonoid glycosides (e.g. apigenin-7-O-glycoside), which are found in *Trigonella foenum-graecum*, were proposed to be responsible for most of its antioxidant properties.[P473]

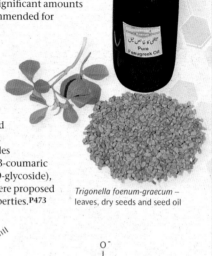

Trigonella foenum-graecum – leaves, dry seeds and seed oil

Diosgenin

Trigonelline

a. *Vepris nobilis (Teclea nobilis)* Indigenous

Common names Teclea, Three-leaved Teclea • **Local names** Munderendu (Kik.), Keryot / Kuriot (Kip.), Mutavo / Kumutare (Luh.), Odar / Ondat / Midat (Luo), Ol-gelai (Maa.), Lugumwa (Mar.), Muteratu (Mer.), Kurion (Pok.), Ekodek (Tur.), Kerionded (Nan.), L'gilai (Sam.), Kurionde (Tug.), Mlimang'ombe (Chag.), Omuzo (Haya), Mwatatsi / Mputsa (Hehe), Mdimudimu / Mulungsigiti (Nyam.), Kilongolo / Nkwaati (Samb.), Mju (Suk.), Muzo (Zin.), Ejorio / Ekude (Ate.), Nzo (Lug.), Lutati (Lugi.), Mudati (Lugw.), Nakamole (Lugwe.), Mugangwe (Luny.), Achacha / Atachogat (Luo-A), Oya (Luo-J), Achacho (Luo-L), Luzu (Luso.), Muzo (Ruki., Runyan., Runy., Ruto.), Gurio (Sebei)

Description and ecology
Evergreen shrub or tree 2–12m tall but reaching 20m in wet forests, with a crooked trunk and spreading crown. **Bark** smooth and grey, with ring marks, branches hairless. **Leaves** alternate, rarely subopposite, 3-foliolately compound, leaflets 5–15cm long, hairless, shiny dark green, tips pointed, edges smooth, leaf stalk 1.5–6(–8)cm long. **Flowers** creamy yellow-green, small, sweetly scented, in loose terminal or axillary sprays 12(–15)cm long. **Fruit** a round or ellipsoid drupe, 6–8 × 5–6mm, in large clusters, orange-red, smooth, becoming wrinkled, 1-seeded. Seed oval, 5–6mm long. Widespread in wet evergreen highland forests but also in bushland, in thickets on rocky hills, in riverine forest and wooded grassland, at 900–2,700m.

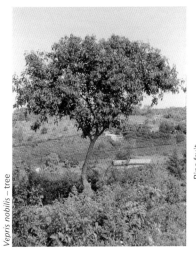

Vepris nobilis – tree

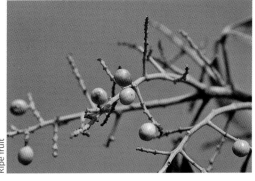

Ripe fruit

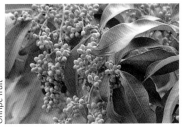

Unripe fruit

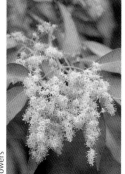

Flowers

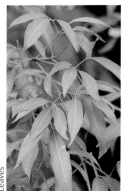

Leaves

PARTS USED Roots, stem bark, leaves and twigs.
TRADITIONAL MEDICINAL USES Bark or leaf decoctions are used to treat malaria.M112 Leaves and twigs are used for treating fever.M70, M115 Roots are taken as an anthelmintic.M115 Decoctions of leaves and roots are used for pneumonia and rheumatism.M1, M70, M115 A decoction of dried twigs is taken for syphilis.M30

PREPARATION AND DOSAGE
FEVER Boil some leaves in water. Inhale the steam vapour.
PNEUMONIA AND RHEUMATISM Boil 5 crushed fresh leaves or 5g of crushed fresh roots in half a litre of water for 10 minutes. Cool and filter the mixture, then sweeten with a little honey or jaggery. Drink a cup twice a day.
ANTHELMINTIC Steep 8g of crushed fresh roots in half a litre of warm water for 15 minutes. Drink a cup 3 times daily after meals.
MALARIA Boil 5g of crushed fresh bark or 5 crushed fresh leaves in half a litre of water for 10 minutes. Cool and filter the mixture, then sweeten with honey or jaggery. Drink a cup twice a day.

b. *Vepris simplicifolia (Teclea simplicifolia)*　　　Indigenous

Common names Teclea, Simple-leaved Teclea • **Local names** Munderendu (Kik.), Mike (Bor.), Muchimi wa tsakani (Dig.), Keryot / Kuriot (Kip., Mar.), Muretu (Mer.), Kurionde (Tug.), Edapalakuyen (Tur.), Ol-gelai (Maa.), Lgelai / Ngolei orok (Sam.)

Description and ecology
Small, much-branched, evergreen shrub or tree 2–5(–12)m tall, much taller in rain forest, with a spreading crown. **Bark** smooth, dark grey, branchlets hairless. **Leaves** simple, smooth, shiny dark green, oblong-elliptic, 5–15cm long, apex pointed, base narrowly cuneate. **Flowers** greenish yellow, small, fragrant, in axillary and terminal panicles. **Fruit** an orange or red drupe, 6–8 × 5–6mm, round or ellipsoid, becoming wrinkled. Seed ovoid, 5.5–6mm long. Common in dry mixed lowland forest, riverine and lower montane thicket or woodland, at 800–2,300m. Commonly associated with *Podocarpus* and *Juniperus*.

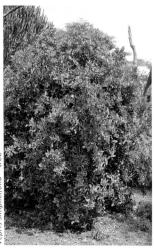

Vepris simplicifolia – tree

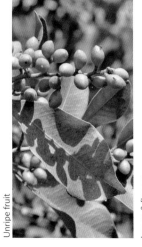

Unripe fruit

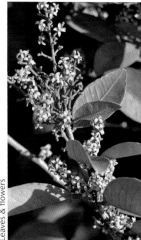

Leaves & flowers

PARTS USED Bark, roots and leaves.
TRADITIONAL MEDICINAL USES Roots are used as an anthelminthic.[M111] Steam inhalation of leaves reportedly cures fever. A bark decoction is drunk to treat chest complaints.[M115] Bark and leaf decoctions are taken for malaria, hepatitis and pleurisy.[M4, M70] A leaf or root decoction mixed with honey can be used for coughs and pneumonia.[M111] Leaf ash is applied externally as treatment against leprosy.[M112, M115] A root decoction may used to treat stomach ache, backache, leprosy and gonorrhoea.[M112, M115]

PREPARATION AND DOSAGE

MALARIA Boil 5g of crushed fresh bark or 5 crushed fresh leaves in half a litre of water for 10 minutes. Cool and filter the mixture, then sweeten with honey or jaggery. Drink a cup twice a day.
ANTHELMINTIC AND STOMACH ACHE Boil 6–8g of crushed fresh roots in half a litre of water for 10 minutes. Cool and filter the mixture, then sweeten with a little honey or jaggery. Drink a cup twice a day after meals.

PHARMACOLOGICAL PROPERTIES

Dried leaf extracts of *Vepris nobilis* (*Teclea nobilis*) show analgesic, anti-inflammatory and antipyretic activities.[P474] Anti-inflammatory activity of the root bark extract of this plant has also been reported.[P475] The alkaloids in species of *Vepris* (*Teclea*) may be partly responsible for these beneficial properties.

COMPOUNDS REPORTED

Numerous alkaloids have been isolated from aerial parts of *V. nobilis* (*T. nobilis*)[P476] and *V. simplicifolia* (*T. simplicifolia*),[P477] including quinoline alkaloids (e.g. isoplatydesmine) and furoquinoline alkaloids (e.g. flindersiamine). *V. nobilis* (*T. nobilis*) also elaborates sesquiterpenes (e.g. teclenone A)[P478] and lupeol, a triterpene.[P479] There is still no reliable published information on the chemistry of the roots and bark. Five new furoquinoline alkaloids were reported from the aerial parts of *V. nobilis* (*T. nobilis*) along with seven known compounds. These compounds were inactive for antimicrobial and antiplasmodial activities.[P480]

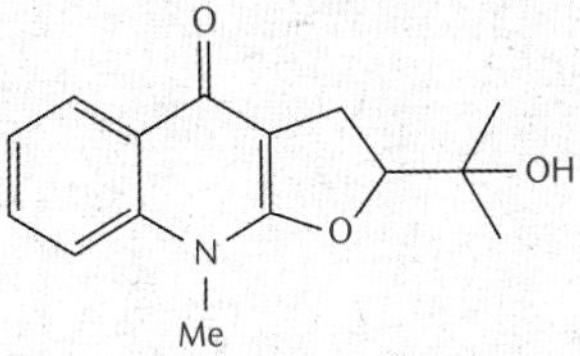

Isoplatydesmine

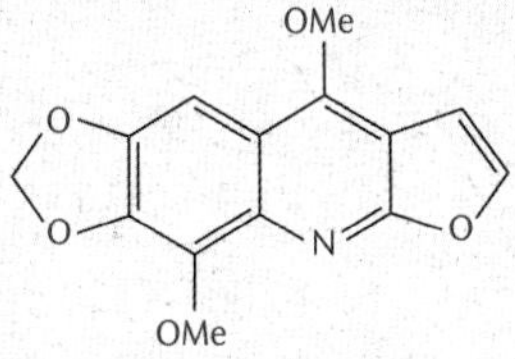

Flindersiamine

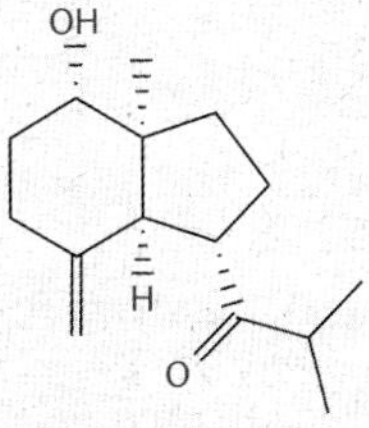

Teclenone A

Vernonia species ASTERACEAE

a. *Vernonia amygdalina* Indigenous

Common names Bitter-leaved Vernonia, Tree Vernonia • **Local names** Omororia (Kis.), Musuritsa / Omulusya / Kumwilulusia / Kumululusia (Luh.), Olusia / Olulusia (Luo), Mtukutu (Swa.), Mululuza (Lug.), Omululisi (Lugb.), Muuluza / Luluza (Lugi.), Labwori / Labori (Luo-A), Okelo-okelo (Luo-L), Olubirizi (Luso.), Kayakaya / Labwore (Madi), Cheburiandet (Nan.), Mubirizi (Runyan.), Kibirizi (Runy.), Omubirizi (Ruto.), Cheburiundet (Sebei)

Description and ecology

Erect, bushy, woody shrub 2–5m high, occasionally a tree 7–10m tall. **Bark** rough and fissured, branches hairy and brittle. **Leaves** ovate or elliptic, 5–10 × 2–6cm, tapering at both ends, dark green above, softly hairy below, margin finely toothed, with short stalk. **Flowers** small, creamy white, sweetly scented, grouped in dense thistle-like heads 5–9mm across, in large, flat, axillary and terminal clusters 15–20cm in diameter. **Fruit** a small achene with bristly hair, brown to black. Common in wooded savanna and pastureland, along rivers and lakes and on forest edges in wetter upland areas, at 900–2,200m.

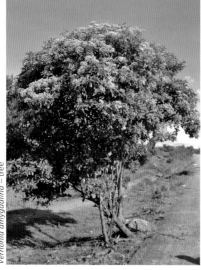

Vernonia amygdalina – tree

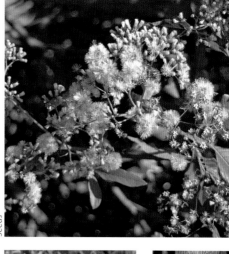

Seeds

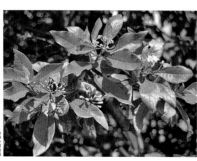

Leaves

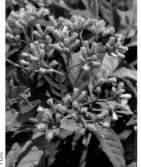

Fruit

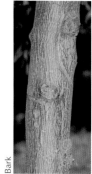

Bark

PARTS USED Leaves and root bark.
TRADITIONAL MEDICINAL USES Root bark and leaves are used to treat malaria,[M6, M70, M71] measles, asthma, diabetes, diarrhoea, tuberculosis, sleeping sickness and some kinds of cancer, while also serving as an anthelmintic agent.[M70, M125] Decoctions of young leaves are used for treating malaria, schistosomiasis, dysentery and for relieving abdominal pain, constipation and gastrointestinal ailments.[M6, M70, M71] A leaf infusion is taken for diabetes and to lower a fever, and also to reduce the persistent fever, headache and joint pain associated with AIDS.[M125] A root decoction is gargled for treating toothache and inflammation of the gums.[M125]

PREPARATION AND DOSAGE
DIABETES, SCHISTOSOMIASIS (BILHARZIA), DYSENTERY, CONSTIPATION, PARASITIC WORMS AND MALARIA Boil a handful of pounded fresh young leaves or 5g of dried root bark in a litre of water for 15 minutes. Filter and drink at intervals during the day. Alternatively, steep a handful of pounded fresh leaves or 5g of dried root bark in a litre of warm water for 20–30 minutes. Drink a cup of the infusion twice a day. For malaria, squeeze the juice from a handful of pounded fresh leaves and take a teaspoon of juice twice daily. For stomach ailments and parasitic worms, take a tablespoon of the juice twice daily.

b. *Vernonia auriculifera* Indigenous

Common name Vernonia • **Local names** Musakwa / Muthakwa (Kik.), Musabakwa (Kis.), Olusia (Luo), Ol-masakwa (Maa.), Turogogwa (Mar.), Tabenguet (Sebei), Tebinguet (Tug.), Kikokooma (Lug.), Ekinyekanyeme (Runyan.)

Description and ecology
Woody, multi-stemmed shrub or small tree 1.8–4(–7)m tall. Stems branching from the base, hairy. **Bark** greyish brown, smooth. **Leaves** narrowly elliptic or oval, densely hairy below, 10–15(–25)cm long, apex pointed, base rounded, margin sharply toothed. **Flowers** purple to violet, fading to pale mauve, borne in large terminal or axillary corymbose, flat or slightly rounded heads. **Fruit** an achene 3–4mm long. **Seeds** dry with stiff white hairs. Common along forest edges, on cleared pastureland, woodland, grassland and beside rivers and lakes, at 1,600–2,650m.

PARTS USED Leaves, stem bark and roots.
TRADITIONAL MEDICINAL USES Leaves are used to treat fever and malaria.[M1, M70] Roots are a known remedy for stomach ache, constipation and colic, and may also be taken as a purgative.[M4, M70, M115] Aerial parts of most species of *Vernonia* are widely used for abdominal pain, dysentery, coughs, bronchitis and indigestion.[M115] Warm leaf decoctions are applied to wounds,[M115] eczema, itching[M9] and other skin afflictions. A drop of fresh juice from crushed stem bark can be used as nasal drops to treat headache.[M115] A root decoction is gargled for inflammation of the gums and for toothache.[M115] Another common species, *V. brachycalyx* (not described here), has similar medicinal uses.

PREPARATION AND DOSAGE
MALARIA, DYSENTERY, COLIC AND STOMACH ACHE Boil a handful of pounded fresh leaves or 5g of dried root bark in a litre of water for 15 minutes. Filter and drink at intervals during the day. Make afresh when needed.

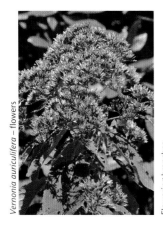

Vernonia auriculifera – flowers

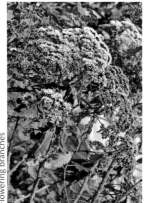

Flowering branches

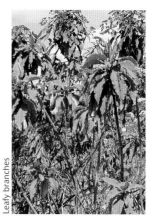

Leafy branches

c. *Vernonia lasiopus*

Indigenous

Common name Vernonia • **Local names** Muvatha (Kam.), Mucatha (Kik.), Kwam-tebenguet (Kip.), Olusia (Luo), Ol-euguru (Maa.), Nkaputi (Sam.)

Description and ecology

Woody herb or shrub 1–3m high. **Bark** greyish brown, smooth, young stems velvety hairy, older stems with raised dark brown lenticels. **Leaves** ovate or elliptic or lanceolate, 2.5–10cm long, densely hairy, apex pointed, base rounded, margin wavy and toothed.

Flowers pale mauve or lilac, often tinged white or fading to white, in flat or slightly rounded heads 5–10mm across. **Fruit** an achene 3.0–3.8mm long, strongly hairy. Found in disturbed areas as well as in bushland, grassland and riverine woodland or forest, at 1,050–2,500m.

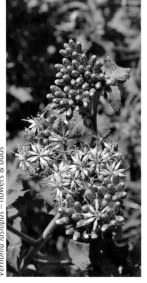

Vernonia lasiopus – flowers & buds

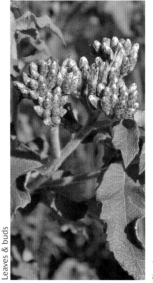

Leaves & buds

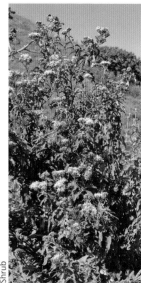

Shrub

USAGE AND TREATMENT

PARTS USED Leaves and roots.

TRADITIONAL MEDICINAL USES Leaf decoctions are used for indigestion,[M71] malaria,[M33] severe stomach ache,[M71] venereal diseases and are also taken as a purgative.[M70, M71] Fresh or dried powdered leaf decoctions are used against malaria.[M71] Root decoctions are a popular remedy for stomach ache[M1, M33, M70] but are also prized as a sexual stimulant for men.

PREPARATION AND DOSAGE

MALARIA, COLIC, STOMACH ACHE AND PURGATIVE USE Boil a handful of pounded fresh leaves or 5g of dried root bark in a litre of water for 15 minutes. Filter and sip at intervals during the day. Alternatively, squeeze the juice from a handful of pounded fresh leaves. Take a teaspoon of this juice twice a day for malaria. For stomach ache and purgative use, take a tablespoon of the juice twice daily.

 WARNING! Species of *Vernonia* contain some cytotoxic compounds such as vernodalin and vernomygdin that may trigger side effects. Excessive dosages should therefore be avoided.

PHARMACOLOGY AND CHEMISTRY

PHARMACOLOGICAL PROPERTIES

Properties that have been widely reported for species of *Vernonia* include antioxidant,[P481] antibacterial,[P13, P210, P482, P483] antifungal,[P96] antitrichomonal,[P102] antihyperglycaemic,[P484] antimalarial,[P485] antigiardiasic,[P211] antiviral,[P486] cytotoxic[P487] and spasmolytic[P488] activities.

COMPOUNDS REPORTED

Sesquiterpenoid lactones (e.g. vernodalin[P489] and 8-deacylvernodalol[P490]), along with flavones (e.g. luteolin[P481]) and saponins, including vernonioside D,[P491] have been isolated from leaves of *Vernonia* species. The bitter leaf taste is due to the presence of sesquiterpenoid lactones. Triterpenoids such as a-amyrin, isolated from *V. auriculifera*, exhibited moderate antibacterial activity. The plant also produced farnesylamine.[P492]

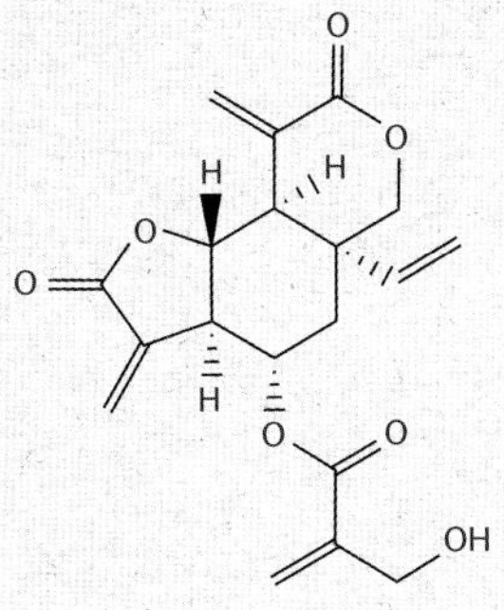

Vernodalin

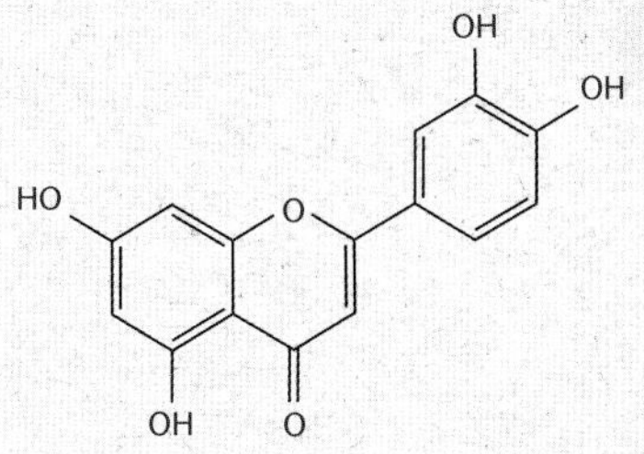

Luteolin

Indigenous

Common names East African Greenheart, Pepper-bark Tree • **Local names** Muthiga / Muthaiga (Kik.), Omenyakige (Kis.), Moissot / Sogoet (Kip.), Apacha / Apachi / Kumusikhu (Luh.), Abaki / Soko (Luo), Osogonoi / Ol-sokonoi (Maa.Ken.), Sekwan (Mar.), Musunui (Mer.), Soget (Nan.), Sorget / Soke (Tug.), Sagonai (Goro.), Muhiya (Haya), Olmsogoni / Msokonoi (Maa.Tan.), Msokonoi (Ran.), Mlifu / Mdee (Samb.), Mukuzanume / Muwiya (Lug.), Balwegira (Luso.), Mwiha (Runyan.), Musizambuzi (Runy.), Muharami (Ruto.).

Description and ecology

Medium-sized to large evergreen tree 6–25m tall, with a dense, rounded or spreading canopy and short bole, all parts with a hot, peppery taste. **Bark** smooth or rough, pale green or black-brown, cracked in rectangular scales. **Leaves** simple, alternate, oblong-lanceolate or elliptic or oblong-elliptic, 3–10(–15)cm long, shiny dark green above, paler below, apex and base tapering, with clear midrib, margin smooth. **Flowers** inconspicuous, greenish yellow or greenish cream, solitary or in small 3- or 4-flowered axillary cymes, less than 1cm across. **Fruit** a hard, round to egg-shaped berry, 3–5cm across, green to purple-black, skin leathery. **Seeds** 2 or more per berry, yellow-brown, 1–1.5cm long. Widespread in wetter low-lying forests and drier highland evergreen forest areas and surrounding secondary bushland and grassland, at 1,000–2,400m.

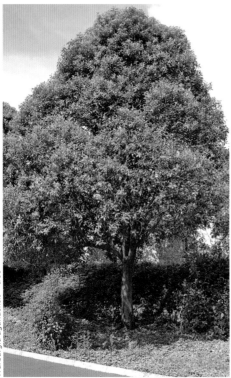

Warburgia ugandensis – tree

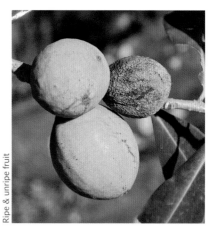

Ripe & unripe fruit

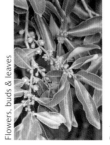

Flowers, buds & leaves

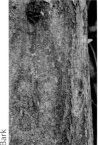

Bark

PARTS USED Roots, stem bark and leaves.
TRADITIONAL MEDICINAL USES An infusion of bark and roots is taken for stomach ache, toothache, malaria, colds and general muscular pain.[M4, M71] Dried bark is a widely used remedy for coughs, colds and chest complaints.[M2, M112] Roots are used to treat diarrhoea.[M115] A decoction of bark, roots or leaves is administered as a treatment for malaria, although it causes violent vomiting.[M4, M71, M112] Dried bark is commonly chewed and the juice swallowed as a remedy for stomach ache, constipation, toothache, coughs, fever, muscle pain, weak joints and general body pain.[M112, M115] Fresh bark provides treatment for the common cold; dried and ground to a snuff, it can be used to clear sinuses.[M112, M115]

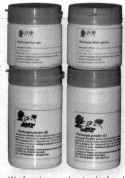

Warburgia ugandensis – leaf and bark powder, and capsules

PREPARATION AND DOSAGE
MALARIA, TOOTHACHE, STOMACH ACHE, CONSTIPATION, AND MUSCULAR PAIN Grind some dried bark and take a teaspoon of the powder twice a day. Or steep a tablespoon of dried bark or root powder in a litre of hot water for 10 minutes, strain and drink a cup of the infusion twice a day.
COUGHS AND COLDS Steep a tablespoon of dried bark powder in a litre of cold boiled water. Take a cup of the cold infusion 2 or 3 times a day as an expectorant. Alternatively, burn the dried bark and inhale the smoke.

PHARMACOLOGY AND CHEMISTRY

PHARMACOLOGICAL PROPERTIES
Species of *Warburgia* are rich in sesquiterpenes. Those with drimane and coloratane skeletons have insect antifeedant, antimicrobial, molluscicidal, antifungal and antimicrobial properties.[P493] Linoleic acid, an unsaturated fatty acid, and muzigadial, a sesquiterpene, show antimicrobial activity and are responsible for the strong antimicrobacterial property of *W. ugandensis*.[P493]

COMPOUNDS REPORTED
The bark contains various sesquiterpenoids such as muzigadial,[P493] and unsaturated fatty acids, including linoleic acid.[P493] Flavonol glycosides (e.g. kaempferol-3,4',7-tri-O-β-D-glucoside) have been reported from the leaves.[P494] Muzigadial, isolated from *W. ugandensis*, showed in vitro trypanocidal activity against *Trypanosoma brucei*. It is also commonly active against the soil pathogens *Fusarium oxysporum, Alternaria passiflorae* and *Aspergillus niger*.[P495]

Muzigadial

Kaempferol-3,7,4'-tri-O-β-D-glucoside

R = glucose

Indigenous

Common names Red Poison Cherry, Poison Gooseberry • **Local names** Hidigaga / Idigaga (Bor.), Idi (Gab.), Murambae (Kik.), Chepterekiat (Kip.), Ofuyaendwa (Luo), Ol-asaiyet (Maa.), Kipkogai (Mar.), Lopotwo (Pok.), Lesayet / Leekurun (Sam.), Kabarra (Tug.), Emotoe (Tur.)

Description and ecology

Woody herb or busy shrub 0.5–2m tall, with silver-grey, velvety hairy stems, branches and leaves. Stems brownish and prostrate to erect, sometimes leafless below. **Leaves** simple, alternate (opposite on flowering shoots), broadly ovate, obovate or oblong, 3–15 × 1.5–8cm, pale green and hairless above, green and densely hairy below, tip pointed, margin smooth. **Flowers** small, yellow-green, bell-shaped, in small axillary clusters at leaf nodes. **Fruit** a hairless, round berry 5–8mm across, orange-red to red, enclosed in an enlarged, papery calyx (sepals). **Seeds** numerous, pale brown, kidney-shaped. Usually found in wetter areas, along rivers or luggas (seasonal watercourses), on black cotton soil, near saline lakes and sometimes as a weed at forest edges, at 450–2,300m.

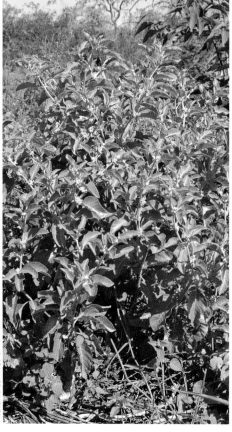

Withania somnifera – shrub

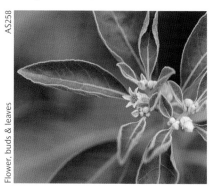

AS258

Flower, buds & leaves

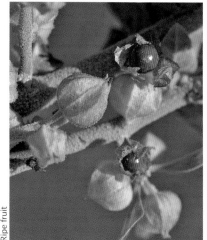

Ripe fruit

USAGE AND TREATMENT

PARTS USED Roots and leaves.

TRADITIONAL MEDICINAL USES Root decoctions or infusions are used to treat gonorrhoea,[M33] stomach ache, gastric ulcers, rheumatism, lumbago, colds and skin rashes,[M45, M70, M116] as well as to confer general immunity or as an aphrodisiac. Heated leaves are applied locally to various parts of the body to reduce pain, swelling and aches.[M7, M45, M70] In South Africa, leaf poultices are used for wounds, cuts, abscesses, haemorrhoids, rheumatic pains and syphilis.[M2, M70, M116]

PREPARATION AND DOSAGE

GONORRHOEA Boil 5–8g of slightly pulped fresh roots in a litre of water for 10 minutes. Cool, filter and drink at intervals during the day for 2 or 3 days.

WOUNDS, RHEUMATIC PAINS, HAEMORRHOIDS AND SYPHILIS Add a little water to some fresh leaves and make a paste. Apply externally to the affected areas, or add oil to make an ointment, which can be rubbed onto the affected areas.

 WARNING! *Withania somnifera* may cause side effects. Excessive dosages, both internally and externally, might trigger side effects such as diarrhoea, a burning sensation of the skin, sedation, liver damage and miscarriage, and should therefore be avoided.

PHARMACOLOGY AND CHEMISTRY

PHARMACOLOGICAL PROPERTIES

Roots of *Withania somnifera* show antibacterial and antifungal activities,[P17] for which the compound withaferin-A is responsible.[P96] The sedative, hypnotic and antiseptic[P496, P497] effects of the plant are widely exploited in Ayurvedic medicine.[P497] Extracts have shown potent antimitotic activity.[P496] Roots show a chemopreventive efficiency against skin and fore-stomach carcinogenesis in mice, with no apparent toxic effects.[P498]

COMPOUNDS REPORTED

W. somnifera contains numerous steroidal lactones, including withaferin-A.[P496, P497] Withanone, a compound isolated from root extract of *W. somnifera*, significantly improved the cognitive impairment in Wistar rats.[P499]

Withaferin-A

Withanone

a. *Zanthoxylum chalybeum* Indigenous

Common names Knobwood, African Knobwood • **Local names** Mudhungu / Mjafari (Gir.),
Mugucua (Emb., Mer.), Mdungu (Chon., Dig.), Gaddaa (Gab.), Mukenea / Mukanu (Kam.),
Sagawaita (Kip.), Roko (Luo), Oloisuki / Oloisugi (Aru., Maa.), Songorurwa / Songoiywa (Mar.),
Mugucwa (Mbe., Mer.), Songowo / Songoogh (Pok.), Loisugi / Loisuki (Sam.), Mjafari (Swa.Ken.),
Muguuchwa (Tha.), Kokian / Kokiin (Tug.), Eusugu (Tur.), Oluisuki (Aru.), Morungi (Goro.), Entare
yeirungo (Haya), Mkunungu (Hehe), Mhunungu (Lugu.), Msele (Pare), Mulungu / Mkunungu /
Mlungu (Ran.), Hombo-muungu / Muuungu-magoma (Samb.), Nungu (Suk.), Mjafari / Mkunungu
(Swa.Tan.), Muuungu-goma (Zig.), Eusuk (Ate.), Ntaleyedungu / Entale y'eddungu (Lug.), Musuku
(Lugwe.), Kichuk / Roki (Luo-A)

Description and ecology
Spiny, deciduous shrub or tree 2–8(–10)m tall,
with a rounded open crown. Bole 15–40cm
in diameter, with characteristic large, conical,
woody knobs with sharp prickles, branches
with scattered black or reddish, recurved spines
up to 2cm long. **Bark** pale grey, fissured or
with ridges. **Leaves** compound, with 5–9(–11)
pairs of shiny leaflets plus a terminal one,
non-hairy, margins entire, lemon-scented
when crushed. **Flowers** yellow-green, in short
racemes or panicles up to 10cm long, produced
immediately below the leaves, male and female
flowers on different trees. **Fruit** ellipsoid,
5–8mm long, red-brown-purple, splitting and
the shiny black seeds then partly protruding.
Found in dry woodland, bushland or wooded
grassland, often on termite mounds and in
rocky areas, on the coast and in dry forest and
closed thicket, at 0–1,800m.

USAGE AND TREATMENT

PARTS USED Roots, bark and leaves.
TRADITIONAL MEDICINAL USES A decoction of leaves, bark or roots can be used to treat
malaria and fever.[M4, M71] A bark or root decoction also serves as a traditional remedy
for influenza, coughs, colds, chest pain and respiratory diseases such as asthma and
tuberculosis.[M3, M4, M71] Juice from fresh bark is added to milk and given to small children
to stimulate appetite.[M4] A decoction of bark and roots can be used as a remedy for
malaria, general body pain, coughs, scorpion stings, snakebites, oedema, anaemia and
body swelling.[M91] Roots and bark are used as toothbrushes and also chewed to relieve
toothache,[M4] also prepared as a gargle for toothache.[M91] A bark decoction can be used as an
emetic, against malaria and also to treat a cough, sore throat and dizziness.[M4] Bark and root
powder mixed with oil is applied externally for pains and sprains.[M91]

PREPARATION AND DOSAGE
MALARIA AND FEVER Boil 3 crushed fresh leaves or 5g of crushed fresh roots or bark in half
a litre of water for 10 minutes. Cool and filter the mixture, adding a little honey or jaggery if
preferred. Drink a cup 2 or 3 times a day.
SORE THROAT, COUGHS, COLDS, INFLUENZA, ASTHMA AND TUBERCULOSIS Boil 5g of crushed
fresh roots or bark, or a tablespoon of root or bark powder or mixed root/bark powder, in half
a litre of water for 10 minutes. Cool and filter the mixture, adding a little honey or jaggery if
preferred. Drink a cup 2 or 3 times a day an hour after meals.
TOOTHACHE Fresh roots and bark can be used as toothbrushes or chewed for relief from
toothache. Alternatively, boil 5–6g of crushed fresh roots or bark for 10 minutes in half a litre
of water and gargle the warm mixture to relieve toothache.

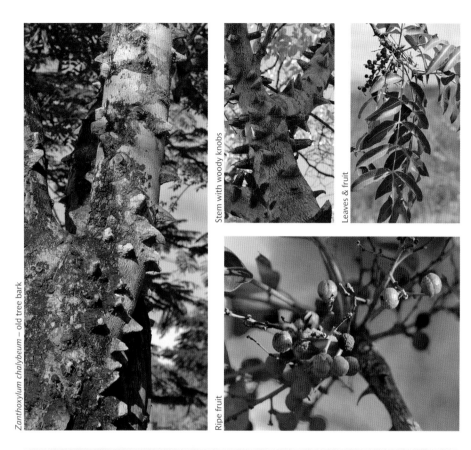

Stem with woody knobs

Leaves & fruit

Zanthoxylum chalybeum – old tree bark

Ripe fruit

b. *Zanthoxylum gilletii*

Indigenous

Common names African Satinwood, East African Satinwood • **Local names** Muchagatha (Kik.), Sagawoita (Kip., Nan.), Shikhuma / Kumusithu (Luh.), Sogo maitha (Luo), Munyenye (Lug.), Shukuma (Lugi.), Omushaga (Ruki.), Mulemankobe (Runyan.), Ntaleye-rungu (Runy.), Mutatembwa (Ruto.), Sagawat (Sebei)

Description and ecology
Semi-evergreen, medium-sized to very large tree 6–20(–35)m tall, with open spreading crown. Bole straight and cylindrical, 0.5–2m in diameter, with straight corky thorns 1–3cm long, larger branches armed with conical prickles up to 8mm long. **Bark:** outer grey to greyish brown, smooth to slightly rough; inner bark granular, yellowish brown, often mottled with orange. **Leaves** alternate, compound, clustered at ends of branches, rachis glabrous but sometimes with prickles, the 13–27(–51) leaflets alternate to nearly opposite, 8–14(–25)cm long, elliptical-oblong, margins entire or sometimes slightly toothed, aromatic when crushed. **Flowers** unisexual, creamy white, in clusters on a terminal or axillary pyramidal panicle 20–35cm long. **Fruit** a round follicle, 3–6mm in diameter, reddish, dehiscent, 1-seeded. Seed round, shiny black, 2.5–3mm in diameter, oil from crushed seed tasting like peppermint. Common in moist evergreen forest, riverine forest, upland rain forest and also found on old farmland and near forest plantations, at 1,500–2,300m.

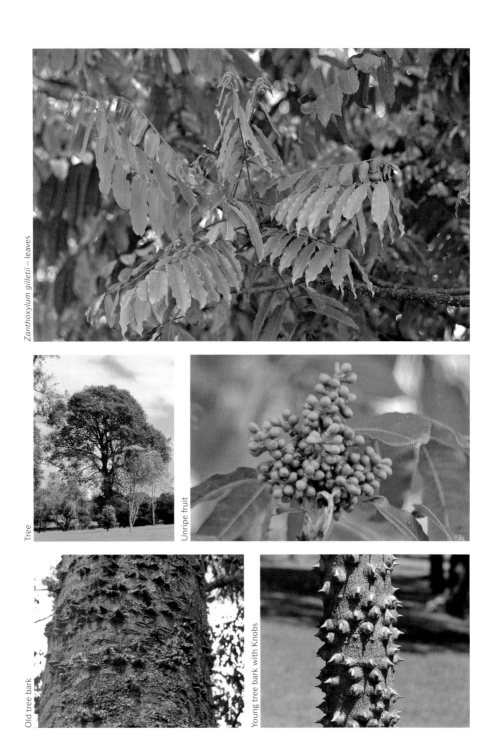

Zanthoxylum gilletii – leaves

Tree

Unripe fruit

Old tree bark

Young tree bark with Knobs

PARTS USED Bark, roots and leaves.
TRADITIONAL MEDICINAL USES A leaf decoction is taken for coughs, gonorrhoea and schistosomiasis, and a leaf maceration to treat diarrhoea and gastritis.[M112, M115] A bark decoction can be used to relieve coughs and colds.[M4] Fresh bark is chewed to treat toothache[M4] and the juice swallowed to deal with stomach ache.[M1] Bark of the stem and roots is an analgesic, aphrodisiac and vermifuge, and is also commonly used as an analgesic, especially to treat burns, rheumatism, headache, stomach ache, toothache and pain after childbirth.[M112, M115]

PREPARATION AND DOSAGE
SCHISTOSOMIASIS (BILHARZIA), GASTRITIS AND DIARRHOEA Boil 3 or 4 crushed fresh leaves in half a litre of water for 10 minutes. Cool and filter the mixture and drink a cup 2 or 3 times a day before meals.
TOOTHACHE, VERMIFUGE, APHRODISIAC AND STOMACH ACHE Chew fresh stem bark for relief from toothache, and swallow the juice to treat stomach ache and to expel intestinal parasites.

PHARMACOLOGY AND CHEMISTRY

PHARMACOLOGICAL PROPERTIES
Root bark extract of *Zanthoxylum chalybeum* is effective in controlling blood glucose in diabetes and protecting pancreatic tissues from diabetic damage.[P500] Good antiplasmodial activities are exhibited by stem bark of *Z. gilletii* against three different strains of *Plasmodium falciparum*.[P501]

COMPOUNDS REPORTED
The presence of the alkaloids chelerythrine, skimmianine, nitidine, N-methylflindersine, arnottianamide and dihydrochelerythrine has been reported from *Z. chalybeum*.[P502] Quaternary alkaloids, including usambanoline, have been identified from *Z. chalybeum* as well as from *Z. usambarense* (not described here), a plant with an alkaloid profile similar to that of *Z. chalybeum*.[P502] The pharmacological activities of these plants may possibly be due to these alkaloids.[P502] The lignan sesamine and the alkaloid 8-acetonyldihydrochelerythrine, isolated from *Z. gilletii*, showed good activity against *Plasmodium falciparum*.[P501] The alkaloids nitidine and norchelerythrine, isolated from the stem bark of *Z. holtzianum* (not described here), were identified as the most active antiplasmodial compounds against the W2 and D6 strains of *P. falciparum*.[P503, P504]

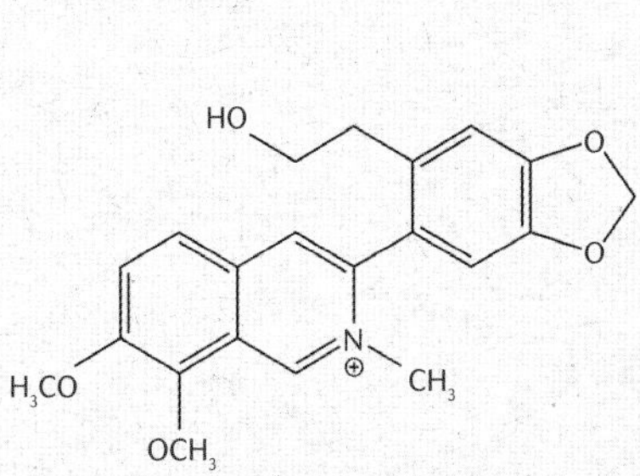

Usambanoline

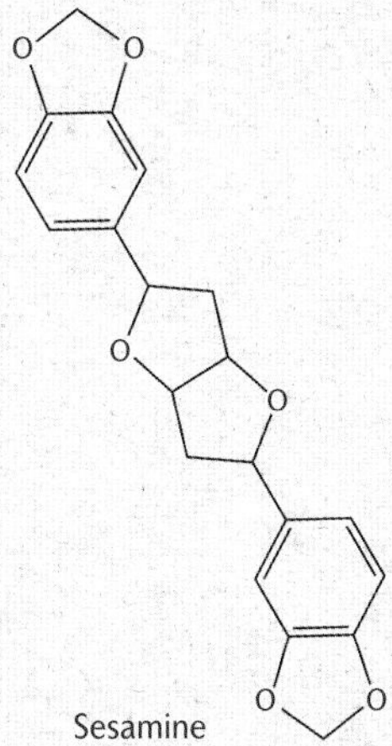

Sesamine

Native to India

Common name Ginger • **Local names** Ntangawizi (Swa.), Adu / Sonth (Guj.), Adrak (Urd., Hind., Punj.)

Description and ecology
Herbaceous perennial up to 1m high. **Leaves** lance-shaped to linear, 1–2 × 15–30cm, resembling those of sugarcane, developing from fleshy, brown, branched, tuberous, underground rhizomes that are highly aromatic and pungent, and used as a spice, especially in Indian curries. **Flowers** in dense cone-shaped spikes, pale yellow, with a purplish lip, resembling orchids, arising on separate shoots of the rhizome. Cultivated commercially throughout East Africa. Grows well in rich, well-drained, loamy soils.

USAGE AND TREATMENT

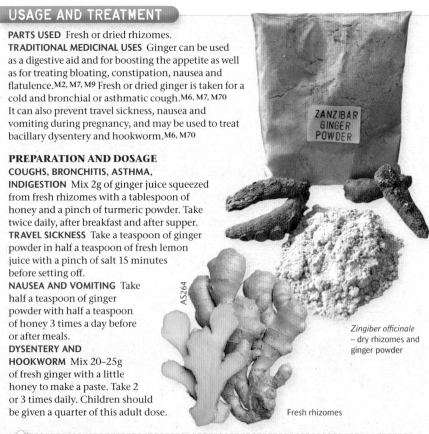

PARTS USED Fresh or dried rhizomes.
TRADITIONAL MEDICINAL USES Ginger can be used as a digestive aid and for boosting the appetite as well as for treating bloating, constipation, nausea and flatulence.[M2, M7, M9] Fresh or dried ginger is taken for a cold and bronchial or asthmatic cough.[M6, M7, M70] It can also prevent travel sickness, nausea and vomiting during pregnancy, and may be used to treat bacillary dysentery and hookworm.[M6, M70]

PREPARATION AND DOSAGE
COUGHS, BRONCHITIS, ASTHMA, INDIGESTION Mix 2g of ginger juice squeezed from fresh rhizomes with a tablespoon of honey and a pinch of turmeric powder. Take twice daily, after breakfast and after supper.
TRAVEL SICKNESS Take a teaspoon of ginger powder in half a teaspoon of fresh lemon juice with a pinch of salt 15 minutes before setting off.
NAUSEA AND VOMITING Take half a teaspoon of ginger powder with half a teaspoon of honey 3 times a day before or after meals.
DYSENTERY AND HOOKWORM Mix 20–25g of fresh ginger with a little honey to make a paste. Take 2 or 3 times daily. Children should be given a quarter of this adult dose.

ZANZIBAR GINGER POWDER

AS264

Zingiber officinale – dry rhizomes and ginger powder

Fresh rhizomes

WARNING! Ginger is not recommended for people with ulcers; in high doses it can trigger gastritis and may cause an anal and abdominal burning sensation.

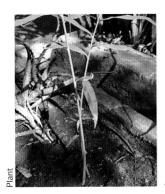

Plant

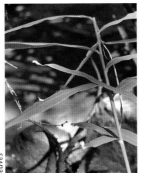

Leaves

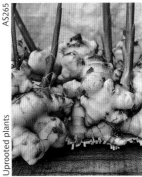

AS265

Uprooted plants

PHARMACOLOGICAL PROPERTIES

Ginger is useful in cases of flatulent colic, dyspepsia and atonic dyspepsia, while also acting as an anti-emetic.[P156, P505] Its role as carminative (in preventing the build-up of gas in the digestive system) is due mainly to the presence of gingerol and α-zingiberene.[P96, P156] Extracts of ginger have anti-inflammatory, antioxidant, antithrombotic and anticancer activities.[P506] Ginger is also effective in alleviating the symptoms of arthritis in humans.[P506] The anti-inflammatory activity of ginger is associated with gingerol and its analogs.[P506]

COMPOUNDS REPORTED

Rhizomes of *Zingiber officinale* contain volatile oils (up to 3%),[P156] comprising terpene derivatives such as monoterpenoids (e.g. camphene, neral and ß-phellandrene) and sesquiterpenoids (e.g. α-zingiberene),[P17, P96, P156, P507] as well as other substances, including resins, gingerols (e.g. [6]-gingerol, [8]-gingerol) and shogaol. The last two substances are pungent.[P17, P156] A number of diarylheptanoids, such as (3R,5S)-1,7-bis-(4-hydroxy-3-ethoxyphenyl)-3,5-diacetylheptane, have also been isolated from ginger rhizomes.[P508] Clinical trials with *Z. officinale* investigated the potential of treating type 2 diabetes through lipid and blood glucose control. (S)-[6]-gingerol, the major compound of ginger, stimulated increase of glucose uptake.[P509]

(3R,5S)-1,7-bis-(4-hydroxy-3-ethoxyphenyl)-3,5-diacetylheptane

[6]-Gingerol

Zingiberene

References for medicinal uses

M1   Kokwaro, J.O. 2009. *Medicinal Plants of East Africa*, edn 3. Nairobi: University of Nairobi Press.

M2   Van Wyk, B.E. *et al.* 2000. *Medicinal Plants of South Africa*, edn 2. Pretoria, South Africa: Briza.

M3   Maundu, P.M. 1999. *Traditional Food Plants of Kenya*. Nairobi: National Museums of Kenya, KENRIK.

M4   Dharani, N. 2019. *Field Guide to Common Trees & Shrubs of East Africa*, edn 3. Cape Town, South Africa: Struik Nature.

M5   Danziel, J.M. 1937. *The Useful Plants of West Tropical Africa*. London: Crown Agents.

M6   Hirt, H.M. & M'Pia, B. 2001. *Natural Medicine in the Tropics*. Winnenden, Germany: Anamed, Action for Natural Medicine.

M7   Hamdard Publications 1959. *Village Physician*. Part 1, pp. 255–256. Delhi, India.

M8   Rao, A.V. 1999. *Improve Your Health with Garlic and Onion: Full of Medicinal Qualities*. New Delhi, India: Diamond Pocket Books.

M9   Pamplona-Roger, M.D.G.D. 2001. *Encyclopaedia of Medicinal Plants*, Vols 1 & 2. Education and Health Library, Inter-American Division Publishing Association.

M10   Ross, I.A. 1999. *Medicinal Plants of the World*: *Chemical Constituents, Traditional and Modern Medicinal Uses*. New Jersey, USA: Humana Press Inc.

M11   Wanjohi, J.M. 2005. Antiplasmodial anthracene derivatives from some Kenyan *Aloe* and *Bulbine* species. PhD thesis, University of Nairobi.

M12   World Agroforestry Centre (ICRAF). Artemisia annua *(handout)*. Available from: www.worldagroforestrycentre. org.

M13   Purcell, K. 2004. WHO approves artemisinin for malaria in Africa. *American Botanical Council HerbalGram* 64, pp. 19–20.

M14   Sofowora, A. 1982. *Medicinal Plants and Traditional Medicine in Africa*. Hoboken, USA: Wiley.

M15   National Research Council, 1992. *Neem: A Tree for Solving Global Problems*.

Washington, DC, USA: The National Academies Press.

M16   Dharani, N. 2006. *Field Guide to Acacias of East Africa*. Cape Town, South Africa: Struik.

M17   Watt, J.M. & Breyer-Brandwijk, M.G. 1962. *The Medicinal and Poisonous Plants of Southern and Eastern Africa*, edn 2. London, UK: Livingstone.

M18   Liu, H.W. & Nakanishi, K. 1982. The structures of balanitins, potent molluscicides isolated from *Balanites aegyptiaca*. *Tetrahedron* 38, pp. 513–519.

M19   Hussein Ayoub, S.M. & Baerheim-Suendsen, A. 1981. Medicinal and aromatic plants in the Sudan: usage and exploration. *Fitoterapia* 52, pp. 243–246.

M20   Samuelsson, G. *et al.* 1991. Inventory of plants used in traditional medicine in Somalia. I: Plants of the families Acanthaceae–Chenopodiaceae. *Journal of Ethnopharmacology* 35, pp. 25–63.

M21   James, J.T. & Dubery, I.A. 2009. Pentacyclic triterpenoids from the medicinal herb *Centella asiatica* (L.) Urban. *Molecules* 14, 3922–3941, doi.10.3390/molecules14103922.

M22   Adesina, S.K. 1982. Studies on some plants used as anticonvulsants in Amerindian and African traditional medicine. *Fitoterapia* 53, pp. 147–162.

M23   Novy, J.W. 1997. Medicinal plants of the eastern region of Madagascar. *Journal of Ethnopharmacology* 55, pp. 119–126.

M24   Tang, C.S. 1979. Macrocyclic piperidine and piperideine alkaloids in *Carica papaya*. *Tropical Foods Chemistry and Nutrition* 1, pp. 55–68.

M25   Stuart, M. 1979. *The Encyclopaedia of Herbs and Herbalism*. London, UK: Orbis.

M26   Johns, T. *et al.* 1990. Herbal remedies of the Luo of Siaya District, Kenya: establishing quantitative criteria for consensus. *Economic Botany* 44, pp. 369–381.

M27   El-Kheir, Y.M. & Salih, M.H. 1980. Investigation of certain plants used in Sudanese folk medicine. *Fitoterapia* 51, pp. 143–147.

M28   Johns, T. *et al.* 1995. Anti-giardial activity of gastrointestinal remedies of the Luo of East Africa. *Journal of Ethnopharmacology* 46, pp. 17–23.

M29 Omino, E.A. & Kokwaro, J.O. 1993. Ethnobotany of Apocynaceae species in Kenya. *Journal of Ethnopharmacology* 40, pp. 167–180.

M30 Hedberg, I. *et al.* 1983. Inventory of plants used in traditional medicine in Tanzania. Part II: Plants of the families Dilleniaceae–Opiliaceae. *Journal of Ethnopharmacology* 9, pp. 105–127.

M31 Hedberg, I. *et al.* 1983. Inventory of plants used in traditional medicine in Tanzania. Part III: Plants of the families Papilionaceae–Vitaceae. *Journal of Ethnopharmacology* 9, pp. 237–260.

M32 Chhabra, S.C. *et al.* 1993. Plants used in traditional medicine in Eastern Tanzania. VI: Angiosperms (Sapotaceae to Zingiberaceae). *Journal of Ethnopharmacology* 39, pp. 83–103.

M33 Beentje, H.J. 1994. *Kenya Trees, Shrubs and Lianas*. Nairobi, Kenya: National Museums of Kenya.

M34 Gill, L.S. & Akinwumi, C. 1986. Nigerian folk medicine: practices and beliefs of the Ondo people. *Journal of Ethnopharmacology* 18, pp. 259–266.

M35 Chhabra, S.C. *et al.* 1987. Plants used in traditional medicine in Eastern Tanzania. I: Pteridophytes and Angiosperms (Acanthaceae to Canellaceae). *Journal of Ethnopharmacology* 21, pp. 253–277.

M36 Ichimaru, J.N.M. *et al.* 1996. Structural elucidation of new flavanones isolated from *Erythrina abyssinica*. *Journal of Natural Products* 59, pp. 1113–1116.

M37 Kamat, V.S. *et al.* 1981. Antimicrobial agents from an East African medicinal plant, *Erythrina abyssinica*. *Heterocycles* 15, pp. 1163–1170.

M38 Kamusiime, H. *et al.* 1996: Kaempferol 3-O-(2-O-β-D-glucopyranosyl-6-O-a-L-rhamnopyranosyl-β-D-glucopyranoside) from the African plant *Erythrina abyssinica*. *International Journal of Pharmacognosy* 34, pp. 370–373, doi. org/10.1076/phbi.34.5.370.13248.

M39 Boily, Y. & Van Puyvelde, L. 1986. Screening of medicinal plants of Rwanda (Central Africa) for antimicrobial activity. *Journal of Ethnopharmacology* 16, pp. 1–13.

M40 Chagnon, M. 1984. General pharmacologic inventory of medicinal plants of Rwanda. *Journal of Ethnopharmacology* 12, pp. 239–251.

M41 Maikere-Faniyo, R. *et al.* 1989. Study of Rwandese medicinal plants used in the treatment of diarrhoea. *Journal of Ethnopharmacology* 26, pp. 101–109.

M42 Muanza, D.N. *et al.* 1994. The antibacterial and antifungal activities of nine medicinal plants from Zaire. *International Journal of Pharmacology* 32, pp. 337–345.

M43 Samuelsson, G. *et al.* 1992. Inventory of plants used in traditional medicine in Somalia. II: Plants of the families Combretaceae–Labiatae. *Journal of Ethnopharmacology* 37, pp. 47–70.

M44 Chhabra, S.C. & Uiso, F.C. 1991. Antibacterial activity of some Tanzanian plants used in traditional medicine. *Fitoterapia* 62, pp. 499–503.

M45 Goraya, G.S. & Somashekhar, B.S. 2005. *Medicinal Plants for Primary Health Care: A Guide*. Bangalore, India: Medplan Conservatory Society.

M46 Chhabra, S.C. *et al.* 1984. Phytochemical screening of Tanzanian medicinal plants. *Journal of Ethnopharmacology* 11, pp. 157–179.

M47 Johns, T. *et al.* 1994. Herbal remedies of the Batemi of Ngorongoro District, Tanzania: a quantitative appraisal. *Economic Botany* 48, pp. 90–95.

M48 Sawhney, A.N. *et al.* 1978. Studies on the rationale of African traditional medicine. Part III: Preliminary screening of medicinal plants for antifungal activity. *Pakistan Journal of Scientific and Industrial Research* 21, pp. 193–196.

M49 Haerdi, F. 1964. Native medicinal plants of Ulanga District of Tanganyika (East Africa). Verlag für Recht und Gesellschaft AG, Basel. PhD dissertation, University of Basel.

M50 Msonthi, J.D. & Magombo, D. 1983. Medicinal herbs in Malawi and their uses. *Hamdard* 26, pp. 94–100.

M51 Hassanali, A. *et al.* 1987. Pedonin, a spiro tetranortriterpenoid insect antifeedant from *Harrisonia abyssinica*. *Phytochemistry* 26, pp. 573–575.

M52 Abebe, W.A. 1986. Survey of prescriptions used in traditional medicine in Gondar Region, northwestern Ethiopia: general pharmaceutical practice. *Journal of Ethnopharmacology* 18, pp. 147–165.

M53 Vlietinck, A.J. *et al.* 1995. The screening of one hundred Rwandese medicinal plants for antimicrobial and antiviral properties. *Journal of Ethnopharmacology* 46, pp. 31–47.

M54 Kloos, H. 1977. Preliminary studies of medicinal plants and plant products in markets of central Ethiopia. *Ethnomedicine* 4, pp. 63–104.

M55 Hakizamungu, E.L. *et al*. 1992. The screening of Rwandese medicinal plants for anti-trichomonas activity. *Journal of Ethnopharmacology* 36, pp. 143–146.

M56 Gladding, S. 1995. *Lantana camara. Australian Journal* of *Medical Herbalism* 7, pp. 5–9.

M57 Mugera, G.M. 1970. Toxic and medicinal plants of East Africa. Part II. *Bulletin of Epizootic Diseases of Africa* 18, pp. 389–403.

M58 Mathias, M.E. 1982. Some medicinal plants of the Hehe (Southern Highlands Province, Tanzania). *Taxon* 31, pp. 488–494.

M59 Kubo, I. *et al.* 1983. Isolation, structure and synthesis of maesanin, a host defense stimulant from an African medicinal plant *Maesa lanceolata. Tetrahedron Letters* 24, pp. 3825–3828.

M60 Lambert D.H. *et al.* 2005. *Capitalizing on the Bio-economic Value of Multipurpose Medicinal Plants for the Rehabilitation of Drylands in Sub-Saharan Africa.* Washington, DC, USA: Global Environment Facility Program. The International Bank for Reconstruction and Development/The World Bank.

M61 Farouk, A. *et al.* 1983. Antimicrobial activity of certain Sudanese plants used in folkloric medicine. Screening for antibacterial activity. *Fitoterapia* 54, pp. 3–7.

M62 Yousif, G. *et al.* 1983. Investigation of the alkaloidal components in the Sudan flora. Part 1. *Fitoterapia* 54, pp. 81–85.

M63 Sawhney, A.N. *et al.* 1978. Studies on the rationale of African traditional medicine. Part II: Preliminary screening of medicinal plants for anti-gonococci activity. *Pakistan Journal of Scientific and Industrial Research* 27, pp. 189–192.

M64 Samuelsson, G. *et al.* 1992. Inventory of plants used in traditional medicine

in Somalia. II: Plants of the families Combretaceae to Labiatae. *Journal of Ethnopharmacology* 37, pp. 47–70.

M65 Desta, B. 1994. Ethiopian traditional herbal drugs. Part III: Anti-fertility activity of 70 medicinal plants. *Journal of Ethnopharmacology* 44, pp. 199–209.

M66 Bhatia, I.S. & Bajaj, K.L. 1975. Chemical constituents of the seeds and bark of *Syzygium cumini. Planta Medica* 28, p. 346.

M67 Kuria, K.A.M. *et al.* 2001. Antimalarial activity of *Ajuga remota* Benth (Labiatae) and *Caesalpinia volkensii* Harms (Caesalpiniaceae): in vitro confirmation of ethnopharmacological use. *Journal of Ethnopharmacology* 74, pp. 141–148.

M68 Newton, L.E. 2006. *Aloe secundiflora* Engl. Record from PROTA4U. Schmelzer, G.H. & Gurib-Fakim, A. (Eds). Wageningen, Netherlands: PROTA (Plant Resources of Tropical Africa / Ressources végétales de l'Afrique tropicale). Available from: prota4u.org/database/protav8. asp?g=pe&p=Aloe+secundiflora+Engl.

M69 Liu, N.Q. *et al.* 2009. *Artemisia afra*: a potential flagship for African medicinal plants? *South African Journal of Botany* 75, 185–195, doi.org/10.1016/j. sajb.2008.11.001.

M70 Dharani, N. & Yenesew, A. 2010. *Medicinal Plants of East Africa: an Illustrated Guide*, edn 1. Nairobi, Kenya: Najma Dharani in association with Drongo Editing & Publishing.

M71 Dharani. N. *et al.* 2011. *Common Antimalarial Trees and Shrubs of East Africa: a Description of Species and a Guide to Cultivation and Conservation Through Use.* Dawson, I. (ed.). Nairobi, Kenya: The World Agroforestry Centre (ICRAF).

M72 Mei, K. 2016. *Asparagus africanus*. PlantZAfrica. Available from: pza.sanbi. org/asparagus-africanus.

M73 Van der Burg, W.J. 2004. *Asparagus flagellaris* (Kunth) Baker. Record from PROTA4U. Wageningen, Netherlands: PROTA (Plant Resources of Tropical Africa / Ressources végétales de l'Afrique tropicale). Available from: www. prota4u.org/search.asp.

M74 Kuria, J.M. 2014. Efficacy of *Aspilia pluriseta* Schweinf in cutaneous wound healing in a mouse model. MSc thesis, University of Nairobi.

M75 Musyimi, D.M. *et al.* 2007. Effects of leaf and root extracts of aspilia plant (*Aspilia mossambicensis*) on some selected micro-organisms. *International Journal of Biological Chemistry* 1, 213–220, doi=ijbc.2007.213.220.

M76 Dharani, N. 2016. Traditional ethnomedicinal uses, phytochemistry and pharmacological properties of *Balanites aegyptiaca* (L.) Del. in East Africa: a review. *Pharm Journal* 2. Kenyatta University Pharmacy Students Association (KUPHSA). Kenyatta University Press.

M77 Bosch, C.H. 2006. *Bulbine abyssinica* A.Rich. Record from PROTA4U. Wageningen, Netherlands: PROTA (Plant Resources of Tropical Africa / Ressources végétales de l'Afrique tropicale). Available from: www. prota4u.org/search.asp.

M78 El-Kamali, H.H. & Bosch, C.H. 2013. *Cadaba farinosa* Forssk. Schmelzer, G.H. & Gurib-Fakim, A. (Eds), *Prota* 11(2): Medicinal plants / Plantes médicinales 2. Wageningen, Netherlands: PROTA (Plant Resources of Tropical Africa / Ressources végétales de l'Afrique tropicale).

M79 Tropical Plants Database. *Capsicum frutescens*. Ken Fern. Available from: https://tropical. theferns.info/viewtropical. php?id=Capsicum+frutescens.

M80 Tropical Plants Database. *Carica papaya*. Ken Fern. Available from: tropical.theferns.info/viewtropical. php?id=Carica+papaya.

M81 Thompson, M. & Refilwe, M. 2012. *Carissa edulis*. PlantZAfrica. Available from: pza.sanbi.org/carissa-edulis.

M82 Dharani, N. 2016. Traditional ethnomedicinal uses and phytochemical compounds of *Carissa spinarum* L. in East Africa: a review. *Pharm Journal* 2. Kenyatta University Pharmacy Students Association (KUPHSA). Kenyatta University Press.

M83 Kawanga, V. 2007. *Cassia abbreviata* Oliv. Schmelzer, G.H. & Gurib-Fakim, A. (Eds). Wageningen, Netherlands: PROTA (Plant Resources of Tropical Africa / Ressources végétales de l'Afrique tropicale).

M84 Tabuti, J.R.S. 2007. *Senna didymobotrya* (Fresen.) H.S.Irwin & Barneby. Schmelzer, G.H. & Gurib-Fakim, A. (Eds). Wageningen, Netherlands: PROTA (Plant Resources of Tropical Africa / Ressources végétales de l'Afrique tropicale).

M85 Schmelzer, G.H. 2007. *Catharanthus roseus* (L.) G.Don. Record from PROTA4U. Schmelzer, G.H. & Gurib-Fakim, A. (Eds). Wageningen, Netherlands: PROTA (Plant Resources of Tropical Africa / Ressources végétales de l'Afrique tropicale).

M86 Lall, N. 2018. (ed.) *Medicinal Plants for Holistic Health and Well-being*. London, UK: Elsevier, Academic Press, doi. org/10.1016/C2016-0-03384-3.

M87 Tropical Plants Database. *Citrus aurantium*. Ken Fern. Available from: tropical.theferns.info/viewtropical. php?id=Citrus+aurantium.

M88 Kamanja I.T. *et al.* 2015. Medicinal plants used in the management of sexually transmitted infections by the Samburu Community, Kenya. *International Journal of Pharmaceutical Research* 7, pp. 44–52.

M89 Tropical Plants Database. *Commiphora africana*. Ken Fern. Available from: tropical.theferns.info/viewtropical. php?id=Commiphora+africana.

M90 Obeng, E.A. 2010. *Cordia africana* Lam. Record from PROTA4U. Lemmens, R.H.M.J., Louppe, D. & Oteng-Amoako, A.A. (Eds). Wageningen, Netherlands: PROTA (Plant Resources of Tropical Africa / Ressources végétales de l'Afrique tropicale).

M91 Ruffo, C.K. *et al.* 2002. *Edible Wild Plants of Tanzania*. Nairobi, Kenya: Regional Land Management Unit.

M92 Encyclopedia of Food Sciences and Nutrition. *Coriander*. Available from: www.sciencedirect.com/topics/ pharmacology-toxicology-and-pharmaceutical-science/coriander.

M93 Maroyi, A. 2010. *Croton megalocarpus* Hutch. Record from PROTA4U. Lemmens, R.H.M.J., Louppe, D. & Oteng-Amoako, A.A. (Eds). Wageningen, Netherlands: PROTA (Plant Resources of Tropical Africa / Ressources végétales de l'Afrique tropicale).

M94 Tropical Plants Database. *Croton macrostachyus*. Ken Fern. Available from: tropical.theferns.info/viewtropical. php?id=Croton macrostachyus.

M95 Committee on Herbal Medicinal Products. *Curcumae longae rhizoma*. Available from: www.ema.europa.eu/ en/medicines/herbal/curcumae-longae-rhizoma.

M96 Bosch, C.H. 2004. *Cyphostemma adenocaule* (Steud. ex A.Rich.) Wild & R.B.Drumm. Record from PROTA4U. Grubben, G.J.H. & Denton, O.A. (Eds). Wageningen, Netherlands: PROTA (Plant Resources of Tropical Africa / Ressources végétales de l'Afrique tropicale).

M97 Priyanka, S. *et al.* 2012. Pharmacological properties of *Datura stramonium* L. as a potential medicinal tree: an overview. *Asian Pacific Journal of Tropical Biomedicine* 2, 1002–1008. Available from: www.ncbi.nlm.nih.gov/pmc/ articles/PMC3621465.

M98 Tropical Plants Database. *Dichrostachys cinerea*. Ken Fern. Available from: tropical.theferns.info/image. php?id=Dichrostachys+cinerea.

M99 Harris, S. 2012. *Dodonaea viscosa*. PlantZAfrica. Available from: pza.sanbi. org/dodonaea-viscosa-var-angustifolia.

M100 Brink, M. 2007. *Dombeya rotundifolia* (Hochst.) Planch. Record from PROTA4U. Louppe, D., Oteng-Amoako, A.A. & Brink, M. (Eds). Wageningen, Netherlands: PROTA (Plant Resources of Tropical Africa / Ressources végétales de l'Afrique tropicale).

M101 Tropical Plants Database. *Ekebergia capensis*. Ken Fern. Available from: tropical.theferns.info/viewtropical. php?id=Ekebergia+capensis.

M102 Tropical Plants Database. *Erythrina abyssinica*. Ken Fern. Available from: tropical.theferns.info/viewtropical. php?id=Erythrina+abyssinica.

M103 WebMD. *Lemon eucalyptus – uses, side effects, and more*. Available from: www.webmd.com/vitamins/ ai/ingredientmono-1108/lemon-eucalyptus.

M104 Tropical Plants Database. *Corymbia maculata*. Ken Fern. Available from: tropical.theferns.info/viewtropical. php?id=Corymbia+maculata.

M105 Al-Fatimi, M. 2019. Antifungal activity of *Euclea divinorum* root and study of its ethnobotany and phytopharmacology. *Processes* 7, p. 680.

M106 Lewis, W.H. 1986. The useful plants of West Tropical Africa. *Economic Botany* 40, 176, doi.org/10.1007/BF02859140.

M107 Manzoor, A.R. *et al.* 2016. *Foeniculum vulgare*: a comprehensive review of its traditional use, phytochemistry, pharmacology, and safety. *Arabian Journal of Chemistry* 9, 1574–1583. Available from: www.sciencedirect.com/ science/article/pii/S1878535212000792.

M108 Agbodjento, E. *et al.* 2018. *Gardenia ternifolia*: review of ethnobotanical, ethnopharmacological, phytochemical and toxicological aspects. *International Journal of Biological and Chemical Sciences* 12, pp. 2922–2932.

M109 Dounias, E. 2006. *Gloriosa superba* L. Record from PROTA4U. Schmelzer, G.H. & Gurib-Fakim, A. (Eds). Wageningen, Netherlands: PROTA (Plant Resources of Tropical Africa / Ressources végétales de l'Afrique tropicale).

M110 Brink, M. 2007. *Grewia bicolor* Juss. Record from PROTA4U. Louppe, D., Oteng-Amoako, A.A. & Brink, M. (Eds). Wageningen, Netherlands: PROTA (Plant Resources of Tropical Africa / Ressources végétales de l'Afrique tropicale). Available from: www. prota4u.org/search.asp.

M111 Orwa, C. *et al.* 2009. *Agroforestree database: a tree reference and selection guide*. Version 4.0. Available from: www. worldagroforestry.org/sites/treedbs/ treedatabases.asp.

M112 Tropical Plants Database. Available from: tropical.theferns.info.

M113 Chopra, R.N. *et al.* 1986. *Glossary of Indian Medicinal Plants (including the Supplement)*. New Delhi, India: Council of Scientific and Industrial Research.

M114 Akhilesh, K. & Tewari, S.K. 2015. Origin, distribution, ethnobotany and pharmacology of *Jatropha curcas*. *Research Journal of Medicinal Plants* 9, pp. 48–59.

M115 PROTA4U. Online database. Available from: www.prota4u.org/database.

M116 PlantZAfrica. Online database. Available from: pza.sanbi.org.

M117 Mzena, T. *et al.* 2018. Antimalarial activity of *Cucumis metuliferus* and

Lippia kituiensis against *Plasmodium berghei* infection in mice. *Research and Reports in Tropical Medicine* 9, pp. 81–88.

M118 Long, H.S. *et al.* 2010. The ethnobotany and pharmacognosy of *Olea europaea* subsp. *africana* (Oleaceae). *South African Journal of Botany* 76, pp. 324–331.

M119 Lukhoba, C.W. *et al.* 2006. *Plectranthus*: a review of ethnobotanical uses. *Journal of Ethnopharmacology* 103, pp. 1–24.

M120 Stewart, K.M. 2003. The African cherry (*Prunus africana*): can lessons be learned from an over-exploited medicinal tree? *Journal of Ethnopharmacology* 89, pp. 3–11.

M121 Naseer, S. *et al.* 2018. The phytochemistry and medicinal value of *Psidium guajava* (guava). *Clinical Phytoscience* 4, p. 32.

M122 Marwat, S.K. *et al.* 2017. Review – *Ricinus communis* – ethnomedicinal uses and pharmacological activities. *Pakistan Journal of Pharmacological Science* 30, pp. 1815–1827, PMID: 29084706.

M123 Dharani, N. 2016. A review of traditional medicinal uses and phytochemical

constituents of exotic *Syzygium* species in East Africa. *Pharmacological Journal of Kenya* 22(4).

M124 Orwa, J.A. *et al.* 2008. The use of *Toddalia asiatica* (L.) Lam. (Rutaceae) in traditional medicine practice in East Africa. *Journal of Ethnopharmacology* 115, pp. 257–262.

M125 Adedapo, A.A. *et al.* 2014. Anti-oxidant, anti-inflammatory and antinociceptive properties of the acetone leaf extract of *Vernonia amygdalina* in some laboratory animals. *Advanced Pharmaceutical. Bulletin* 4(Suppl. 2), pp. 591–598, PMCID: PMC4312410; PMID: 25671194.

M126 Indravathi, G. *et al.* 2013. *Albizia amara* – a potential medicinal plant: a review. *International Journal of Science and Research* 5, pp. 621–627.

M127 Kweyamba, P.A. *et al.* 2019. In vitro and in vivo studies on anti-malarial activity of *Commiphora africana* and *Dichrostachys cinerea* used by the Maasai in Arusha region, Tanzania. *Malaria Journal* 18, 119, doi.org/10.1186/s12936-019-2752-8.

References for pharmacology & chemistry

P1 Farouk, A. *et al.* 1983. Antimicrobial activity of certain Sudanese plants used in folkloric medicine. Screening for antibacterial activity (I). *Fitoterapia* 54, pp. 3–7.

P2 Hussein, G. *et al.* 1999. Inhibitory effects of Sudanese plant extracts on HIV-1 replication and HIV-1 protease. *Phytotherapy Research* 13, pp. 31–36.

P3 Gupta, S.C. & Bilgrami, R.S. 1970. Inhibitory effect of some plant decoctions on the production and activity of cellulolytic (GX) enzyme of three pathogenic fungi. *Proceedings of the National Academy of Sciences, India Section B: Biological Sciences* 40, pp. 6–8.

P4 Al-Yahya, M.A. *et al.* 1985. Phytochemical studies on Saudi plants used for the treatment of fever. *45th International Congress of Pharmaceutical Sciences of F.I.P.*, held in Montreal Canada. Amsterdam, Netherlands; New York, USA: Elsevier Science Publishers.

P5 El Tahir, A. *et al.* 1999. Antiplasmodial activity of selected Sudanese medicinal plants with emphasis on *Acacia nilotica*. *Phytotherapy Research* 13, pp. 474–478.

P6 Dhawan, B.N. *et al.* 1977. Screening of Indian plants for biological activity. VI. *Indian Journal of Experimental Biology* 15, pp. 208–219.

P7 Uzunuigbe E.O. et *al.* 2019. Phytochemical constituents and antioxidant activities of crude extracts from *Acacia senegal* leaf extracts. *Pharmacognosy Journal* 11, 1409–1414, doi:10.5530/pj.2019.11.218.

P8 Ayoub, S.M.H. 1984. Polyphenolic molluscicides from *Acacia nilotica*. *Planta Medica* 50, p. 532.

P9 Ayoub, S.M.H. 1985. Flavanol molluscicides from the Sudan acacias. *International Journal of Crude Drug Research* 23, pp. 87–90.

P10 Saharia, G.S. & Sharma, M. 1981. Chemical examination of *Acacia senegal* Willd. *Indian Journal of Forestry* 4, p. 63.

P11 Jain, R. *et al.* 2012. Phytochemical investigation and antimicrobial activity of *Acacia senegal* root heartwood. *Journal of Pharmacy Research* 5, pp. 4934–4938.

P12 Mettam, R.W.M. 1930. Poisonous plants of Kenya. Part I. *Kenya Department of Agriculture Annual Report* 1929, p. 377.

P13 Desta, B. 1993. Ethiopian traditional herbal drugs. Part II. Antimicrobial activity of 63 medicinal plants. *Journal of Ethnopharmacology* 39, pp. 129–139.

P14 Martindale. 1958. *The Extra Pharmacopoeia*. London: Pharmaceutical Press.

P15 Mohammed, T. *et al.* 2014. Evaluation of antimalarial activity of leaves of *Acokanthera schimperi* and *Croton macrostachyus* against *Plasmodium berghei* in Swiss albino mice. *BMC Complementary and Alternative Medicine* 14, p. 314.

P16 Tesfaye, S. *et al.* 2021. Ethiopian medicinal plants traditionally used for the treatment of cancer. Part 3. Selective cytotoxic activity of 22 plants against human cancer cell lines. *Molecules* 26, p. 3658.

P17 Trease, G.E. & Evans, W.C. 1987. *Pharmacognosy*, edn 12. Oxford, Great Britain: ELBS Alden Press.

P18 Thudium, F. *et al.* 1959. The glycosides of *Acokanthera schimperi*. Glycosides and aglycones. CXCIII. 3. The seeds of the form the Wa-Giriama use for preparing arrow poisons. *Helvetica Chimica Acta* 42, pp. 2–49.

P19 Neuwinger, H.D. 1994. *Afrikanische Arzneipflanzen und Jagdgifte*. Stuttgart: Wissenschaftliche Verlagsgesellschaft.

P20 Matebie, A.W. *et al.* 2019. Triterpenoids from *Acokanthera schimperi* in Ethiopia. *Records of Natural Products* 13, pp. 182–188

P21 Adesanya, S.A. *et al.* 1988. Anti-sickling activity of *Adansonia digitata*. *Planta Medica* 54, p. 374.

P22 Ramadan, A. *et al.* 1994. Anti-inflammatory, analgesic and antipyretic effects of the fruit pulp of *Adansonia digitata*. *Fitoterapia* 65, pp. 418–422.

P23 Gessler, M.C. *et al.* 1994. Screening Tanzanian medicinal plants for anti-malarial activity. *Acta Tropica* 56, pp. 65–77.

P24 Ismail, B.B. *et al.* 2021. Investigating the effect of in vitro gastrointestinal digestion on the stability, bioaccessibility, and biological activities of baobab (*Adansonia digitata*) fruit polyphenolics. *Food Science and Technology* 145, 111348, doi.org/10.1016/j.lwt.2021.111348.

P25 Braca, A. *et al.* 2018. Phytochemical profile, antioxidant and antidiabetic activities of *Adansonia digitata* L. (baobab) from Mali, as a source of health-promoting compounds. *Molecules* 23, p. 3104.

P26 Watt, J.M. & Breyer-Brandwijk, M.G. 1962. *The Medicinal and Poisonous Plants of Southern and Eastern Africa*, edn 2. London: Livingstone.

P27 Chauban, J.S. *et al.* 1984. A new flavanone glycoside from the roots of *Adansonia digitata*. *Planta Medica* 50, 113, doi:10.1055/s-2007-969642.

P28 Ibraheem, S. *et al.* 2021. Phytochemical profile and biological activities of Sudanese baobab (*Adansonia digitata* L.) fruit pulp extract. *International Food Research Journal* 28, pp. 31–43.

P29 Mumtaz, T. *et al.* 2016. Phytochemical screening and standardization profile of *Adansonia digitata* L. – a universal remedial plant. *Hamdard Medicus* 59, p. 4.

P30 Shahat, A.A. 2006. Procyanidins from *Adansonia digitata*. *Pharmaceutical Biology* 44, pp. 445–450.

P31 Kariba, R.M. 2001. Antifungal activity of *Ajuga remota*. *Fitoterapia* 72, pp. 177–178.

P32 Odek-Ogunde, M. *et al.* 1993. Blood pressure responses to an extract of *Ajuga remota* in experimentally hypertensive rats. *Planta Medica* 59, pp. 573–574.

P33 Kuria, K.A.M. *et al.* 2001. Antimalarial activity of *Ajuga remota* Benth. (Labiatae) and *Caesalpinia volkensii* Harms (Caesalpiniaceae): in vitro confirmation of ethnopharmacological use. *Journal of Ethnopharmacology* 74, pp. 141–148.

P34 Abbasi, B.H. *et al.* 2020. Exogenous application of salicylic acid and gibberellic acid on biomass accumulation, antioxidant and anti-inflammatory secondary metabolites production in multiple shoot culture of *Ajuga integrifolia* Buch. Ham. ex D.Don. *Industrial Crops & Products* 145, 112098, doi.org/10.1016/j.indcrop.2020.112098.

P35 Tafesse, T.B. *et al.* 2017. Antidiabetic activity and phytochemical screening

of extracts of the leaves of *Ajuga remota* Benth. on alloxan-induced diabetic mice. *BMC Complementary and Alternative Medicine* 17, 243, doi.org/10.1186/s12906-017-1757-5.

P36 Yacob, T. *et al.* 2016. Antidiarrheal activity of 80% methanol extract of the aerial part of *Ajuga remota* Benth. (Lamiaceae) in mice. *BMC Complementary and Alternative Medicine* 16, p. 303.

P37 Mukungu, N. *et al.* 2016. Medicinal plants used for management of malaria among the Luhya community of Kakamega East sub-County, Kenya. *Journal of Ethnopharmacology* 194, pp. 98–107.

P38 Kubo, I. *et al.* 1983. Structure of ajugarin-V. *Chemistry Letters* 2, pp. 223–224.

P39 Kubo, I. *et al.* 1981. Insect ecdysis inhibitors from the East African medicinal plant *Ajuga remota* (Labiatae). *Agricultural and Biological Chemistry* 45, pp. 1925–1927.

P40 Cocquyt, K. *et al.* 2011. *Ajuga remota* Benth.: from ethnopharmacology to phytomedical perspective in the treatment of malaria. *Phytomedicine* 18, pp. 1229–1237.

P41 Pezzuto, J.M. *et al.* 1991. DNA as an affinity probe useful in the detection and isolation of biologically active natural products. *Journal of Natural Products* 54, pp. 1522–1530.

P42 Ayoub, S.M.H. & Yankov, L.K. 1986. The molluscicidal factor of tannin-bearing plants. *International Journal of Crude Drug Research* 24, pp. 16–18.

P43 Freiburghaus, F. *et al.* 1996. In vitro antitrypanosomal activity of African plants used in traditional medicine in Uganda to treat sleeping sickness. *Tropical Medicine & International Health* 1, 765–771, doi:10.1111/j.1365-3156.1996.tb00108.x.

P44 Lipton, A. 1959. Physiological activity in extracts of *Albizia* species. *Nature* 184, 822–823, doi:10.1038/184822b0.

P45 Rukunga, G.M. *et al.* 2007. The antiplasmodial activity of spermine alkaloids isolated from *Albizia gummifera*. *Fitoterapia* 78, pp. 455–459.

P46 Gradé, J.T. *et al.* 2008. Anthelmintic efficacy and dose determination of *Albizia anthelmintica* against gastrointestinal nematodes in naturally infected Ugandan sheep. *Veterinary Parasitology* 157, pp. 267–274.

P47 Pezzuto, J.M. *et al.* 1991. DNA-based isolation and the structure elucidation of the budmunchiamines, novel macrocyclic alkaloids from *Albizia amara*. *Heterocycles* 32, pp. 1961–1967.

P48 Chandra, I. *et al.* 1956. Oil from the seeds of *Albizia amara*. *Journal of Scientific and Industrial Research-B* 15, p. 196.

P49 Deshpande, V.H. & Shastri, R.K. 1977. Phenolics of *Albizia lebbeck*, *A. amara* and *A. procera*. *Indian Journal of Chemistry* 15B, pp. 201–205.

P50 Rukunga, G.M. & Waterman, P.G. 2001. A new oleanane glycoside from the stem bark of *Albizia gummifera*. *Fitoterapia* 72, pp. 140–145.

P51 Mohamed, T.K. *et al.* 2013. Secondary metabolites and bioactivities of *Albizia anthelmintica*. *Pharmacognosy Research* 5, pp. 80–85.

P52 Pratt, D.E. & Watts, B.M. 1964. The antioxidant activity of vegetable extracts I. flavone aglycones. *Journal of Food Science* 29, 27–33, doi. org/10.1111/j.1365-2621.1964.tb01689.x.

P53 Jain, R.C. & Vyas, C.R. 1974. Hypoglycaemia action of onion on rabbits. *British Medical Journal* 2, p. 730.

P54 Badria, F.A. 1994. Is man helpless against cancer? An environmental approach: anti-mutagenic agents from Egyptian food and medicinal preparations. *Cancer Letters* 84, 1–5, doi:10.1016/0304-3835(94)90351-4.

P55 Amla, V. *et al.* 1981. Clinical study of *Allium cepa* Linn. in patients of bronchial asthma. *Indian Journal of Pharmacology* 13, pp. 63–64.

P56 Abdullah, T.H. *et al.* 1988. Garlic revisited: therapeutic for the major diseases of our times? *Journal of the National Medical Association* 80, pp. 439–445.

P57 Yin, M.C. & Cheng, W.S. 1998. Inhibition of *Aspergillus niger* and *Aspergillus flavus* by some herbs and spices. *Journal of Food Protection* 61, 123–125, doi:10.4315/0362-028x-61.1.123.

P58 Lund, B.M. & Lyon, G.D. 1975. Detection of inhibitors of *Erwinia*

carotovora and *E. herbicola* on thin-layer chromatograms. *Journal of Chromatography* 110, 193–196, doi:10.1016/s0021-9673(00)91229-9.

P59 Khan, M.R. & Omoloso, A.D. 1998. *Momordica charantia* and *Allium sativum*: broad spectrum antibacterial activity. *Korean Journal of Pharmacognosy* 29, 155–158. Available from: www.koreascience. or.kr/article/JAKO199803041271489.pdf.

P60 Yin, M.C. & Cheng, W.S. 1998. Antioxidant activity of several *Allium* members. *Journal of Agricultural and Food Chemistry* 46, pp. 4097–4101.

P61 Yeh, Y.Y. & Yeh, S.M. 1994. Garlic reduces plasma lipids by inhibiting hepatic cholesterol and triacylglycerol synthesis. *Lipids* 29, pp. 189–193.

P62 Okekhov, A.N. & Grunwald, J. 1997. Effects of garlic on atherosclerosis. *Nutrition* 13, pp. 656–663.

P63 DiPaolo, J. & Carruthers, C. 1960. The effect of allicin from garlic on tumor growth. *Cancer Research* 20, p. 431.

P64 Hsu, W.C. 1977. Garlic slice in repairing eardrum perforation. *Chinese Medical Journal* 3, pp. 204–205.

P65 Steerenberg, P.A. *et al.* 1997. The effect of oral quercetin on UVB-induced tumor growth and local immunosuppression in SKH-1. *Cancer Letters* 114, pp. 187–189.

P66 Sharaf, A. 1969. Food plants as a possible factor in fertility control. *Qualitas Plantarum et Materiae Vegetabiles* 17, pp. 153–160.

P67 Banerjee, S.K. *et al.* 2001. Garlic-induced alteration in rat liver and kidney morphology and associated changes in endogenous antioxidant status. *Food and Chemical Toxicology* 39, pp. 793–797.

P68 Raj, R. 1975. Screening of indigenous plants for anthelmintic action against human *Ascaris lumbricoides*. Part II. *Indian Journal of Physiology and Pharmacology* 19, pp. 47–49.

P69 Schwikkard, S. & Van Heerden, F. 2002. Antimalarial activity of plant metabolites. *Natural Products Report* 19, pp. 675–692.

P70 Singh, U.P. *et al.* 1990. Antifungal activity of ajoene, a constituent of garlic (*Allium sativum*). *Canadian Journal of Botany* 68, doi/10.1139/b90-172.

P71 Donne, R.H. *et al.* 1997. Separation and characterization of simple and malonylated anthocyanins in red onions, *Allium cepa* L. *Food Research International* 30, pp. 647–643.

P72   Singh, U.P. *et al.* 1992. Effect of ajoene, a compound derived from garlic (*Allium sativum*), on *Phytophthora drechsleri* f. sp. *cajani*. *Mycologia* 84, 105–108, doi:10.1080/00275514.1992.12026110.

P73   Inagaki, M. *et al.* 1998. Isolation and structure determination of cerebrosides from garlic, the bulbs of *Allium sativum* L. *Chemical and Pharmaceutical Bulletin* 46, 1153–1156, doi.org/10.1248/cpb.46.1153.

P74   Koch, H.P. *et al.* 1993. Carbohydrates from garlic bulbs (*Allium sativum* L.) as inhibitors of adenosine deaminase enzyme activity. *Phytotherapy Research* 7, pp. 387–389.

P75   Maenthaisong, R. *et al.* 2007. The efficacy of *Aloe vera* used for burn wound healing: a systematic review. *Burns* 33, pp. 713–718.

P76   Sahu, P.K. *et al.* 2013. Therapeutic and medicinal uses of *Aloe vera*: a review. *Pharmacology & Pharmacy* 4, 599–610, doi.org/10.4236/pp.2013.48086.

P77   Qiu, Z. *et al.* 2000. Modified *Aloe barbadensis* polysaccharide with immunoregulatory activity. *Planta Medica* 66, 152–156, doi:10.1055/s-2000-11125.

P78   Suga, T. & Hirata, T. 1983. The efficacy of the aloe plant's chemical constituents and biological activities. *Cosmetics & Toiletries* 98, pp. 105–108.

P79   Ross, I.A. 1999. *Medicinal Plants of the World: Chemical Constituents, Traditional and Modern Medicinal Uses*. New Jersey, USA: Humana Press.

P80   Wanjohi, J.M. 2005. Antiplasmodial anthracene derivatives from some Kenyan *Aloe* and *Bulbine* species. PhD thesis, University of Nairobi, Kenya.

P81   Mohsin, A. *et al.* 1989. Analgesic antipyretic activity and phytochemical screening of some plants used in traditional Arab system of medicine. *Fitoterapia* 60, pp. 174–177.

P82   Suvitayavat, W. *et al.* 2004. Effects of *Aloe* preparation on the histamine-induced gastric secretion in rats. *Journal of Ethnopharmacology* 90, pp. 239–247.

P83   Msoffe, P.L. & Mbilu, Z.M. 2009. The efficacy of crude extract of *Aloe secundiflora* on *Candida albicans*. *African Journal of Traditional, Complementary and Alternative Medicine* 6, pp. 592–595.

P84   Pamplona-Roger, M.D.G.D. 2001. *Encyclopaedia of Medicinal Plants*, Vol. 1. Madrid, Spain. Editorial Safeliz.

P85   Saccu, D. *et al.* 2001. *Aloe* exudate: characterization by reversed phase HPLC and headspace GC-MS. *Journal of Agricultural and Food Chemistry* 49, pp. 4526–4530.

P86   Rauwald, H.W. & Niyonzima, D.D. 1991. A new investigation on constituents of *Aloe* and *Rhamnus* species, XV (1). Homonataloin A and B from *Aloe lateritia*: isolation, structure and configurational determination of the diastereomers. *Zeitschrift fuer Naturforschung* C 46, pp. 177–182.

P87   Dagne, E. *et al.* 1994. Anthraquinones, pre-anthraquinones and isoeleutherol in the roots of *Aloe* species. *Phytochemistry* 35, pp. 401–406.

P88   Newton, L.E. 2006. *Aloe secundiflora* Engl. Record from PROTA4U. Schmelzer, G.H. & Gurib-Fakim, A. (Eds). Wageningen, Netherlands: PROTA (Plant Resources of Tropical Africa / Ressources végétales de l'Afrique tropicale). Available from: https://uses.plantnetproject.org/en/Aloe_secundiflora_(PROTA) [Accessed 3 July 2021].

P89   Induli, M. *et al.* 2012. Naphthoquinones from the roots of *Aloe secundiflora* (Asphodelaceae). *Phytochemistry Letters* 5, pp. 506–509.

P90   Sharma, R. 2004. *Agrotechniques of Medicinal Plants*, pp. 3–8. New Delhi: Daya Publishing House.

P91   Kaur, G.J. & Arora, D.S. 2009. Antibacterial and phytochemical screening of *Anethum graveolens*, *Foeniculum vulgare* and *Trachyspermum ammi*. *BMC Complementary and Alternative Medicine* 9, 30, doi.org/10.1186/1472-6882-9-30.

P92   Jana, S. & Shekhawat, G.S. 2010. *Anethum graveolens*: an Indian traditional medicinal herb and spice. *Pharmacognosy Review* 4, 179–184, doi:10.4103/0973-7847.70915.

P93   Kaur, V. *et al.* 2020. A review on dill essential oil and its chief compounds as natural biocide. *Flavour and Fragrance Journal* 36, 412–431, doi.org/10.1002/ffj.3633.

P94 Graven, E.H. *et al.* 1992. Antimicrobial and antioxidative properties of the volatile (essential) oil of *Artemisia afra* Jacq. *Flavour and Fragrance Journal* 7, 121–123, doi.org/10.1002/ffj.2730070305.

P95 Liu, N.Q. *et al.* 2009. *Artemisia afra*: a potential flagship for African medicinal plants? *South African Journal of Botany* 75, 185–195, doi:10.1016/j.sajb.2008.11.001.

P96 Bruneton, J. 1995. *Pharmacognosy. Phytochemistry. Medicinal Plants.* Hampshire: Intercept.

P97 Hutchings, A. 1989. Observations on plant usage in Xhosa and Zulu medicine. *Bothalia* 19, pp. 225–235.

P98 Yang, S.L. *et al.* 1995. Flavonoids and chromenes from *Artemisia annua*. *Phytochemistry* 38, pp. 255–257.

P99 Nigam, M. *et al.* 2019. Bioactive compounds and health benefits of *Artemisia* species. *Natural Product Communications*, 1–17, doi.org/10.1177/1934578X19850354

P100 Oketch-Rabah, H.A. *et al.* 1997. Antiprotozoal compounds from *Asparagus africanus*. *Journal of Natural Products* 60, pp. 1017–1022.

P101 Mfengwana, P-M-A.H. & Mashele, S.S. 2019. *Medicinal properties of selected Asparagus species: a review*, doi:10.5772/intechopen.87048. Available from: www.intechopen.com/chapters/67855 [Accessed 25 August 2021].

P102 Hakizamungu, E. *et al.* 1992. Screening of Rwandese medicinal plants for anti-trichomonas activity. *Journal of Ethnopharmacology* 36, pp. 143–146.

P103 Cos, P. *et al.* 2002. Antiviral activity of Rwandan medicinal plants against human immunodeficiency virus type-1 (HIV-1). *Phytomedicine* 9, pp. 62–68.

P104 Lasure, A. *et al.* 1995. Screening of Rwandese plant extracts for their influence on lymphocyte proliferation. *Phytomedicine* 1, pp. 303–307.

P105 Rodriguez, E. *et al.* 1985. Thiarubrine A, a bioactive constituent of *Aspilia* (Asteraceae) consumed by wild chimpanzees. *Experientia* 41, pp. 419–420.

P106 Bohlmann, F. *et al.* 1983. Steiractinolides, a new group of sesquiterpene lactones. *Liebigs Annalen der Chemie* 6, pp. 962–973.

P107 Yaouba, S. *et al.* 2018. Crystal structures and cytotoxicity of ent-Kaurane-Type diterpenoids from two *Aspilia* species. *Molecules* 23, 3199, doi:10.3390/molecules23123199.

P108 Devi, C.U. *et al.* 2001. Anti-plasmodial effect of three medicinal plants: a preliminary study. *Current Science* 80, pp. 917–919.

P109 Bandyopadhyay, U. *et al.* 2002. Gastroprotective effect of neem (*Azadirachta indica*) bark extract: possible involvement of H+-K+-ATPase inhibition and scavenging of hydroxyl radical. *Life Sciences* 71, pp. 2845–2865.

P110 Shimizu, M. *et al.* 1985. *China tree bark extract with antineoplastic action*. Patent-Swiss-650,404, 12pp.

P111 Okpanyi, S.N. & Ezeukwu, G.C. 1981. Anti-inflammatory and antipyretic activities of *Azadirachta indica*. *Planta Medica* 41, pp. 34–39.

P112 Ahmad, I. *et al.* 1998. Screening of some Indian medicinal plants for their antimicrobial properties. *Journal of Ethnopharmacology* 62, pp. 183–193.

P113 Lucantoni, L. *et al.* 2010. Transmission blocking activity of a standardized neem (*Azadirachta indica*) seed extract on the rodent malaria parasite *Plasmodium berghei* in its vector *Anopheles stephensi*. *Malaria Journal* 9, 66, doi.org/10.1186/1475-2875-9-66.

P114 Shin-Foon, C. 1989. Studies on plants as a source of insect growth regulators for crop protection. *Journal of Applied Entomology* 107, pp. 185–192.

P115 Biswas, K. *et al.* 2002. Biological activities and medicinal properties of neem (*Azadirachta indica*). *Current Science* 82, pp. 1336–1345.

P116 Kraus, W. *et al.* 1981. Tetranortriterpenoids from the seed of *Azadirachta indica*. *Phytochemistry* 20, pp. 117–120.

P117 Sarah, R. *et al.* 2019. Bioactive compounds isolated from neem tree and their applications in Akhtar, M.S. *et al.* (Eds), *Natural Bio-active Compounds, Vol. 1: Production and Applications*. Singapore: Springer.

P118 Taniguchi, M. *et al.* 1978. Screening of East African plants for antimicrobial activity. I. *Chemical and Pharmaceutical Bulletin* 26, pp. 2910–2913.

P119 Chothani, D.L. & Vaghasiya, H.U. 2011. A review on *Balanites aegyptiaca* Del (desert date): phytochemical constituents, traditional uses, and pharmacological activity. *Pharmacognosy Reviews* 5, 55–62, doi:10.4103/0973-7847.79100.

P120 Archibald, R.G. 1933. The use of the fruit of the tree *Balanites aegyptiaca* in the control of schistosomiasis in the Sudan. *Transactions of the Royal Society of Tropical Medicine and Hygiene* 27, pp. 207–210.

P121 Liu, H.W. & Nakanishi, K. 1982. The structures of balanitins, potent molluscicides isolated from *Balanites aegyptiaca. Tetrahedron* 38, pp. 513–519.

P122 Jaiprakash, B. *et al.* 2003. Hepatoprotective activity of bark of *Balanites aegyptiaca* Linn. *Journal of Natural Remedies* 3, pp. 205–207.

P123 Nakanishi, K. 1982. Recent studies on bioactive compounds from plants. *Journal of Natural Products* 45, pp. 15–26.

P124 Mahato, S.B. *et al.* 1982. Steroidal saponins. *Phytochemistry* 21, p. 959.

P125 Saleh, N.A.M. & El-Hadidi, M.N. 1977. An approach to the chemosystematics of the Zygophyllaceae. *Biochemical Systematics and Ecology* 5, pp. 121–128.

P126 Kupchan, S.M. *et al.* 1971. Tumor inhibitors. LXV. Bersenogenin, bersicillogenin, and 3-epibersicillogenin, three new cytotoxic bufadienolides from *Bersama abyssinica. The Journal of Organic Chemistry* 36, p. 2611.

P127 Taniguchi, M. & Kubo, I. 1993. Ethnobotanical drug discovery based on medicine men's trials in the African savanna: screening of East African plants for antimicrobial activity. II. *Journal of Natural Products* 56, pp. 1539–1546.

P128 Asres, K. *et al.* 2001. Antiviral activity against human immunodeficiency virus type 1 (HIV-1) and type 2 (HIV-2) of ethnobotanically selected Ethiopian medicinal plants. *Phytotherapy Research* 15, pp. 62–69.

P129 Kupchan, S.M. *et al.* 1971. Tumor inhibitors. LXIV. isolation and structural elucidation of novel bufadienolides, the cytotoxic principles of *Bersama abyssinica. Bioorganic Chemistry* 1, pp. 13–31.

P130 Kubo, I. & Matsumoto, T. 1985. Potent insect antifeedants from the African medicinal plant *Bersama abyssinica. ACS Symposium Series* 276, pp. 183–200.

P131 Nyamboki, D.K. *et al.* 2021. Cytotoxic compounds from the stem bark of two subsp. of *Bersama abyssinica. Journal of Natural Products* 84, pp. 1453–1458.

P132 Hassan, S.W. *et al.* 2006. Evaluation of antibacterial activity and phytochemical analysis of root extracts of *Boscia angustifolia. African Journal of Biotechnology* 5, pp. 1602–1607.

P133 Theddeus, M. & Kiswii, T.M. 2014. Efficacy of selected medicinal plants from eastern Kenya against *Aspergillus flavus. Journal of Plant Sciences* 2, 226–231, doi:10.11648/j.jps.20140205.22.

P134 Morgan, A.M.A. *et al.* 2014. A new flavonol glycoside from the leaves of *Boscia senegalensis. Bulletin of the Korean Chemical Society* 35, pp. 3447–3452.

P135 Pather, N. *et al.* 2011. A biochemical comparison of the in vivo effects of *Bulbine frutescens* and *Bulbine natalensis* on cutaneous wound healing. *Journal of Ethnopharmacology* 133, pp. 364–370

P136 Bringmann, G. *et al.* 2008. Joziknipholones A and B: the first dimeric phenylanthraquinones from the roots of *Bulbine frutescens. Chemistry – A European Journal* 14, pp. 1420–1429.

P137 Abegaz, B.M. *et al.* 2002. Gaboroquinones A and B and 4'-O-demethylknipholone-4'-O-b-D-glucopyranoside, phenylanthrquinones from the roots of *Bulbine frutescens. Journal of Natural Products* 65, pp. 1117–1121.

P138 Bringmann, G. *et al.* 2002. Bulbine-knipholone, a new, axially chiral phenylanthraquinone from *Bulbine abyssinica* (Asphodelaceae): isolation, structural elucidation, synthesis, and antiplasmodial activity. *European Journal of Organic Chemistry* 2002, pp. 1107–1111.

P139 Van Staden, L.F. & Drewes, S.E. 1994. Knipholone from *Bulbine latifolia* and *Bulbine frutescens. Phytochemistry* 35, pp. 685–686.

P140 Wanjohi, J.M. *et al.* 2005. Three dimeric anthracene derivatives from *Bulbine abyssinica. Tetrahedron* 61, pp. 2667–2674.

P141 Olusola, B.O. & Prinsloo, G. 2020. Ethnobotany, phytochemistry and pharmacological significance of the genus *Bulbine* (Asphodelaceae). *Journal of Ethnopharmacology* 260, 112986, doi.org/10.1016/j.jep.2020.112986.

P142 Telrandhe, U. & Uplanchiwar, V. 2013. Phyto-pharmacological perspective of *Cadaba farinosa* Forssk. *American Journal of Phytomedicine and Clinical Therapeutics* 1, pp. 011–022.

P143 Ahmad, V.U. *et al.* 1990. Cadabicilone, a sesquiterpene lactone from *Cadaba farinosa*. *Zeitschrift fuer Naturforschung* B 45, 1100–1102, doi:10.1002/CHIN.199042299.

P144 Ahmad, V.U. *et al.* 1987. Cadabicine and cadabicine diacetate from *Crataeva nurvala* and *Cadaba farinosa*. *Journal of Natural Products* 50, p. 1186.

P145 Gohar, A.A. 2002. Flavonol glycosides from *Cadaba glandulosa Zeitschrift fuer Naturforschung* C 57, 216–220, doi:10.1515/znc-2002-3-403.

P146 Monjane, J.A. *et al.* 2016. Novel metabolites from the roots of *Cadaba natalensis. Phytochemistry Letters* 16, pp. 283–286.

P147 Misra, P. *et al.* 1991. Antimalarial activity of traditional plants against erythrocytic stages of *Plasmodium berghei. International Journal of Pharmacology* 29, 19–33, doi:10.3109/13880209109082843.

P148 Sharma, P. & Sharma, J.D. 2001. In vitro hemolysis of human erythrocytes – by plant extracts with antiplasmodial activity. *Journal of Ethnopharmacology* 74, pp. 239–243.

P149 Mossa, J.S. *et al.* 1991. Pharmacological studies on aerial parts of *Calotropis procera. The American Journal of Chinese Medicine* 19, pp. 223–231.

P150 Tariq, M. *et al.* 1984. Studies on Saudi plants causing neuromuscular blockade. Abstr. *9th International Congress of Pharmacology, London (1984)* Abstr-2030p.

P151 Kumar, V.L. & Shivkar, Y.M. 2004. In vivo and in vitro effect of latex of *Calotropis procera* on gastrointestinal smooth muscles. *Journal of Ethnopharmacology* 93, pp. 377–379.

P152 Srivastava, G.N. *et al.* 1962. Studies on anticoagulant therapy. 3. In vitro screening of some Indian plant latices for fibrinolytic and anticoagulant activity. *Indian Journal of Medical Sciences* 16, pp. 873–877.

P153 Alrheam, A.I. 2015. Biochemical effects of *Calotropis procera* on hepatotoxicity. *Biomedical Research and Therapy* 2, pp. 446–453.

P154 Bhutani, K.K. *et al.* 1992. Occurrence of D/E trans stereochemistry isomeric to ursane (cis) series in a new pentacyclic triterpene from *Calotropis procera. Tetrahedron Letters* 33, pp. 7593–7596.

P155 Gaurav Parihar, G. & Balekar, N. 2016. *Calotropis procera*: a phytochemical and pharmacological review. *Thai Journal of Pharmaceutical Sciences* 40, pp. 115–131.

P156 Stuart, M. 1979. *The Encyclopaedia of Herbs and Herbalism*. London: Orbis Publishing.

P157 National Academies of Sciences, Engineering, and Medicine. 2017. *The Health Effects of Cannabis and Cannabinoids: the Current State of Evidence and Recommendations for Research*. Washington, DC: The National Academies Press, doi:10.17226/24625.

P158 Saleh, B.K. *et al.* 2018. Medicinal uses and health benefits of chili pepper (*Capsicum* spp.): a review. *MOJ Food Processing & Technology* 6, 325–328, doi:10.15406/mojfpt.2018.06.00183.

P159 Hirt, H.M. & M'Pia, B. 2001. *Natural Medicine in the Tropics*. Winnenden, Germany: Anamed, Action for Natural Medicine.

P160 Antonio, A.S. *et al.* 2018. The genus *Capsicum*: a phytochemical review of bioactive secondary metabolites. *RSC Advances* 8, 25767, doi:10.1039/c8ra02067a.

P161 Osato, J.A. *et al.* 1993. Antimicrobial and antioxidant activities of unripe papaya. *Life Sciences* 53, pp. 1383–1389.

P162 Chen, C.F. *et al.* 1981. Protective effects of *Carica papaya* Linn on the exogenous gastric ulcer in rats. *The American Journal of Chinese Medicine* 9, pp. 205–212.

P163 Tecelão, C. *et al.* 2011. *Carica papaya* latex: a low-cost biocatalyst for human milk fat substitutes production. *European Journal of Lipid Science and Technology* 114, 266–276, doi.org/10.1002/ejlt.201100226.

P164 Giri, J. *et al.* 1980. Evaluation of the nutritive content of five varieties of papaya in different stages of ripening.

The Indian Journal of Nutrition and Dietetics 17, pp. 319–325.

P165 Strocchi, A. *et al.* 1977. Composition of papaya seed oil. *Rivista Italiana delle Sostanze Grasse* 54, pp. 429–431.

P166 Ghosh, S. *et al.* 2017. Extraction, isolation and characterization of bioactive compounds from chloroform extract of *Carica papaya* seed and its in vivo antibacterial potentiality in *Channa punctatus* against *Klebsiella* PKBSG14. *Microbial Pathogenesis* 111, pp. 508–518.

P167 El-Fiky, F.K. *et al.* 1996. Effect of *Luffa aegyptiaca* (seeds) and *Carissa edulis* (leaves) extracts on blood glucose levels of normal and streptozotocin diabetic rats. *Journal of Ethnopharmacology* 50, pp. 43–47.

P168 Omer, M.E.A. *et al.* 1998. Sudanese plants used in folkloric medicine: screening for antibacterial activity. Part IX. *Fitoterapia* 69, pp. 542–545.

P169 Elsheikh, S.H. *et al.* 1990. Toxicity of certain Sudanese plant extracts on cercariae and miracidia of *Schistosoma mansoni*. *International Journal of Crude Drug Research* 28, pp. 241–245.

P170 Achenbach, H. *et al.* 1983. Constituents of West African medicinal plants. 12 Lignans and other constituents from *Carissa edulis*. *Phytochemistry* 22, pp. 749–753.

P171 Bentley, M.D. & Brackett, S.R. 1984. 2-Hydroxyacetophenone: principal root volatile of the East African medicinal plant, *Carissa edulis*. *Journal of Natural Products* 47, pp. 1056–1057.

P172 Wangteeraprasert, R. *et al.* 2012. Bioactive compounds from *Carissa spinarum*. *Phytotherapy Research* 26, 1496–1499, doi:10.1002/ptr.4607.

P173 Dharani, N. 2016. Traditional ethnomedicinal uses and phytochemical compounds of *Carissa spinarum* L. in East Africa: a review. *Pharm Journal* 2. Kenyatta University Pharmacy Students Association (KUPHSA). Kenyatta University Press.

P174 Connelly, M.P.E. *et al.* 1996. Anti-malarial activity in crude extacts of Malawian medicinal plants. *Annals of Tropical Medicine and Parasitology* 90, pp. 597–602.

P175 Sawhney, A.N. *et al.* 1978. Studies on the rationale of African traditional medicine. Part II. Preliminary screening of medicinal plants for anti-gonococci activity. *Pakistan Journal of Scientific and Industrial Research* 21, pp. 189–192.

P176 Mutasa, S.L. & Kahn, M.R. 1995. Phytochemical investigations of *Cassia abbreviata*. *Fitoterapia* 66, p. 184.

P177 Nel, R.J.J. *et al.* 1999. The novel flavan-3-ol, (2R,3S)-guibourtinidol and its diastereomers. *Phytochemistry* 52, pp. 1153–1158.

P178 Yang, X. *et al.* 2021. Chemical constituents of *Cassia abbreviata* and their anti-HIV-1 activity. *Molecules* 26, 2455, doi.org/10.3390/molecules26092455.

P179 Kalix, P. 1991. The pharmacology of psychoactive alkaloids from *Ephedra* and *Catha*. *Journal of Ethnopharmacology* 32, pp. 201–208.

P180 Crombie, L. *et al.* 1990. Alkaloids of khat (*Catha edulis*) in Brossi, A. (ed.), *The Alkaloids, Chemistry and Pharmacology* 39, pp. 139–164. San Diego: Academic Press.

P181 Getasetegn, M. 2016. Chemical composition of *Catha edulis* (khat): a review. *Phytochemistry Reviews* 15, 907–920, doi.org/10.1007/s11101-015-9435-z.

P182 Marles, R.J. & Farnsworth, N.R. 1995. Antidiabetic plants and their active constituents. *Phytomedicine* 2, pp. 137–189.

P183 Sofowora, A. 1982. *Medicinal Plants and Traditional Medicine in Africa*. Hoboken, USA: Wiley.

P184 Tiong, S.H. *et al.* 2015. Vindogentianine, a hypoglycemic alkaloid from *Catharanthus roseus* (L.) G.Don (Apocynaceae). *Fitoterapia* 102, 182–188, doi:10.1016/j.fitote.2015.01.019.

P185 Sunilkumar, S.P. & Shivakumar, H.G. 1998. Evaluation of topical formulations of aqueous extract of *Centella asiatica* on open wounds in rats. *Indian Journal of Experimental Biology* 36, pp. 569–572.

P186 Adesina, S.K. 1982. Studies on some plants used as anticonvulsants in Amerindian and African traditional medicine. *Fitoterapia* 53, pp. 147–162.

P187 Morante, J.M.O. *et al.* 1998. Contact dermatitis allergy from *Centella asiatica* extract: report of a new case. *Acta Dermo-Sifiliográficas* 89, pp. 341–343.

P188 Ray, P.G. & Majumdar, S.K. 1976. Antimicrobial activity of some Indian plants. *Economic Botany* 30, pp. 317–320.

P189 Yang, H.C. *et al.* 1953. Influence of several Chinese drugs on the growth of some pathologic organisms. Preliminary report. *Journal of the Formosan Medical Association* 52, pp. 109–112.

P190 Ponglux, D. *et al* (Eds). 1987. *Medicinal Plants.* Bangkok, Thailand: The First Princess Chulabhom Science Congress.

P191 Yoshinori, A. *et al.* 1982. Mono- and sesquiterpenoids from *Hydrocotyle* and *Centella* species. *Phytochemistry* 21, pp. 2590–2592.

P192 Wong, K.C. & Tan, G.L. 1994. Essential oil of *Centella asiatica* (L.) Urb. *Journal of Essential Oil Research* 6, pp. 307–309.

P193 Somchit, M.N. *et al.* 2004. Antinociceptive and antiinflammatory effects of *Centella asiatica. Indian Journal of Pharmacology* 36, p. 377.

P194 Hashim, P. *et al.* 2011. Triterpene composition and bioactivities of *Centella asiatica. Molecules* 16, 1310–1322, doi:10.3390/molecules16021310.

P195 Morganti, P. *et al.* 1999. Extraction and analysis of cosmetic active ingredients from an anti-cellulitis transdermal delivery system by high-performance liquid chromatography. *Journal of Chromatographic Science* 37, pp. 51–55.

P196 Babu, T.D. *et al.* 1995. Cytotoxic and anti-tumor properties of certain taxa of Umbelliferae with special reference to *Centella asiatica* (L.) Urban. *Journal of Ethnopharmacology* 48, pp. 53–57.

P197 Roy, D.C. *et al.* 2013. Current updates on *Centella asiatica*: phytochemistry, pharmacology and traditional uses. *Medicinal Plant Research* 3, pp. 20–36.

P198 Rui Wang, R. *et al.* 2008. Extraction of essential oils from five cinnamon leaves and identification of their volatile compound compositions. *Innovative Food Science & Emerging Technologies* 10, pp. 289–292.

P199 Benarroz, M.O. *et al.* 2008. *Cinnamomum zeylanicum* extract on the radiolabelling of blood constituents and the morphometry of red blood cells: in vitro assay. *Applied Radiation and Isotopes* 66, pp. 139–146.

P200 Khan, A. *et al.* 2003. Cinnamon improves glucose and lipids of people with type 2 diabetes. *Diabetes Care* 26, pp. 3215–3218.

P201 Murcia, M.A. *et al.* 2004. Antioxidant evaluation in dessert spices compared with common food additive. Influence of irradiation procedure. *Journal of Agricultural and Food Chemistry* 57, pp. 1872–1881.

P202 Singh, N. *et al.* 2020. Phytochemical and pharmacological review of *Cinnamomum verum* J. Presl – a versatile spice used in food and nutrition. *Food Chemistry* 338, 127773, doi.org/10.1016/j.foodchem.2020.127773.

P203 Audicana, M. & Bernaola, G. 1994. Occupational contact dermatitis from citrus fruits: lemon essential oils. *Contact Dermatitis* 31, pp. 183–185.

P204 Hammer, K.A. *et al.* 1998. In-vitro activity of essential oils, in particular *Melaleuca alternifolia* (tea tree) oil and tea tree oil products, against *Candida* spp. *The Journal of Antimicrobial Chemotherapy* 42, pp. 591–595.

P205 Simard, J.P. 1986. *Antiobesity agent.* Patent-Fr Demande-2,576, 212.

P206 De Blasi, V. *et al.* 1990. Amoebicidal effect of essential oils in vitro. *Journal de Toxicologie Clinique et Experimentale* 10, pp. 361–373.

P207 Otero, R. *et al.* 2000. Snakebites and ethnobotany in the northwest region of Colombia. Part III. Neutralization of the haemorrhagic effect of *Bothrops atrox* venom. *Journal of Ethnopharmacology* 73, pp. 233–241.

P208 Viana, M.D.M. *et al.* 2016. Anxiolytic-like effect of *Citrus limon* (L.) Burm f. essential oil inhalation on mice. *Revista Brasileira de Planta Medicinais* 18, pp. 96–104.

P209 Eureka, T.F. *et al.* 1978. Flavonoids in flowers of *Citrus limon* cv. *Proceedings of the International Society of Citriculture* 1978, pp. 74–76.

P210 Hussain, H.S.N. & Deeni, Y.Y. 1991. Plants in Kano ethnomedicine; screening for antimicrobial activity and alkaloids. *International Journal of Pharmacognosy* 29, pp. 51–56.

P211 Johns, T. *et al.* 1995. Anti-giardial activity of gastrointestinal remedies of the Luo of East Africa. *Journal of Ethnopharmacology* 46, pp. 17–23.

P212   Ayedoun, M.A. *et al*. 1998. Aromatic plants of tropical West Africa. VI. Alpha-oxobisabolene as main constituent of the leaf essential oil of *Commiphora africana* (A. Rich.) Engl. from Benin. *Journal of Essential Oil Research* 10, pp. 105–107.

P213   Ma, J. *et al*. 2005. A dihydroflavonol glucoside from *Commiphora africana* that mediates DNA strand scission. *Journal of Natural Products* 68, pp. 115–117.

P214   Dinku, W. *et al*. 2020. Anti-proliferative activity of a novel tricyclic triterpenoid acid from *Commiphora africana* resin against four human cancer cell lines. *Applied Biological Chemistry* 63, 16, doi. org/10.1186/s13765-020-00499-w.

P215   Sertié, J.A.A. *et al*. 2005. Pharmacological assay of *Cordia verbenacea* V: oral and topical anti-inflammatory activity, analgesic effect and fetus toxicity of a crude leaf extract. *Phytomedicine* 12, pp. 338–344.

P216   Alhadi, E.A. *et al*. 2015. Antimicrobial and phytochemical screening of *Cordia africana* in Sudan. *World Journal of Pharmaceutical Research* 4, pp. 257–269.

P217   Menezes, J.E.S.A. *et al*. 2001. Trichotomol, a new cadinenediol from *Cordia trichotoma*. *Journal of the Brazilian Chemical Society* 12, pp. 787–790.

P218   Moir, M. & Thomson, R.H. 1973. Naturally occurring quinones. Part XXII. Terpenoid quinones in *Cordia* spp. *Journal of the Chemical Society, Perkin Transactions 1* 1973, 1352–1357, doi:10.1039/P19730001352.

P219   Kamau, R.W. *et al*. 2019. Oleanolic acid and other compounds isolated from *Cordia africana* Lam which inhibit vancomycin resistant *Enterococcus*. *Pharmacognosy Communications* 9, 91–95, doi:10.5530/pc.2019.3.19.

P220   Masahiko Taniguchi, M. *et al*. 1996. Three isocoumarins from *Coriandrum sativum*. *Phytochemistry* 42, pp. 843–846.

P221   Hamdard Publication. 1959. *Village Physician*. Part 1. Delhi, India.

P222   Msaada, K. *et al*. 2007. Changes on essential oil composition of coriander (*Coriandrum sativum* L.) fruits during three stages of maturity. *Food Chemistry* 102, pp. 1131–1134.

P223   Eguale, T. *et al*. 2007. In vitro and in vivo anthelmintic activity of crude extracts of *Coriandrum sativum* against *Haemonchus contortus*. *Journal of Ethnopharmacology* 110, 428–433, doi:10.1016/j.jep.2006.10.003.

P224   Matasyoh, J.C. *et al*. 2009. Chemical composition and antimicrobial activity of the essential oil of *Coriandrum sativum*. *Food Chemistry* 113, pp. 526–529.

P225   Tachibana, Y. *et al*. 1993. Mitogenic activities in African traditional herbal medicines. *Planta Medica* 59, pp. 354–358.

P226   Kloos, H. *et al*. 1987. Preliminary evaluation of some wild and cultivated plants for snail control in Machakos District, Kenya. *The Journal of Tropical Medicine and Hygiene* 90, pp. 197–204.

P227   De Paula, A.C.B. *et al*. 2008. The antiulcer effect of *Croton cajucara* Benth in normoproteic and malnourished rats. *Phytomedicine* 15, p. 815.

P228   Stuart, K.L. 1970. Chemical and biological investigations of *Croton* genus. *Revista Latinoamericana de Química* 1, pp. 140–147.

P229   Addae-Mensah, I. *et al*. 1989. A clerodane diterpene and other constituents of *Croton megalocarpus*. *Phytochemistry* 28, pp. 2759–2761.

P230   Addae-Mensah, I. *et al*. 1992. Epoxychiromodine and other constituents of *Croton megalocarpus*. *Phytochemistry* 31, pp. 2055–2058.

P231   Aldhaher, A. *et al*. 2017. Diterpenoids from the roots of *Croton dichogamus* Pax. *Phytochemistry* 144, pp. 1–8.

P232   Chainani-Wu, N. 2003. Safety and anti-inflammatory activity of curcumin: a component of turmeric (*Curcuma longa*). *The Journal of Alternative and Complementary Medicine* 9, pp. 161–168.

P233   Ramsewak, R.S. *et al*. 2000. Cytotoxicity, antioxidant and anti-inflammatory activities of curcumins I–III from *Curcuma longa*. *Phytomedicine* 7, pp. 303–308.

P234   Bello, O.M. *et al*. 2019. Phytochemistry, pharmacology and perceived health uses of non-cultivated vegetable *Cyphostemma adenocaule* (Steud. ex A. Rich.) Desc. ex Wild and R.B. Drumm.: a review. *Scientific African* 2, e00053, doi. org/10.1016/j.sciaf.2019.e00053.

P235 Chouna, J.R. *et al.* 2016. Ceanothane-type triterpenoids from *Cyphostemma adenocaule*. *Archives of Pharmacal Research*, doi.org/10.1007/s12272-016-0801-1.

P236 Soni, P. *et al.* 2012. Pharmacological properties of *Datura stramonium* L. as a potential medicinal tree: an overview. *Asian Pacific Journal of Tropical Biomedicine* 2012 Dec., 2(12), 1002–1008, doi:10.1016/S2221-1691(13)60014-3.

P237 Eisa, M.M. *et al.* 2000. Antibacterial activity of *Dichrostachys cinerea*. *Fitoterapia* 71, pp. 324–327.

P238 Kweyamba P.A. *et al.* 2019. In vitro and in vivo studies on anti-malarial activity of *Commiphora africana* and *Dichrostachys cinerea* used by the Maasai in Arusha region, Tanzania. *Malaria Journal* 18, 119, doi.org/10.1186/s12936-019-2752-8.

P239 Joshi, K.C. & Sharma, T. 1974. Triterpenoids and some other constituents from *Dichrostachys cinerea*. *Phytochemistry* 13, pp. 2010–2011.

P240 Rao, R.J. *et al.* 2003. Novel 3-O-acyl mesquitol analogues as free-radical scavengers and enzyme inhibitors: synthesis, biological evaluation and structure–activity relationship. *Bioorganic & Medicinal Letters* 13, pp. 2777–2780.

P241 Mbaveng, A.T. *et al.* 2019. Cytotoxicity of crude extract and isolated constituents of the *Dichrostachys cinerea* bark towards multifactorial drug-resistant cancer cells. *Evidence-Based Complementary and Alternative Medicine*, 2019, 8450158, doi. org/10.1155/2019/8450158.

P242 Khalil, N.M. *et al.* 2006. Anti-inflammatory activity and acute toxicity of *Dodonaea viscosa*. *Fitoterapia* 77, pp. 478–480.

P243 Getie, M. *et al.* 2003. Evaluation of the anti-microbial and anti-inflammatory activities of the medicinal plants *Dodonaea viscosa*, *Rumex nervosus* and *Rumex abyssinicus*. *Fitoterapia* 74, pp. 139–143.

P244 Amabeoku, G.J. *et al.* 2001. Analgesic and antipyretic effects of *Dodonaea*

angustifolia and *Salvia africana-lutea*. *Journal of Ethnopharmacology* 75, pp. 117–124.

P245 Van Heerden, A.M. *et al.* 2000. The major flavonoids of *Dodonaea angustifolia*. *Fitoterapia* 71, p. 602.

P246 Sachev, K. & Kulshreshtha, D.K. 1983. Flavonoids from *Dodonaea viscosa*. *Phytochemistry* 22, pp. 1253–1256.

P247 Sachev, K. & Kulshreshtha, D.K. 1984. Dodonic acid, a new diterpenoid from *Dodonaea viscosa*. *Planta Medica* 50, pp. 448–449.

P248 Kaigongi, M.M. *et al.* 2020. LC-MS-based metabolomics for the chemosystematics of Kenyan *Dodonaea viscosa* Jacq (Sapindaceae) populations. *Molecules* 25, 4130, doi:10.3390/molecules25184130.

P249 Reid, K.A. *et al.* 2001. Pharmacological and phytochemical properties of *Dombeya rotundifolia*. *South African Journal of Botany* 67, pp. 349–353.

P250 Maroyi, A. 2018. *Dombeya rotundifolia* (Hochst.) Planch.: review of its botany, medicinal uses, phytochemistry, and biological activities. *Journal of Complementary Medicine Research* 9, pp. 74–82.

P251 Irungu, B. *et al.* 2014. Constituents of the roots and leaves of *Ekebergia capensis* and their potential antiplasmodial and cytotoxic activities. *Molecules* 19, 14235–14246, doi:10.3390/ molecules190914235.

P252 Taylor, D.A.H. 1981. Ekebergin, a limonoid extractive from *Ekebergia capensis*. *Phytochemistry* 20, pp. 2263–2265.

P253 Olajide, O.A. & Alada, A.R.A. 2001. Studies on the anti-inflammatory properties of *Entada abyssinica*. *Fitoterapia* 72, pp. 492–496.

P254 Vlietinck, A.J. *et al.* 1995. Screening of hundred Rwandese medicinal plants for antimicrobial and antiviral properties. *Journal of Ethnopharmacology* 46, pp. 31–47.

P255 Freiburghaus, F. *et al.* 1998. Bioassy-guided isolation of a diastereoisomer of kolavenol from *Entada abyssinica* active on *Trypanosama brucei rhodesiense*. *Journal of Ethnopharmacology* 61, pp. 179–183.

P256 Fabry, W. *et al.* 1998. Antibacterial activity of East African medicinal plants. *Journal of Ethnopharmacology* 60, pp. 79–84.

P257 Cos, P. *et al.* 2002. Further evaluation of Rwandan medicinal plant extracts for their antimicrobial and antiviral activities. *Journal of Ethnopharmacology* 79, pp. 155–163.

P258 Dzoyem, J.P. *et al.* 2017. Cytotoxicity, antimicrobial and antioxidant activity of eight compounds isolated from *Entada abyssinica* (Fabaceae). *BMC Research Notes* 10, 118, doi.org/10.1186/s13104-017-2441-z.

P259 Maikere-Faniyo, R. *et al.* 1989. Study of Rwandese medicinal plants used in the treatment of diarrhoea I. *Journal of Ethnopharmacology* 26, pp. 101–109.

P260 Kamat, V.S. *et al.* 1981. Antimicrobial agents from an East African medicinal plant *Erythrina abyssinica*. *Heterocycles* 15, pp. 1163–1170.

P261 Yenesew, A. *et al.* 2003. Flavonoids and isoflavonoids with anti-plasmodial activities from the roots of *Erythrina abyssinica*. *Planta Medica* 69, pp. 658–661.

P262 Barakat, I. *et al.* 1977. Further studies of *Erythrina* alkaloids. *Lloydia* 40, pp. 471–475.

P263 Juma, B. & Majinda, R.R.T. 2004. Erythrinaline alkaloids from the flowers and pods of *Erythrina lysistemon* and their DPPH radical scavenging properties. *Phytochemistry* 65, p. 1397.

P264 Nguyen, P.H. *et al.* 2009. Cytotoxic and PTP1B inhibitory activities from *Erythrina abyssinica*. *Bioorganic & Medicinal Chemistry Letters* 19, pp. 6745–6749.

P265 Safaei-Ghomi, J. & Ahd, A.A. 2010. Antimicrobial and antifungal properties of the essential oil and methanol extracts of *Eucalyptus largiflorens* and *Eucalyptus intertexta*. *Pharmacognosy Magazine* 6, 172–175, doi:10.4103/0973-1296.66930.

P266 Dethier, M. *et al.* 1994. Aromatic plants of tropical Central Africa. XVI. Studies on essential oils of five *Eucalyptus* species grown in Burundi. *Journal of Essential Oil Research* 6, 469–473, doi.org/10.1080/10412905.1994.9698428.

P267 Zrira, S.S. *et al.* 1992. Essential oils of twenty-seven *Eucalyptus* species grown in Morocco. *Journal of Essential Oil Research* 4, pp. 259–264, doi.org/10.1080/10412905.1992.9698059.

P268 Hanghang Lou, H. *et al.* 2021. A review on preparation of betulinic acid and its biological activities. *Molecules* 26, 5583, doi.org/10.3390/molecules26185583.

P269 Abdel-Sattar, E. *et al.* 2000. Phenolic compounds from *Eucalyptus maculata*. *Pharmazie* 55, pp. 623–624.

P270 Mazumder, A. *et al.* 2020. Bactericidal activity of essential oil and its major compound from leaves of *Eucalyptus maculata* Hook. against two fish pathogens. *Journal of Essential Oil Bearing Plants* 23, 149–155, doi:10.1080/0972060X.2020.1729248.

P271 Sparg, S.G. *et al.* 2000. Efficiency of traditionally used South African plants against schistosomiasis. *Journal of Ethnopharmacology* 73, pp. 209–214.

P272 Homer, K.A. *et al.* 1990. Inhibition of protease activities of periodontopathic bacteria by extracts of plants used in Kenya as chewing sticks (mswaki). *Archives of Oral Biology* 35, pp. 421–424.

P273 More, G. *et al.* 2008. Antimicrobial activity of medicinal plants against oral microorganisms. *Journal of Ethnopharmacology* 119, pp. 473–477.

P274 Bringmann, G. *et al.* 2008. Antitumoral and antileishmanial dioncoquinones and ancistroquinones from cell cultures of *Triphyophyllum peltatum* (Dioncophyllaceae) and *Ancistrocladus abbreviatus* (Ancistrocladaceae). *Phytochemistry* 69, pp. 2501–2509.

P275 Dagne, E. *et al.* 1993. Flavonoids from *Euclea divinorum*. *Bulletin of the Chemical Society of Ethiopia* 7, pp. 87–92.

P276 Mebe, P.P. *et al.* 1998. Pentacyclic triterpenes and naphthoquinones from *Euclea divinorum*. *Phytochemistry* 47, pp. 311–313.

P277 Kim, S.S. *et al.* 2003. Eugenol suppresses cyclooxygenase-2 expression in lipopolysaccharide-stimulated mouse macrophage RAW264.7 cells. *Life Sciences* 73, pp. 337–348.

P278 Mohaddese Mahboubi, M. & Mahboubi, M. 2015. Chemical composition, antimicrobial and antioxidant activities of *Eugenia caryophyllata* essential oil. *Journal of Essential Oil Bearing Plants* 18, 967–975, doi:10.1080/097206 0X.2014.884779.

P279 Runyoro, K.B.D *et al.* 2006. Screening of Tanzanian medicinal plants for anti-

Candida activity. *BMC Complementary and Alternative Medicine* 6, 11, doi. org/10.1186/1472-6882-6-11

P280   Ajaib, M. *et al.* 2018. Phytochemical screening and anthelmintic activity of *Flueggea virosa. Chemical Society of Pakistan* 40, pp. 702–706.

P281   Gan, L.-S. *et al.* 2006. Flueggenines A and B, two novel C,C-linked dimeric indolizidine alkaloids from *Flueggea virosa. Organic Letters* 8, pp. 2285–2288.

P282   Qiu-Jie, X. *et al.* 2020. Alkaloid constituents from the fruits of *Flueggea virosa. Chinese Journal of Natural Medicines* 18, 385–392, doi:10.1016/S1875-5364(20)30045-5.

P283   Saad, El-Z. *et al.* 2006. Acaricidal activities of some essential oils and their monoterpenoidal constituents against house dust mite, *Dermatophagoides pteronyssinus* (Acari: Pyroglyphidae). *Journal of Zhejiang University. Science. B.* 7, 957–962, doi:10.1631/jzus.2006. B0957.

P284   Bogucka-Kocka, A. *et al.* 2008. Apoptotic activities of ethanol extracts from some Apiaceae on human leukaemia cell lines. *Fitoterapia* 79, pp. 487–497.

P285   Türkyilmaz, Z. *et al.* 2008. A striking and frequent cause of premature thelarche in children: *Foeniculum vulgare. Journal of Pediatric Surgery* 43, pp. 2109–2111.

P286   Yaralizadeh, M. *et al.* 2016. Effect of *Foeniculum vulgare* (fennel) vaginal cream on vaginal atrophy in postmenopausal women: a double-blind randomized placebo-controlled trial. *Maturitas* 84, 75–80, doi. org/10.1016/j.maturitas.2015.11.005 0378-5122.

P287   Koch, A. *et al.* 2006. An antimalarial abietane diterpene from *Fuerstia africana. Biochemical Systematics and Ecology* 34, pp. 270–272.

P288   Karanatsios, D. *et al.* 1966. Structure of fuerstion. *Helvetica Chimica Acta* 49, pp. 1151–1172.

P289   Achola, K.J. *et al.* 1995. Pharmacological activities of *Gardenia ternifolia* var. *jovis-tonantis. International Journal of Pharmacognosy* 33, pp. 250–252.

P290   Ibrahim, A.M. 1992. Anthelmintic activity of some Sudanese medicinal plants. *Phytotherapy Research* 6, pp. 155–157.

P291   Agbodjento, E. *et al.* 2018. *Gardenia ternifolia*: review of ethnobotanical, ethnopharmacological, phytochemical and toxicological aspects. *International Journal of Biological and Chemical Sciences* 12, pp. 2922–2932.

P292   Babady-Bila & Tandu, K.R. 1988. Triterpenoids of *Gardenia ternifolia* var. *jovis-tonantis. Planta Medica* 54, p. 86.

P293   Jose, J. & Ravindran, M. 1988. A rare case of poisoning by *Gloriosa superba. The Journal of the Association of Physicians of India* 36, pp. 451–452.

P294   Pandey, D.K. *et al.* 2021. Screening the elite chemotypes of *Gloriosa superba* L. in India for the production of anticancer colchicine: simultaneous microwave-assisted extraction and HPTLC studies. *BMC Plant Biology* 21, 77, doi.org/10.1186/s12870-021-02843-8.

P295   Dvorackova, S. *et al.* 1984. Alkaloids of *Gloriosa superba* L. *Collection of Czechoslovakia Chemical Communications* 49, pp. 1536–1542.

P296   Ullah, W. *et al.* 2012. Ethnic uses, pharmacological and phytochemical profile of genus *Grewia. Journal of Asian Natural Products Research* 14, pp. 186–195.

P297   Almagboul, A.Z. *et al.* 1985. Antimicrobial activity of certain Sudanese plants used in folkloric medicine. Screening for antibacterial activity (IV). *Fitoterapia* 56, pp. 331–337.

P298   Almagboul, A.Z. *et al.* 1988. Antimicrobial activity of certain Sudanese plants used in folkloric medicine. Screening for antifungal activity (VI). *Fitoterapia* 59, pp. 393–396.

P299   Jaspers, M.W.J.M. *et al.* 1986. Investigation of *Grewia bicolor* Juss. *Journal of Ethnopharmacology* 17, pp. 205–211.

P300   Tariq, M. 1985. Anti-inflammatory studies on *Grewia populifolia. Fitoterapia* 56, pp. 178–180.

P301   Ahmed, E. *et al.* 2011. Phytochemical and antimicrobial studies of *Grewia tenax. Journal of the Chemical Society of Pakistan* 33, pp. 676–681.

P302   Di Giorgio, C. *et al.* 1988. In vitro activity of the β-carboline alkaloids harmane, harmine, and harmaline toward parasites of the species *Leishmania infantum. Experimental Parasitology* 106, pp. 67–74.

P303   El Tahir, A. *et al*. 1999. Antiplasmodial activity of selected Sudanese medicinal plants with emphasis on *Maytenus senegalensis* (Lam.) Exell. *Journal of Ethnopharmacology* 64, pp. 227–233.

P304   Baldé, A.M. *et al*. 1995. Biological investigations on *Harrisonia abyssinica. Phytomedicine* 1, pp. 299–302.

P305   Rajab, M.S. *et al*. 1999. 11β,12β-Diacetoxyharrisonin, a tetranortriterpenoid from *Harrisonia abyssinica. Phytochemistry* 52, pp. 127–133.

P306   Baldé, A.M. *et al*. 1999. Oumarone, bissaone, and aissatone, unusual prenylated polyketides from *Harrisonia abyssinica. Journal of Natural Products* 62, pp. 364–366.

P307   Liu, H.W. *et al*. 1981. A hydroperoxychroman with insect antifeedant properties from an African shrub. Characterization of fully-substituted aromatic structures. *Chemical Communications* 1981, pp. 1271–1272.

P308   Baldé, A.M. *et al*. 2001. Cycloabyssinone, a new cycloterpene from *Harrisonia abyssinica. Fitoterapia* 72, pp. 438–440.

P309   Mayaka, R. *et al*. 2012. Antimicrobial prenylated acetophenones from berries of *Harrisonia abyssinica. Planta Medica* 78, pp. 383–386

P310   Vasudeva, N. & Sharma, S.K. 2008. Biologically active compounds from the genus *Hibiscus. Pharmaceutical Biology* 46, 145–153, doi:10.1080/13880200701575320.

P311   Li, L. *et al*. 2006. Structure elucidation of a new friedelane triterpene from the mangrove plant *Hibiscus tiliaceus. Magnetic Resonance in Chemistry* 44, pp. 624–628.

P312   Desta, B. 1995. Ethiopian traditional herbal drugs. Part 1. Studies on the toxicity and therapeutic activity of local taenicidal medications. *Journal of Ethnopharmacology* 45, pp. 27–33.

P313   Komen, C. *et al*. 2005. Efficacy of *Jasminum abyssinicum* treatment against *Haemonchus contortus* in sheep. *African Journal of Traditional,*

Complementary and Alternative Medicine 2, pp. 264–268.

P314   Harborne, J.B. & Green, P.S. 1980. A chemotaxonomic survey of flavonoids in leaves of the Oleaceae. *Botanical Journal of the Linnean Society* 81, pp. 155–167.

P315   Gallo, F.R. *et al*. 2006. Oligomeric secoiridoid glucosides from *Jasminum abyssinicum. Phytochemistry* 67, pp. 504–510.

P316   Arivoli, S. *et al*. 2018. Phytochemical constituents of *Jasminum fluminense* Linnaeus (Oleaceae): an additional tool in the ecofriendly management of mosquitoes? *Journal of Pharmacognosy and Phytochemistry* 7, pp. 548–556.

P317   El-Shiek, R.A. *et al*. 2021. Anti-inflammatory activity of *Jasminum grandiflorum* L. subsp. *floribundum* (Oleaceae) in inflammatory bowel disease and arthritis models. *Biomedicine & Pharmacotherapy* 140, 111770, doi.org/10.1016/j.biopha.2021.111770.

P318   Dekker, T.G. *et al*. 1987. Studies of South African medicinal plants. Part 4. Jaherin, a new daphnane diterpene with antimicrobial properties from *Jatropha zeyheri. South African Journal of Chemistry* 40, pp. 74–76.

P319   Hirota, M. *et al*. 1988. A new tumour promoter from the seed oil from *Jatropha curcas* L. *Cancer Research* 48, pp. 5800–5804.

P320   Adolf, W. *et al*. 1984. Irritant phorbol derivatives from four *Jatropha* species. *Phytochemistry* 23, pp. 129–132.

P321   Joubert, P.H. *et al*. 1984. Acute poisoning with *Jatropha curcas* (purging nut tree) in children. *South African Medical Journal* 65, pp. 729–730.

P322   Mujumdar, A.M. & Misar, A.V. 2004. Anti-inflammatory activity of *Jatropha curcas* roots in mice and rats. *Journal of Ethnopharmacology* 90, pp. 11–15.

P323   Van Wyk, B.E. *et al*. 2000. *Medicinal Plants of South Africa*, edn 2. Pretoria, South Africa: Briza.

P324   Akunyili, D.N. *et al*. 1991. Anti-microbial activities of the stem bark of *Kigelia africana. Journal of Ethnopharmacology* 35, pp. 173–178.

P325   Govindachari, T.R. *et al*. 1971. Isolation and structure of two new dihydroisocoumarins from *Kigelia pinnata*. *Phytochemistry* 10, pp. 1603–1606.

P326 Picerno, P. *et al.* 2005. Anti-inflammatory activity of verminoside from *Kigelia africana* and evaluation of cutaneous irritation in cell cultures and reconstituted human epidermis. *Journal of Natural Products* 68, pp. 1610–1614.

P327 Nabatanzi, A. *et al.* 2020. Ethnobotany, phytochemistry and pharmacological activity of *Kigelia africana* (Lam.) Benth. (Bignoniaceae). *Plants* 9: 753, doi:10.3390/plants9060753.

P328 Deena, M.J. & Thoppil, J.E. 2000. Antimicrobial activity of the essential oil of *Lantana camara*. *Fitoterapia* 71, pp. 453–455.

P329 Occhiuto, F. *et al.* 1989. Studies on some medicinal plants on Senegal: effects on isolated guinea pig ileum. *Journal of Ethnopharmacology* 26, pp. 205–210.

P330 Achola, K.J. & Munenge, R.W. 1996. Pharmacological activities of *Lantana trifolia* on isolated guinea pig trachea and rat phrenic nerve diaphragm. *International Journal of Pharmacognosy* 34, pp. 273–276.

P331 Weyerstahl, P. *et al.* 1999. Constituents of commercial Brazilian lantana oil. *Flavour and Fragrance Journal* 14, pp. 15–28.

P332 Ahmed, Z.F. *et al.* 1972. Phytochemical study of *Lantana camara*. Terpenes and lactones. II. *Planta Medica* 22, pp. 34–37.

P333 Taoubi, K. *et al.* 1997. Phenylpropanoid glycosides from *Lantana camara* and *Lippia multiflora*. *Planta Medica* 63, pp. 192–193.

P334 Rwangabo, P.C. *et al.* 1988. Umuhengerin, a new antimicrobially active flavonoid from *Lantana trifolia*. *Journal of Natural Products* 51, pp. 966–968.

P335 Subhalakshmi Ghosh, S. *et al.* 2010. Anti-inflammatory and anticancer compounds isolated from *Ventilago madraspatana* Gaertn., *Rubia cordifolia* Linn. and *Lantana camara* Linn. *Journal of Pharmacy and Pharmacology* 62, 1158–1166, doi.org/10.1111/j.2042-7158.2010.01151.x.

P336 David, J.P. *et al.* 2007. Radical scavenging, antioxidant and cytotoxic activity of Brazilian *Caatinga* plants. *Fitoterapia* 78, 215–218, doi:10.1016/j.fitote.2006.11.015.

P337 Kaplan, E.R. & Rivett, D.E.A. 1968. The structures of compounds X and Y, two labdane diterpenoids from *Leonotis leonurus*. *Journal of the Chemistry Society C Organic*, pp. 262–266.

P338 He, F. *et al.* 2012. Leonurenones A–C: labdane diterpenes from *Leonotis leonurus*. *Phytochemistry* 83, pp. 168–172.

P339 De Oliveira, D.P. *et al.* 2019. Exploring the bioactivity potential of *Leonotis nepetifolia*: phytochemical composition, antimicrobial and antileishmanial activities of extracts from different anatomical parts. *Natural Product Research* 35, 3120–3125, doi:10.1080/14786419.2019.1686367.

P340 Habtemariam, S. *et al.* 1994. Diterpenes from the leaves of *Leonotis ocymifolia* var. *raineriana*. *Journal of Natural Products* 57, pp. 1570–1574.

P341 Oladimeji, F.A. *et al.* 2004. Physical properties and antimicrobial activities of leaf essential oil of *Lippia multiflora* Moldenke. *International Journal of Aromatherapy* 14, pp. 162–168.

P342 Manenzhe, N.J. *et al.* 2004. Composition and antimicrobial activities of volatile components of *Lippia javanica*. *Phytochemistry* 65, pp. 2333–2336.

P343 Martins, G.R. *et al.* 2019. Antifungal phenylpropanoid glycosides from *Lippia rubella*. *Journal of Natural Products* 82, 566–572, doi.org/10.1021/acs.jnatprod.8b00975.

P344 Mwangi, J.W. *et al.* 1991. Essential oils of Kenyan *Lippia* species. Part III. *Flavour and Fragrance Journal* 6, pp. 221–224.

P345 Viljoen, A.M. *et al.* 2005. The composition, geographical variation and antimicrobial activity of *Lippia javanica* (Verbenaceae) leaf essential oils. *Journal of Ethnopharmacology* 96, pp. 271–277.

P346 Olivier, D.K. *et al.* 2010. Phenylethanoid glycosides from *Lippia javanica*. *South African Journal of Botany* 76, 58–63, doi.org/10.1016/j.sajb.2009.07.002.

P347 Chagnon, M. 1984. General pharmacologic inventory of medicinal plants of Rwanda. *Journal of Ethnopharmacology* 12, pp. 239–251.

P348 Boily, Y. & Van Puyvelde, L. 1986. Screening of medicinal plants of Rwanda (Central Africa) for antimicrobial activity. *Journal of Ethnopharmacology* 16, pp. 1–13.

P349   Jang, D.S. 2004. Potential cancer chemopreventive constituents of the leaves of *Macaranga triloba*. *Phytochemistry* 65, pp. 345–350.

P350   Suffness, M. *et al*. 1988. The utility of P388 leukemia compared to B16 melanoma and colon carcinoma 38 for in vivo screening of plant extracts. *Phytotherapy Research* 2, pp. 89–97.

P351   Hashim, I. *et al*. 2021. Antibacterial activities and phytochemical screening of crude extracts from Kenyan *Macaranga* species towards MDR phenotypes expressing efflux pumps. *Pharmacognosy Communications* 11, pp. 119–126.

P352   Midiwo, J.O. *et al*. 2002. Bioactive compounds from some Kenyan ethnomedicinal plants: Myrsinaceae, Polygonaceae and *Psiadia punctulata*. *Phytochemistry Reviews* 1, pp. 311–323.

P353   Midiwo, J.O. *et al*. 1988. Distribution of benzoquinone pigments in Kenyan Myrsinaceae. *Bulletin of the Chemical Society of Ethiopia* 2, pp. 83–85.

P354   Manguro, L.O.A. *et al*. 2002. Flavonol glycosides of *Maesa lanceolata* leaves. *Natural Products Sciences* 8, 77–82. Available from: www.koreascience.or.kr/article/JAKO200203041137937.pdf.

P355   Sindambiwe, J.B. *et al*. 1998. Evaluation of biological activities of triterpenoid saponins from *Maesa lanceolata*. *Journal of Natural Products* 61, pp. 585–590.

P356   Shin, S.Y. *et al*. 2014. Identification of an anticancer compound contained in seeds of *Maesa lanceolata*, a medicinal plant in Ethiopia. *Journal of the Korean Society of Applied Biological Chemistry* 57, 519–522, doi:10.1007/s13765-014-4177-y.

P357   Rogers, L.L. *et al*. 1998. Volkensinin: a new limonoid from *Melia volkensii*. *Tetrahedron Letters* 39, pp. 4623–4626.

P358   Srivastava, S.K. & Mishra, M. 1985. New anthraquinone pigments from the stem bark of *Melia azedarach* Linn. *Indian Journal of Chemistry* 24B, 7, pp. 793–794.

P359   Gupta, H.O. & Srivastava, S.K. 1985. Apigenin-5-O-galactoside from the roots of *Melia azedarach* Linn. *Current Science* 54, pp. 570–571.

P360   Nakatani, M. *et al*. 1998. Degraded limonoids from *Melia azedarach*. *Phytochemistry* 49, pp. 1773–1776.

P361   Ervina, M. *et al*. 2020. Bio-selective hormonal breast cancer cytotoxic and antioxidant potencies of *Melia azedarach* L. wild type leaves. *Biotechnology Reports* 25, doi.org/10.1016/j.btre.2020.e00437.

P362   Wachsman, M. *et al*. 1982. Antiviral activity of a *Melia azedarach* plant extract. *Fitoterapia* 53, pp. 167–170.

P363   Carpinella, M.C. *et al*. 2003. Antifungal effects of different organic extracts from *Melia azedarach* L. on phytopathogenic fungi and their isolated active components. *Journal of Agricultural and Food Chemistry* 51, 2506–2511, doi:10.1021/jf026083f.

P364   Cantrell, C.L. *et al*. 1999. Antimycobacterial triterpenes from *Melia volkensii*. *Journal of Natural Products* 62, pp. 546–548.

P365   Jaoko, V. *et al*. 2020. The phytochemical composition of *Melia volkensii* and its potential for insect pest management. *Plants 9*, 143, doi.org/10.3390/plants9020143.

P366   Dhar, M.L. *et al*. 1968. Screening of Indian plants for biological activity. Part I. *Indian Journal of Experimental Biology* 6, pp. 232–247.

P367   Kusamba, C. *et al*. 1991. Antibacterial activity of *Mirabilis jalapa* seed powder. *Journal of Ethnopharmacology* 35, pp. 197–199.

P368   Wang, Y.F. *et al*. 2002. New rotenoids from roots of *Mirabilis jalapa*. *Helvetica Chimica Acta* 85, pp. 2342–2348.

P369   Saha, S. *et al*. 2020. Review on *Mirabilis jalapa* L. (Nyctaginaceae): a medicinal plant. *International Journal of Herbal Medicine* 8, pp. 14–18.

P370   Walker, C.I.B *et al*. 2008. Antinociceptive activity of *Mirabilis jalapa* in mice. *Journal of Ethnopharmacology* 120, pp. 169–175.

P371   Piattelli, M. & Minale, L. 1964. Pigments of Centrospermae-II. Distribution of betacyanins. *Phytochemistry* 3, pp. 547–557.

P372   Makonnen, E. *et al*. 1997. Hypoglycaemic effect of *Moringa stenopetala* aqueous extract in rabbits. *Phytotherapy Research* 11, pp. 147–148.

P373 Mekonnen, Y. 1999. Effects of ethanol extract of *Moringa stenopetala* leaves on guinea pig and mouse smooth muscle. *Phytotherapy Research* 13, pp. 442–444.

P374 Mekonnen, Y. *et al.* 1999. In vitro antitrypanosomal activity of *Moringa stenopetala* leaves and roots. *Phytotherapy Research* 13, pp. 538–539.

P375 Mekonnen, Y. & Dräger, B. 2003. Glucosinolates in *Moringa stenopetala*. *Planta Medica* 69, 380–382, doi:10.1055/s-2003-38881.

P376 Mekonen, A. & Gebreyesus, T. 2000. Chemical investigation of the leaves of *Moringa stenopetala*. *Bulletin of the Chemical Society of Ethiopia* 14, pp. 51–55.

P377 Waterman, C. *et al.* 2014. Stable, water extractable isothiocyanates from *Moringa oleifera* leaves attenuate inflammation in vitro. *Phytochemistry* 103, 114–122, doi:10.1016/j. phytochem.2014.03.028.

P378 Chokechaijaroenporn, O. *et al.* 1994. Mosquito repellent activities of *Ocimum* volatile oils. *Phytomedicine* 1, pp. 135–139.

P379 Akhtar, M.S. *et al.* 1992. Anti-ulcerogenic effects of *Ocimum basilicum* extracts, volatile oils and flavonoid glycosides in albino rats. *International Journal of Pharmacognosy* 30, pp. 97–104.

P380 Economou, K.D. *et al.* 1991. Antioxidant activity of some plant extracts of the family Labiatae. *Journal of the American Oil Chemists Society* 68, pp. 109–113.

P381 Akhtar, M.S. & Munir, M. 1989. Evaluation of the gastric antiulcerogenic effects of *Solanum nigrum*, *Brassica oleracea* and *Ocimum basilicum* in rats. *Journal of Ethnopharmacology* 27, pp. 163–176.

P382 Pino, J.A. *et al.* 1994. The essential oil of *Ocimum basilicum* L. from Cuba. *Journal of Essential Oil Research* 6, pp. 89–90.

P383 Charles, D.J. & Simon, J.E. 1992. Essential oil constituents of *Ocimum kilimandscharicum* Guerke. *Journal of Essential Oil Research* 4, 125–128.

P384 Fleisher, Z. & Fleisher, A. 1992. Volatiles of *Ocimum basilicum* traditionally grown in Israel. Aromatic plants of the Holy Land and the Sinai. Part VIII. *Journal of Essential Oil Research* 4, pp. 97–99.

P385 Maurya, P. *et al.* 2009. Evaluation of the toxicity of different phytoextracts of *Ocimum basilicum* against *Anopheles stephensi* and *Culex quinquefasciatus*. *Journal of Asia-Pacific Entomology* 12, pp. 113–115.

P386 Joshi, R.K. 2013. Chemical composition of the essential oil of camphor basil (*Ocimum kilimandscharicum* Guerke). *Global Journal of Medicinal Plant Research* 1, pp. 207–209.

P387 Janssen, A.M. *et al.* 1986. Screening for antimicrobial activity of some essential oils by the agar overlay technique. *Pharmaceutisch Weekblad*, scientific edn 8, pp. 289–292.

P388 Prasad, G. *et al.* 1986. Antimicrobial activity of essential oils of some *Ocimum* species and clove oil. *Fitoterapia* 57, pp. 429–432.

P389 Bekele, J. & Hassanali, A. 2001. Blend effects in the toxicity of the essential oil constituents of *Ocimum kilimandscharicum* and *Ocimum kenyense* (Labiatae) on two post-harvest insect pests. *Phytochemistry* 57, pp. 385–391.

P390 Panchal, P. & Parvez, N. 2019. Phytochemical analysis of medicinal herb (*Ocimum sanctum*). *International Journal of Nanomaterial, Nanotechnology and Nanomedicine* 5, 008–011, doi. org/10.17352/2455-3492.000029.

P391 Terreaux, C. *et al.* 1994. Analysis of the fungicidal constituents from the bark of *Ocotea usambarensis* Engl. (Lauraceae). *Phytochemical Analysis* 5, pp. 233–238.

P392 Tjitraresmi, A. *et al.* 2020. Antimalarial activity of Lamiaceae family plants: review. *Systematic Reviews in Pharmacy* 11, 324–333, doi:10.31838/srp.2020.7.51.

P393 Carnmalm, B. 1956. Constitution of resin phenols and their biogenetic relations. XX. Identity of pseudocubebin and D-sesamin. *Acta Chemica Scandinavica* 10, 134. Available from: actachemscand.org/pdf/acta_vol_10_p0134-0135.pdf.

P394 Hansen, K. *et al.* 1996. Isolation of an angiotension converting enzymes (ACE) inhibitor from *Olea europaea* and *Olea lancea*. *Phytomedicine* 2, pp. 319–325.

P395 Somova, L.I. *et al.* 2004. Cardiotonic and antidysrhythmic effects of oleanolic and ursonic acids, methyl maslinate and uvaol. *Phytomedicine* 11, pp. 121–129.

P396 Somova, L.I. *et al.* 2003. Antihypertensive, antiatherosclerotic and antioxidant activity of triterpenoids isolated from *Olea europaea* subspecies *africana* leaves. *Journal of Ethnopharmacology* 84, 299–305, doi.org/10.1016/s0378-8741(02)00332-x.

P397 Matu, E.N. & Van Staden, J. 2003. Antibacterial and anti-inflammatory activities of some plants used for medicinal purposes in Kenya. *Journal of Ethnopharmacology* 87, pp. 35–41.

P398 Camara, C.C. *et al*. 2003. Antispasmodic effect of the essential oil of *Plectranthus barbatus* and some major constituents on the guinea-pig ileum. *Planta Medica* 69, pp. 1080–1085.

P399 Gupta, P.P. *et al*. 1993. Anti-allergic activity of some traditional Indian medicinal plants. *International Journal of Pharmacognosy* 31, pp. 15–18.

P400 Lukhoba, C.W. *et al*. 2006. *Plectranthus*: a review of ethnobotanical uses. *Journal of Ethnopharmacology* 103, pp. 1–24.

P401 Alasbahi, R.H. & Melzig, M.F. 2010. *Plectranthus barbatus*: a review of phytochemistry, ethnobotanical uses and pharmacology. Part 2. *Planta Medica* 76, pp. 753–765.

P402 Tilak, J.C. *et al*. 2004. Antioxidant properties of *Plumbago zeylanica*, an Indian medicinal plant and its active ingredient, plumbagin. *Redox Report* 9, 219–227, doi:10.1179/135100004225005976.

P403 Mehdi, H. *et al*. 1997. Cell culture assay system for the evaluation of natural product-mediated anti-hepatitis B virus activity. *Phytomedicine* 3, pp. 369–377.

P404 Xiu-Li, Q. *et al*. 1980. Chemical investigation of *Plumbago zeylanica* Linn. II. Structural determination of plumbagic acid. *Acta Chimica Sinica* 38, pp. 377–380.

P405 Gupta, A. *et al*. 2000. A new anthraquinone glycoside from the roots of *Plumbago zeylanica*. *Indian Journal of Chemistry*, Section B 39, 796–798. Available from: hdl.handle.net/123456789/22586.

P406 Nguyen, A.T. *et al*. 2004. Cytotoxic constituents from *Plumbago zeylanica*. *Fitoterapia* 75, pp. 500–504.

P407 Singh, K. *et al*. 2018. A comprehensive review on the genus *Plumbago* with focus on *Plumbago auriculata*

(Plumbaginaceae). *African Journal of Traditional, Complementary and Alternative Medicines* 15, 199–215, doi:10.21010/ajtcam.v15i1.21.

P408 Fourneau, C. *et al*. 1996. Triterpenes from *Prunus africana* bark. *Phytochemistry* 42, pp. 1387–1389.

P409 Mutuma, G.G. *et al*. 2020. Phytochemical and anti-inflammatory analysis of *Prunus africana* bark extract. *Research Journal of Pharmacognosy* 7, 31–38, doi:10.22127/rjp.2020.229941.1583.

P410 Nyamai, D.W. *et al*. 2015. Phytochemical profile of *Prunus africana* stem bark from Kenya. *Journal of Pharmacognosy and Natural Products* 1, 110–118, doi:10.4172/jpnp.1000110.

P411 Ngbolua, K.-te-N. *et al*. 2018. A review on the phytochemistry and pharmacology of *Psidium guajava* L. (Myrtaceae) and future direction. *Discovery Phytomedicine* 5, 7–13, doi:10.15562/phytomedicine.2018.58.

P412 El-Toumy, S.A.A. & Rauwald, H.W. 2002. Two ellagitannins from *Punica granatum* heartwood. *Phytochemistry* 61, pp. 971–974.

P413 Singh, B. *et al*. 2018. Phenolic compounds as beneficial phytochemicals in pomegranate (*Punica granatum* L.) peel: a review. *Food Chemistry* 261, 75–86, doi.org/10.1016/j.foodchem.2018.04.039.

P414 Ilavarasan, R. *et al*. 2006. Anti-inflammatory and free radical scavenging activity of *Ricinus communis* root extract. *Journal of Ethnopharmacology* 103, pp. 478–480.

P415 Audi, J. *et al*. 2005. Ricin poisoning: a comprehensive review. *The Journal of the American Medical Association* 294, pp. 2342–2351.

P416 Wei, C.H. 1973. Two phytotoxic antitumor proteins: ricin and abrin. Isolation, crystallization, and preliminary x-ray study. *Journal of Biological Chemistry* 248, pp. 3745–3747.

P417 Ahn, B.T. *et al*. 1995. A chemotaxonomic study on Euphorbiaceae in Korea. *Natural Product Sciences* 1, pp. 86–98.

P418 Hall, S.M. & Medlow, G.C. 1974. Identification of IAA in phloem and root pressure saps of *Ricinus communis* L. by mass spectrometry. *Planta* 119, pp. 257–261.

P419 Ribeiro, P.R. *et al.* 2016. Chemical constituents of the oilseed crop *Ricinus communis* and their pharmacological activities: a review. *Industrial Crops and Products* 91, pp. 358–376.

P420 Njeru, S.N. *et al.* 2016. Antimicrobial and cytotoxicity properties of the organic solvent fractions of *Clerodendrum myricoides* (Hochst.) R. Br. ex Vatke: Kenyan traditional medicinal plant. *Journal of Intercultural Ethnopharmacology* 5, 226–232, doi:10.5455/jice.20160416122003.

P421 Bashwira, S. & Hootele, C. 1988. Myricoidine and dihydromyricoidine, two new macrocyclic spermidine alkaloids from *Clerodendrum myricoides*. *Tetrahedron* 44, pp. 4521–4526.

P422 Bashwira, S. *et al.* 1989. Cleromyrine I, a new cyclohexapeptide from *Clerodendrum myricoides*. *Tetrahedron* 45, pp. 5845–5852.

P423 Machumi, F. *et al.* 2010. Antimicrobial and antiparasitic abietane diterpenoids from the roots of *Clerodendrum eriophyllum*. *Natural Product Communications* 5, pp. 853–858.

P424 Zhu, J.J. *et al.* 2006. Anthraquinones and chromones from *Rumex dentatus*. *Biochemical Systematics and Ecology* 34, pp. 753–756.

P425 Kuob, I. & Kinst-Hori, I. 1999. 2-Hydroxy-4-methoxybenzaldehyde: a potent tyrosinase inhibitor from African medicinal plants. *Planta Medica* 65, pp. 19–22.

P426 Lee, J-D. *et al.* 2009. Flavonol-rich RVHxR from *Rhus verniciflua* Stokes and its major compound fisetin inhibits inflammation-related cytokines and angiogenic factor in rheumatoid arthritic fibroblast-like synovial cells and in vivo models. *International Immunopharmacology* 9, 268–276, doi:10.1016/j.intimp.2008.11.005.

P427 Matata, D.Z. *et al.* 2020. Isolation of a new cytotoxic compound, 3-((Z)-heptadec-14-enyl)benzene-1-ol from *Rhus natalensis* root extract. *Phytochemistry Letters* 36, 120–126, doi.org/10.1016/j.phytol.2020.01.024.

P428 Ahir, K.B. *et al.* 2013. Effect of *Solanum nigrum* L. on blood glucose concentration and lipid profile in normal and STZ-induced diabetic rats.

Pharmacognosy Communications 3, 6–11, doi:10.5530/pc.2013.2.3.

P429 Wang, K.R. *et al.* 1982. Effects of traditional Chinese herbs, toad tincture and adenosine 3',5' cAMP on Ehrlich ascites tumor cells in mice. *Chinese Medical Journal* 95, pp. 527–532.

P430 Potawale, S.E. *et al.* 2008. *Solanum nigrum* Linn: a phytopharmacological review. *PharmacologyOnLine* 3, pp. 140–163.

P431 Patel, K. *et al.* 2012. A review on pharmacological and analytical aspects of diosgenin: a concise report. *Natural Products and Bioprospecting* 2, 46–52, doi:10.1007/s13659-012-0014-3.

P432 Son, K.H. *et al.* 1991. Neochlorogenin from the fruits of *Solanum nigrum*. *Korean Journal of Pharmacognosy* 22, pp. 142–143.

P433 Lin, Y.L. *et al.* 2000. Nonsteroidal constituents from *Solanum incanum* L. *Journal of the Chinese Chemical Society* 47, 247–251, doi.org/10.1002/jccs.200000029.

P434 Nawaz, R. & Sorensen, H. 1977. Distribution of saccharopine and 2-aminoadipic acid in higher plants. *Phytochemistry* 16, pp. 599–600.

P435 Grace, M.H. & Saleh, M.M. 1996. Hepato-protective effect of daturaolone isolated from *Solanum arundo*. *Pharmazie* 51, pp. 593–595.

P436 Hameed, I.H. *et al.* 2017. A review: *Solanum nigrum* L. antimicrobial, antioxidant properties, hepatoprotective effects and analysis of bioactive natural compounds. *Research Journal of Pharmacy and Technology* 10, 4063–4068, doi:10.5958/0974-360X.2017.00737.5.

P437 Duraipandiyan, V. *et al.* 2006. Antimicrobial activity of some ethnomedicinal plants used by Paliyar tribe from Tamil Nadu, India. *BMC Complementary and Alternative Medicine* 6, 35, doi.org/10.1186%2F1472-6882-6-35.

P438 Braga, F.G. *et al.* 2007. Antileishmanial and antifungal activity of plants used in traditional medicine in Brazil. *Journal of Ethnopharmacology* 111, pp. 396–402.

P439 Teixeira, C.C. & Fuchs, F.D. 2006. The efficacy of herbal medicines in clinical models: The case of jambolan. *Journal of Ethnopharmacology* 108, pp. 16–19.

P440 Banerjee, A. *et al.* 2005. In vitro study of antioxidant activity of *Syzygium cuminii* fruit. *Food Chemistry* 90, pp. 727–733.

P441 Djoukeng, J.D. *et al.* 2005. Antibacterial triterpenes from *Syzygium guineense* (Myrtaceae). *Journal of Ethnopharmacology* 101, pp. 283–286.

P442 Musabayane, C.T. *et al.* 2005. Effects of *Syzygium cordatum* (Hochst.) [Myrtaceae] leaf extract on plasma glucose and hepatic glycogen in streptozotocin-induced diabetic rats. *Journal of Ethnopharmacology* 97, pp. 485–490.

P443 Simirgiotis, M.J. *et al.* 2008. Cytotoxic chalcones and antioxidants from the fruits of *Syzygium samarangense* (Wax Jambu). *Food Chemistry* 107, pp. 813–819.

P444 Ramya, S. *et al.* 2012. Profile of bioactive compounds in *Syzygium cumini* – a review. *Journal of Pharmacy Research* 5, pp. 4548–4553.

P445 Dharani, N. 2016. A review of traditional medicinal uses and phytochemical constituents of exotic *Syzygium* species in East Africa. *Pharmaceutical Journal of Kenya* 22, pp. 123–127.

P446 Sudjaroen, Y. *et al.* 2005. Isolation and structure elucidation of phenolic antioxidants from tamarind (*Tamarindus indica* L.) seeds and pericarp. *Food and Chemical Toxicology* 43, pp. 1673–1682.

P447 Okoh, O.O. *et al.* 2007. Ethanol extract and chromatographic fractions of *Tamarindus indica* stem bark inhibits Newcastle disease virus replication. *Pharmaceutical Biology* 55, 1806–1808, doi:10.1080/13880209.2017.1331364.

P448 Garcia, L.C. 2011. A comparative study on the antifungal effects of tamarind (*Tamarindus indica*) and garlic (*Allium sativum*) extracts on banana anthracnose. *Journal of Nature Studies* 10, pp. 96–107.

P449 Srinivasan, D. *et al.* 2001. Antimicrobial activity of certain Indian medicinal plants used in folkloric medicine. *Journal of Ethnopharmacology* 74, pp. 217–220.

P450 Tsuda, T. *et al.* 1994. Antioxidative components isolated from the seed of tamarind (*Tamarindus indica* L.). *Journal of Agricultural and Food Chemistry* 42, pp. 2671–2674.

P451 Sagrero-Nieves, L. *et al.* 1994. Supercritical fluid extraction of the volatile constituents from tamarind (*Tamarindus indica* L.). *Journal of Essential Oil Research* 6, pp. 547–548.

P452 Zhang, Y.G. *et al.* 1990. Volatile flavor components of tamarind (*Tamarindus indica* L.). *Journal of Essential Oil Research* 2, pp. 197–198.

P453 Matasyoh, J.C. *et al.* 2006. Chemical composition and antimicrobial activity of the essential oil of *Tarchonanthus camphoratus*. *Food Chemistry* 101, pp. 1183–1187.

P454 *Dictionary of Organic Compounds on CD Rom*. 2008. CRC Press.

P455 Mwangi, J.W. *et al.* 1994. Volatile constituents of essential oil of *Tarchonanthus camphoratus* L. *Journal of Essential Oil Research* 6, pp. 183–185.

P456 Kimani, N.M. *et al.* 2018. Antiprotozoal sesquiterpene lactones and other constituents from *Tarchonanthus camphoratus* and *Schkuhria pinnata*. *Journal of Natural Products* 81, 124–130, doi.org/10.1021/acs.jnatprod.7b00747.

P457 Saxena, V.K. & Sharma, R.N. 1999. Antimicrobial activity of the essential oil of *Toddalia asiatica*. *Fitoterapia* 70, pp. 64–66.

P458 Lin, T.-T. *et al.* 2014. Prenylated coumarins: natural phosphodiesterase-4 inhibitors from *Toddalia asiatica*. *Journal of Natural Products* 77, pp. 955–962.

P459 Weenen, H. *et al.* 1990. Antimalarial activity of Tanzanian medicinal plants. *Planta Medica* 56, pp. 368–370.

P460 Combes, G. & Gaignault, J.C. 1984. On the coumarins of *Toddalia asiatica*. *Fitoterapia* 55, pp. 161–170.

P461 Gakunju, D.M.N. *et al.* 1995. Potent antimalarial activity of the alkaloid nitidine isolated from a Kenyan herbal remedy. *Antimicrobial Agents and Chemotherapy* 39, pp. 2606–2609.

P462 Tsai, I.-L. *et al.* 1998. Anti-platelet aggregation constituents from Formosan *Toddalia asiatica*. *Phytochemistry* 48, pp. 1377–1382.

P463 Ishii, H. *et al.* 1991. Studies on the chemical constituents of rutaceous plants. LXVI. The chemical constituents of *Toddalia asiatica* (L.) Lam. (*T. aculeata* Pers.). 1. Chemical constituents of root bark. *Yakugaku Zasshi* 111, 365–375, doi:10.1248/yakushi1947.111.7_365.

P464 Zeng, Z. *et al.* 2021. A systematic review on traditional medicine

Toddalia asiatica (L.) Lam.: chemistry and medicinal potential. *Saudi Pharmaceutical Journal* 29, 781–798, doi:10.1016/j.jsps.2021.05.003.

P465 Oketch-Rabah, H.A. *et al.* 2000. A new antiplasmodial coumarin from *Toddalia asiatica* roots. *Fitoterapia* 71, pp. 636–640.

P466 Duraipandiyan, V. & Ignacimuthu, S. 2009. Antibacterial and antifungal activity of flindersine isolated from the traditional medicinal plant, *Toddalia asiatica* (L.) Lam. *Journal of Ethnopharmacology* 123, pp. 494–498.

P467 Nakatani, M. *et al.* 1981. Isolation and structures of trichilins, antifeedants against the southern army worm. *Journal of the American Chemical Society* 103, pp. 1228–1230.

P468 Diallo, D. *et al.* 2003. The Malian medicinal plant *Trichilia emetica*; studies on polysaccharides with complement fixing ability. *Journal of Ethnopharmacology* 84, pp. 279–287.

P469 Sanogo, R. *et al.* 2001. *Trichilia roka* Chiov. (Meliaceae): pharmacognostic researches. *Farmaco* 56, 357–360, doi:10.1016/s0014-827x(01)01051-5.

P470 Nakatani, M. *et al.* 1985. Structure of limonoid antifeedant from *Trichilia roka*. *Phytochemistry* 24, pp. 195–196.

P471 Taylor, D.A.H. 1984. The chemistry of limonoids from Meliaceae in Herz, W. *et al.* (Eds), *Progress in Chemistry of Organic Natural Products* 45, pp. 2–92. New York: Springer-Verlag.

P472 Komane, B.M. *et al.* 2011. *Trichilia emetica* (Meliaceae) – a review of traditional uses, biological activities and phytochemistry. *Phytochemistry Letters* 4, pp. 1–9.

P473 Kenny, O. *et al.* 2013. Antioxidant properties and quantitative UPLC-MS analysis of phenolic compounds from extracts of fenugreek (*Trigonella foenum-graecum*) seeds and bitter melon (*Momordica charantia*) fruit. *Food Chemistry* 141, pp. 4295–4302.

P474 Mascolo, N. *et al.* 1988. Antipyretic and analgesic studies of the ethanolic extract of *Teclea nobilis* Delile. *Phytotherapy Research* 2, pp. 154–156.

P475 Omujal, F. 2020. Phytochemistry and anti-inflammatory activity of ethanolic root bark extract of *Vepris nobilis* Mziray

(Rutaceae family). *Scientific African* 9, e00484, doi.org/10.1016/j.sciaf.2020.e00484.

P476 Yenesew, A. & Dagne, E. 1988. Alkaloids of *Teclea nobilis*. *Phytochemistry* 27, pp. 651–653.

P477 Wondimu, A. *et al.* 1988. Quinoline alkaloids from the leaves of *Teclea simplicifolia*. *Phytochemistry* 27, pp. 959–960.

P478 Al-Rehaily, A.J. *et al.* 2002. New axane and oppositane sesquiterpenes from *Teclea nobilis*. *Journal of Natural Products* 65, pp. 1374–1376.

P479 Al-Rehaily, A.J. *et al.* 2001. Pharmacological studies of various extracts and the major constituent, lupeol, obtained from hexane extract of *Teclea nobilis* in rodents. *Natural Product Sciences* 7, pp. 76–82.

P480 Al-Rehaily, A.J. *et al.* 2003. Furoquinoline alkaloids from *Teclea nobilis*. *Phytochemistry* 64, pp. 1405–1411.

P481 Igile, G.O. *et al.* 1994. Flavonoids from *Vernonia amygdalina* and their antioxidant activities. *Journal of Agricultural and Food Chemistry* 42, pp. 2445–1448.

P482 Fadulu, S.O. 1975. The antibacterial properties of the buffer extracts of chewing sticks used in Nigeria. *Planta Medica* 27, pp. 122–126.

P483 Taniguchi, I. *et al.* 1978. Screening of East African plants for antimicrobial activity. *Chemical and Pharmaceutical Bulletin* 26, pp. 2910–2913.

P484 Akah, P.A. & Okafor, C.L. 1992. Blood sugar lowering effect of *Vernonia amygdalina* Del, in an experimental rabbit model. *Phytotherapy Research* 6, pp. 171–173.

P485 Madureira, M.D.C. *et al.* 2002. Antimalarial activity of medicinal plants used in traditional medicine in S. Tomé and Príncipe Islands. *Journal of Ethnopharmacology* 81, pp. 23–29.

P486 Kaij-A-Kamb, M. *et al.* 1992. Search for new antiviral agents of plant origin. *Pharmaceutica Acta Helvetiae* 67, pp. 130–147.

P487 Kupchan, S.M. *et al.* 1969. Tumor inhibitors. XLVII. Vernodalin and vernomygdin, two new cytotoxic sesquiterpene lactones from *Vernonia*

amygdalina. *Journal of Organic Chemistry* 34, pp. 3908–3911.

P488 Kambu, K. *et al.* 1990. Antispasmodic activity of extracts proceeding of plant antidiarrheic traditional preparations used in Kinshasa, Zaire. *Annales Pharmaceutiques Francaises* 48, pp. 200–208.

P489 Ganjian, I. *et al.* 1983. Insect antifeedant elemanolide lactones from *Vernonia amygdalina*. *Phytochemistry* 22, pp. 2525–2529.

P490 Keriko, J.M. *et al.* 1995. A plant growth regulator from *Vernonia auriculifera* (Asteraceae). *Zeitschrift fuer Naturforschung* C 50, pp. 455–458.

P491 Igile, G. *et al.* 1995. Vernoniosides D and E, two novel saponins from *Vernonia amygdalina*. *Journal of Natural Products* 58, pp. 1438–1443.

P492 Kiplimo, J.J. *et al.* 2011. Triterpenoids from *Vernonia auriculifera* Hiern exhibit antimicrobial activity. *African Journal of Pharmacy and Pharmacology* 5, pp. 1150–1156.

P493 Woube, A.A. *et al.* 2005. Sesquiterpenes from *Warburgia ugandensis* and their antimycobacterial activity. *Phytochemistry* 66, pp. 2309–2315.

P494 Manguro, L.O.A. *et al.* 2003. Flavonol glycosides of *Warburgia ugandensis* leaves. *Phytochemistry* 64, pp. 891–896.

P495 Dharani, N. 2020. A review of phytochemical constituents and pharmacological activities of ethnomedicinal *Warburgia ugandensis* Sprague ssp. *ugandensis* in East Africa. *Pharmaceutical Journal of Kenya* 24, pp. 67–71.

P496 Kala, C.P. *et al.* 2006. Developing the medicinal plants sector in northern India: challenges and opportunities. *Journal of Ethnobiology and Ethnomedicine* 2, 32, doi. org/10.1186/1746-4269-2-32.

P497 Cowan, M.M. 1999. Plant products as antimicrobial agents. *Clinical Microbiology Reviews* 12, pp. 564–582.

P498 Padmavathi, B. *et al.* 2005. Roots of *Withania somnifera* inhibit forestomach and skin carcinogenesis in mice. *Evidence-based Complementary and Alternative Medicine* 2, pp. 99–105.

P499 Pandey, A. *et al.* 2018. Multifunctional neuroprotective effect of withanone, a compound from *Withania somnifera* roots in alleviating cognitive dysfunction. *Cytokine* 102, pp. 211–221.

P500 Agwaya, M.S. *et al.* 2016. Hypoglycemic activity of aqueous root bark extract *Zanthoxylum chalybeum* in alloxan-induced diabetic rats. *Journal of Diabetes Research* 2016, Article ID 8727590, doi. org/10.1155/2016/8727590.

P501 Omosa, L.O. & Okemwa, E.K. 2017. Antiplasmodial activities of the stem bark extract and compounds of *Zanthoxylum gilletii* (De Wild) P.G. Waterman. *Pharmacognosy Communications* 7, pp. 41–46.

P502 Kato, A. *et al.* 1996. Isolation of alkaloidal constituents of *Zanthoxylum usambarense* and *Zanthoxylum chalybeum* using ion-pair HPLC. *Journal of Natural Products* 59, pp. 316–318.

P503 Akampurira, D. *et al.* 2022. A new C—C-linked benzophenathridine—2-quinoline dimer, and the antiplasmodial activities of alkaloids from *Zanthoxylum holtzianum*. *Natural Product Research*, pp. 1–11.

P504 Akampurira, D. 2013. Phytochemical investigation of *Zanthoxylum holtzianum* for antiplasmodial, larvicidal and antinociceptive principles. Doctoral dissertation, University of Nairobi, Kenya.

P505 Phillip, S. *et al.* 1993. *Zingiber officinale* (ginger) – an anti-emetic for day case surgery. *Anaesthesia* 48, pp. 715–717.

P506 Lantz, R.C. *et al.* 2007. The effect of extracts from ginger rhizome on inflammatory mediator production. *Phytomedicine* 14, pp. 123–128.

P507 Van Beek, T.A. 1991. Special methods for essential oil of ginger in Linskens, H.F. & Jackson, J.F. (Eds), *Essential Oils and Waxes*, pp. 79–97. Berlin: Springer-Verlag.

P508 Ma, J. *et al.* 2004. Diarylheptanoids from the rhizomes of *Zingiber officinale*. *Phytochemistry* 65, pp. 1137–1143.

P509 Roufogalis, B.D. 2014. *Zingiber officinale* (ginger): a future outlook on its potential in prevention and treatment of diabetes and prediabetic states. *New Journal of Science* 2014, 674684, doi. org/10.1155/2014/67468

Glossary of medical terms

Bold formatting in a definition indicates that the term is defined elsewhere in this glossary.

abortifacient agent that induces abortion.

abscess swelling on the body in which a thick yellowish liquid, pus, accumulates.

acne common pustular eruption from inflamed sebaceous glands in the pores of the skin.

amenorrhea abnormal absence or suppression of menstruation.

anaemia condition in which the red blood cell count is abnormally low, leading to weakness and pallor.

analgesic agent or medication that reduces or eliminates pain.

anorexia severe eating disorder characterised by abnormally repressed appetite.

anthelmintic drug that kills or causes the expulsion of parasitic intestinal worms.

anthrax splenic fever and infectious disease of animals (mainly herbivores) caused by the presence of *Bacillus anthracis* in the blood.

anti-allergic having the capacity to counteract allergies.

anti-asthmatic relieving **asthma**; see also **bronchodilator**.

antibacterial killing bacteria or stopping their growth.

anticonvulsant agent that helps to counter violent, involuntary muscular contractions.

antidote substance that neutralises a poison or counteracts its effects.

antiflatulent drug or agent that helps to relieve flatulence.

antifungal with the capacity to kill or eliminate fungal growth or infection.

antihistamines variety of drugs used to treat allergies, especially hay fever.

antihyperglycaemic antidiabetic.

antihypertensive with the capacity to reduce high blood pressure.

anti-inflammatory with the capacity to reduce swellings and limit painful reactions following injury or infection.

anti-leukaemic with the capacity to help to counter leukaemia.

antimicrobial with the capacity to kill or inhibit the growth of micro-organisms.

antipyretic drug or agent that reduces fever.

antischistosomal capable of affecting the viability of the parasitic worms that cause schistosomiasis (**bilharzia**).

antiscorbutic remedy for scurvy.

antiseptic substance that helps to kill or prevent the growth of harmful micro-organisms (germs) on the skin or in the mucosa.

antispasmodic substance that relaxes cramps and stops spasms of internal organs such as the stomach, gall bladder or urinary bladder, thus preventing colic.

antitumour with the capacity to prevent the formation of malignant cancer tumours.

antiviral substance or drug effective against the growth or spread of a virus.

aphrodisiac substance that stimulates sexual desire.

appendicitis medical condition in which the appendix swells and becomes extremely painful (dangerous if left untreated)

appetiser agent that stimulates the appetite.

arteriosclerosis condition characterised by hardening of the arteries.

arthritis inflammation of the joints.

asthma breathing difficulty caused by constriction of, or spasms in, the air passages, usually as a result of an allergic reaction in the bronchi and trachea to external stimuli.

astringent substance that causes contraction, shrinkage or firming of living tissues of the body, facilitating healing; also applied to cosmetic preparations that tighten the skin.

atherosclerosis a build-up of fats, cholesterol and other substances in and on the artery walls, causing narrowing of the arteries and blocking blood flow

Ayurveda (adj. Ayurvedic) traditional system of Indian folk medicine that, translated literally, means 'a knowledge of how to live'.

bilharzia disease caused by parasites (schistosomes) in infected lakes and rivers; the two common forms in East Africa are genito-urinary bilharzia, which is caused by *Schistosoma haematobium*, and intestinal bilharzia, caused by *S. mansoni*; also known as **schistosomiasis**.

boil infection originating in a hair follicle, often very painful.

bronchitis inflammation of mucous membranes in the bronchial tubes of the lungs.

bronchodilator agent that relaxes and opens the bronchi; see also **anti-asthmatic**.

candida white, yeast-like fungus sometimes

found in the mouths of babies; in adults suffering from weakness and low immunity, an overgrowth may form white lesions in the mouth, vagina, digestive tract or on the skin.

carminative substance or drug that relieves gastric and intestinal flatulence.

cerebral relating to the foremost part of the brain.

chemotherapy treatment of disease with chemicals; often used to treat cancer.

colic spasmodic pain in the abdomen or severe intestinal pain.

colitis inflammation of the large intestine (the bowels).

conjunctivitis inflammation of the mucous membranes of the eyes.

decoction a 'tea' produced through sustained boiling of the hard parts of plants (roots, bark, seeds or rhizomes) in order to liberate their active principles.

decongestant drug or medicine that breaks up blockages, especially of fluid in the sinuses.

depurative substance or drug that eases the draining (in the liver and through urine or sweat) of toxic substances circulating in the blood; depurative agents are usually also **diuretic** and **sudorific**.

dermatitis inflammation of the skin.

diabetes condition characterised by too much sugar in the blood.

diabetes mellitus carbohydrate metabolism disorder, associated with disruption of the body's insulin-regulating mechanism resulting in excess sugar in the blood.

diaphoretic substance that causes perspiration.

diarrhoea abnormally frequent discharge of more or less fluid faecal matter from the bowels.

diuretic agent that increases the flow of urine.

dysentery serious bacterial or parasitic infection of the bowels resulting in severe diarrhoea or in watery stools often passed along with blood, pus or mucus.

dysmenorrhoea difficult and painful menstruation, often with cramps.

dyspepsia upset stomach or indigestion.

dyspnoea difficulty in breathing or in catching the breath.

eczema inflammation of the skin associated with allergic reactions causing redness, rashes, lesions and itching.

embrocation liquid for rubbing on the body to relieve pain from sprains and strains.

emetic drug or substance that causes vomiting.

emmenagogue substance that regulates the menstrual cycle.

emollient substance that helps to soothe or calm irritations of the skin and the mucosa; see also **anti-inflammatory**.

enema liquid injected into the rectum in order to clean out the bowels.

epilepsy brain condition characterised by fits and loss of consciousness, caused by abnormal brain activity.

euphoria feeling of intense elation or extreme excitement.

expectorant substance that promotes secretion or expulsion of mucus and other fluids from the respiratory system, particularly the lungs.

fatigue condition characterised by extreme tiredness from physical or mental exertion.

flatulence build-up of excessive gas in the stomach or intestine.

flu see also **influenza**.

furuncles painful, pus-filled bumps that develop under the skin, usually caused by the bacterium *Staphylococcus aureus* (staph infection).

galactogogue (adj. **galactogenic**) agent that induces the secretion of milk, stimulating lactation in breast-feeding women.

gastritis illness in which the stomach lining becomes swollen and painful.

glaucoma disease of the eye resulting in gradual loss of sight.

gonorrhoea contagious disease of the sexual organs spread by sexual contact.

gout inflammation of the smaller joints.

haemorrhage abnormal loss of blood, internally or externally.

haemorrhoids swollen or twisted veins around the anus or lower rectum that may cause bleeding and discomfort; also known as **piles**.

hepatic relating to the liver, also to any of a class of substances used to enhance liver function.

hepatitis inflammation of the liver.

hernia protrusion of an organ or part of an organ through the wall of the cavity that normally contains it, a rupture.

herpes viral infection that causes cold sores on the skin and mucous membranes; different herpes viruses cause infections around the genitals (*Herpes genitalis*), the trunk and buttocks (*H. zoster*, or **shingles**) or the nose and mouth (*H. labialis*).

hyperglycaemia increase in the level of sugar in the blood; opposite of **hypoglycaemia**.

hypertensive relating to increased arterial blood pressure; opposite of **hypotensive**.

hyperthermia dangerous condition in which the body has an abnormally high temperature; opposite of **hypothermia**.

hypoglycaemia decrease in the level of sugar in the blood; opposite of **hyperglycaemia**.

hypoglycaemic substance or agent that decreases the sugar levels in the blood; used for treating **diabetes**.

hypotensive relating to low arterial blood pressure; opposite of **hypertensive**.

hypothermia dangerous condition in which the body develops an abnormally low temperature; elderly people sometimes die of hypothermia in cold weather; opposite of **hyperthermia**.

immunostimulant agent that stimulates the immune system of the body, usually when it is weak; also known as an immunoregulator.

impotence inability in men to perform sexual intercourse.

influenza contagious feverish illness characterised by inflammation of the mucous membranes, usually in the head and neck, resulting in copious discharge; widely known simply as **flu**.

infusion product derived from steeping a substance in water to extract its soluble principles; see also **steep**.

insomnia sleeplessness or inability to sleep.

intoxicant substance such as alcohol whose consumption results in a loss of control, reflected in states ranging from heightened excitement to stupor.

jaundice yellowness of the skin, eyes and mucous membranes triggered by high levels of bilirubin (a component of bile) in the blood; a common cause is viral **hepatitis**.

kwashiorkor disease of malnutrition, mainly in children, caused by severe protein and vitamin deficiency and characterised by retarded growth.

lactation secretion of milk in mothers after childbirth.

laryngitis inflammation of the mucous membranes of the larynx.

laxative substance that by loosening the contents of the lower gut stimulates evacuation of the bowels.

leprosy infectious disease that destroys the nerves, causing painful white patches to appear on the skin.

leucoderma any area of skin that is white from congenital albinism or acquired absence or loss of melanin pigmentation.

leucorrhoea white or yellowish vaginal discharge, often indicating infection.

leukaemia cancer of the blood, uncontrolled proliferation of leucocytes.

lumbago painful condition of the lower back or rheumatic pain of the lumbar region.

malnutrition weakened state caused by a lack of food or by a deficient or unbalanced diet.

measles infectious disease, especially in children, with fever-like symptoms and small red spots that cover the entire body.

meningitis infection and inflammation of the fluid and membranes (meninges) protecting the brain and spinal cord.

menorrhagia excessive and prolonged bleeding at menstruation.

migraine severe form of headache, usually on one side of the head or face and often accompanied by nausea and unsettled vision.

mucolytic easing the expulsion of mucus by making it more fluid.

neuralgia (adj. neuralgic) pain manifest along the course of one or more nerves.

obesity accumulation of excessive body fat.

oedema swelling of tissue due to an accumulation of fluid.

ophthalmia inflammation of the inner parts of the eye.

ophthalmic relating to the eye and its diseases, such as infections and substances used to alleviate such infections.

palpitation pulsating of the heart with increased frequency, with or without an irregular rhythm.

Parkinson's disease severe wasting condition in which the muscles become weak, causing the limbs to shake.

parturition childbirth; the act of giving birth.

peptic ulcer ulcer of the stomach / duodenum.

piles see also **haemorrhoids**.

pleurisy inflammation of the tissues that line the lungs and chest cavity.

pneumonia inflammation of the lungs.

postpartum phase immediately after childbirth.

poultice moist dressing applied to an infected area of the body.

prostatitis inflammation of the prostate gland, which surrounds the neck of the bladder and urethra in men.

psychotic psychiatric condition characterised by abnormal, often violent, behaviour.

purgative agent that causes evacuation of the bowels.

rheumatism acute disease characterised by painful inflammation and swelling of the joints, muscles or connective tissues.

scabies contagious skin disease caused by the mite *Sarcoptes scabiei*, resulting in scabs and itching.

schistosomiasis disease caused by parasitic worms; also known as **bilharzia**.

sciatica pain on or near the sciatic nerves running through the pelvis and the thighs.

scorbutus disease caused by lack of vitamin C.

sedative having a soothing, tranquillising or calming effect on the nervous system.

shingles a viral infection that causes a painful rash, most often appearing as a single stripe of blisters around the left or right side of the torso.

sinusitis inflammation of the sinuses, especially in the nasal area.

steep to soak an object (e.g. roots, bark or leaves) in water or another liquid for a period of time to soften it or extract substances from it.

stimulant substance that raises levels of physiological or nervous activity in the body.

styptic a substance that, when applied to a wound, is capable of causing bleeding to stop.

sudorific substance that stimulates sweating; see also **diaphoretic**.

syphilis infectious sexually transmitted disease.

thrombosis serious condition caused by the formation of blood clots.

tonsillitis inflammation of the tonsils, especially the palatine tonsils.

toxaemia condition characterised by the presence of bacterial toxins in the blood (usually absorbed via a local lesion).

trachoma contagious and chronic inflammation of the eyes, marked by the formation of greyish or yellowish, translucent granules of adenoid tissue.

trypanosomiasis sleeping sickness.

tuberculosis infectious bacterial disease affecting the lungs and sometimes the bones, caused by *Mycobacterium tuberculosis*.

typhoid acute gastrointestinal disease commonly spread in contaminated water, caused by *Salmonella typhi*.

varicose veins dilated superficial veins that become prominent, mainly on the legs.

vasodilator agent causing the dilation of the walls of the blood vessels.

venereal disease blanket term for any number of infectious diseases that are transmitted through sexual intercourse.

vermifuge drug that expels parasitic worms.

vertigo dizziness.

water extract mixture made by soaking ground-up plant material in water, which is then filtered or decanted before use.

Glossary of botanical terms

Bold formatting in a definition indicates that the term is defined elsewhere in this glossary.

achene small, dry, single-seeded fruit that does not split open.

alternate relating to leaves or flowers arranged singly at different heights on either side of a stem.

annuals plants that do not live longer than one year.

anther part of a flower that produces **pollen**.

aril an appendage on certain seeds, often brightly coloured and fleshy.

aromatic having a pleasant distinctive smell.

axil upper angle between a leaf and the stem on which it is borne.

axillary arising from an **axil**.

axis the real or imaginary line that divides a regular shape into two equal parts (vertical or horizontal axis).

berry many-seeded fleshy fruit without a hard layer, the seeds immersed in pulp.

biennial attaining full vegetative growth in the first year; producing flowers and fruits in the second year, after which the plant dies.

bipinnate relating to a compound leaf that is further divided (twice **pinnate**).

bisexual having both male and female parts (**stamens** and **carpels**) of a flower present.

bract small, leaf-like organ or modified leaf with a single flower or inflorescence growing in its **axil**.

branchlet small branch.

calyx lowermost whorl of a flower, consisting of a number of green leafy **sepals**.

capsule dry, dehiscent, 1- to many-chambered fruit, developing from a **syncarpous pistil**.

cladode leaf-like stem having the form and function of a leaf, but arising in the **axil** of a minute, bract-like true leaf that drops off very early.

climbers plants that climb neighbouring plants or other objects by means of special attachment organs.

compound relating to a leaf that is broken up into a number of segments, called '**leaflets**', that are free from one another.

coryomb (adj. **coryombose**) the shape of an **inflorescence**, being a flat-topped flower cluster with older flowers situated at the periphery.

cuneate wedge-shaped.

cyme (adj. **cymose**) **inflorescence** in which the main **axis** ends in a flower and the lateral axis does the same; the terminal flower is always older, opening earlier than the lateral one.

deciduous with leaves lasting only one season.

decompound relating to a leaf having divisions that are themselves **compound**.

dehiscent relating to a fruit that bursts open to liberate the seeds when mature.

dentate with a toothed edge.

digitate with **leaflets** (generally five or more) radiating from a common point in the form of a spread hand.

dimorphic of two forms.

dioecious relating to a species with male and female reproductive organs in separate flowers borne on different plants.

drupe fleshy, non-opening (**indehiscent**) fruit, usually 1-seeded, in which the seed is contained by a hard, stony coating.

elliptic with a more or less oval shape.

entire having an even and smooth **margin** or edge, without teeth or **lobes**.

evergreen relating to a plant whose leaves persist for more than one season.

filament stalk of a **stamen** of a flower.

follicle dry, 1-chambered fruit that splits on one side.

glabrous hairless, without any outgrowths.

head an **inflorescence** in which the main **axis** is suppressed, becoming almost flat, bearing a mass of small **sessile** flowers (**florets**) on its surface.

herb plant of which the aerial parts do not persist above ground after the end of the growing season; a soft, non-woody plant.

herbaceous see also **herb**.

hesperidium fleshy, many-celled fruit (notably of citrus plants), protected by separable skin or rind.

higher plants plants with developed vascular tissues having veins to transport resources in the plant.

indehiscent relating to a fruit that remains closed when ripe.

inflorescence flowering part of a plant with the flowers arranged on it.

internode portion of a stem between two successive **nodes**.

irregular relating to a flower that is symmetrical in one plane only.

lanceolate lance-shaped.

latex liquid substance secreted by certain plants.

leaf base the part of a leaf attached to the stem.

leaf blade the flat, green, expanded portion of a leaf.

leaflet a single division of a **compound** leaf.

legume dry, 1-chambered fruit, developing from a simple **pistil** and dehiscing along both **margins**.

lenticel (adj. **lenticellate**) breathing pore in a plant stem.

liana woody climbing plant, capable of climbing to the top of a large tree.

linear long, narrow and flat.

lobe division of a leaf, **perianth** or **anther**.

lugga seasonal watercourse

margin edge of a leaf, which may be smooth, toothed or spiny.

midrib strong vein that runs centrally through a **leaf blade** from its base to the apex.

monoecious relating to a species with male and female reproductive organs in separate flowers but borne on the same plant.

naturalised relating to a plant that has been so successfully introduced into a foreign region/country that it reproduces naturally.

node joint or point on a stem or branch at which a leaf or another branch is produced or borne.

nut non-opening (**indehiscent**), single-celled, single-seeded, hard fruit with a woody **pericarp**.

nutlet small **nut**, especially an **achene**.

oblong much longer than broad, with nearly parallel sides.

obovate egg-shaped but inversely so, with the broader end towards the tip.

obovoid egg-shaped, with the narrow end at the base

obtuse blunt or rounded at the tip.

opposite (1) arranged in pairs on either side of the stem (e.g. opposite leaves), (2) with one organ arising at the base of another (e.g. **stamen** in front of a **petal**).

ovate shaped like the outline of an egg, with the broader end at the base.

palmate divided into **lobes**, like the outspread fingers of a hand (as in palms).

panicle compound **raceme** in which the flowers are borne on the lateral branches of the main **axis** or on further branches of these.

pappus tuft or ring of hairs or scales around the fruits of plants of the family Asteraceae, helping with dispersal by wind.

paripinnate relating to a compound leaf with an even number of **leaflets**.

pedicel stalk of a flower.

perennial plant that lives for more than two years.

pericarp wall of a fruit that develops from the ovary wall and encloses the seeds.

petal any of the separate parts of the **corolla** of a flower.

pinna (pl. **pinnae**) primary division of any **pinnate** leaf.

pinnate having **leaflets** arranged along each side of a common **rachis**.

pubescent covered with short soft hair.

raceme (adj. **racemose**) inflorescence with an elongated main axis laterally bearing a number of flowers on long stalks, the flowers towards the tip being the youngest and last to open, and the inflorescence continuing to grow and give off flowers laterally at the tip.

rachis the axis of an inflorescence or of a pinnately compound leaf.

recurved (**reclinate**) bending backwards or downwards.

regular radially symmetrical, relating to a flower that can be divided into two exactly equal halves (mirror images) by any vertical section passing through the centre.

resins a group of substances, often sticky, found mainly in the stems of conifers; when present in the wood, resin adds to its strength and durability.

rhizome thickened, prostrate, underground stem with distinct **nodes** and **internodes**.

sepal any of the separate parts of the **calyx** of a flower.

serrate relating to a margin cut like the teeth of a saw, the teeth directed upwards.

sessile without a stalk.

simple relating to a leaf consisting of a single unbranched, undivided leaf blade.

solitary borne singly.

spathe a large, shading bract enclosing a flower spike (called a spadix) on certain plants.

spike an inflorescence with the flowers **sessile** along an elongated, undivided main axis, older flowers at the base, younger ones towards the tip.

spines sharp-pointed, hardened structures modified from another organ (e.g. leaf, branch, stipule) or from part of an organ, having a defensive function.

stamen male organ of a flower, usually consisting of pollen sacs (**anthers**) and a stalk (**filament**).

stellate star-shaped.

stem main axis of a plant.

stigma small rounded or lobed head of the pistil which receives the pollen.

tapering pointed.

terminal at the end or tip of a branch or stalk.

throat (of a flower with a united corolla) the somewhat expanded portion between the corolla tube and the rest of the united corolla.

tripinnate relating to a **compound** leaf with **bipinnate** leaflets that are themselves pinnately divided, making the leaf thrice **pinnate**.

umbel umbrella-shaped **inflorescence** in which all the **pedicels** of the flowers are more or less of equal length and arise in a group at the tip of the main **axis**.

unisexual bearing only male or only female reproductive organs, not both.

whorl (1) a group of three or more parts (e.g. leaves, branches) at a **node**, (2) a circle of organs (e.g. **stamens**, **petals**, **sepals**) in a flower.

winged relating to (1) seeds or fruits that have developed one or more thin, membranous expansions for dispersal by wind, (2) stems or leaf stalks with a thin flange of tissue that extends beyond the normal outline.

List of East African languages & abbreviations

ABBREVIATION	LANGUAGE	COUNTRY
Ach.	Acholi	Uganda
Aru.	Arusha	Tanzania
Ate.	Ateso	Uganda
Ate.T.	Ateso, Tororo	Uganda
Baj.	Bajun	Kenya
Bon.	Boni	Kenya
Bor.	Boran	Kenya
Buk.	Bukusu	Uganda
Chag.	Chagga	Tanzania
Chon.	Chonyi	Kenya
Dig.	Digo	Kenya
Emb.	Embu	Kenya
Gab.	Gabbra	Kenya
Gir.	Giriama	Kenya
Gogo	Gogo	Tanzania
Goro.	Gorowa	Tanzania
Guj.	Gujarati	Indian (EA)
Haya	Haya	Tanzania
Hehe	Hehe	Tanzania
Hind.	Hindi	Indian (EA)
Ilw.	Ilwana	Kenya
Kam.	Kamba	Kenya
Kik.	Kikuyu	Kenya
Kip.	Kipsigis	Kenya
Kis.	Kisii	Kenya
Lan.	Langi	Uganda
Lug.	Luganda	Uganda
Lugb.	Lugbara	Uganda
Lugi.	Lugishu	Uganda
Lugu.	Luguru	Tanzania
Lugw.	Lugwe	Uganda
Lugwe.	Lugwere	Uganda
Luh.	Luhya	Kenya
Luny.	Lunyoro	Uganda
Lunya.	Lunyankole	Uganda
Luo	Luo	Kenya
Luo-A	Luo, Acholi	Uganda
Luo-J	Luo, Japadora	Uganda
Luo-L	Luo, Lango	Uganda
Luo-Ug.	Luo	Uganda
Luso.	Lusoga	Uganda
Maa.	Maasai	Kenya/Tanzania
Maa.Ken.	Maasai	Kenya
Maa.Tan.	Maasai	Tanzania
Madi	Madi	Uganda
Mar.	Marakwet	Kenya

ABBREVIATION	LANGUAGE	COUNTRY
Mbe.	Mbeere	Kenya
Mbu.	Mbulu	Tanzania
Mbug.	Mbugwe	Tanzania
Mer.	Meru	Kenya
Mer.Ken.	Meru	Kenya
Mer.Tan.	Meru	Tanzania
Mwe.	Mwera	Tanzania
Nan.	Nandi	Kenya
Ngaka.	Ngakarimojong	Uganda
Ngu.	Nguu	Tanzania
Nyak.	Nyakyusa	Tanzania
Nyam.	Nyamwezi	Tanzania
Nyan.	Nyankore	Tanzania
Nyat.	Nyaturu	Tanzania
Nyir.	Nyiramba	Tanzania
Orm.	Orma	Kenya
Pare	Pare	Tanzania
Pok.	Pokot	Kenya
Punj.	Punjabi	Indian (EA)
Ran.	Rangi	Tanzania
Ren.	Rendille	Kenya
Ruki.	Rukiga	Uganda
Ruko.	Rukonjo	Uganda
Runy.	Runyoro	Uganda
Runyan.	Runyankore	Uganda
Runyar.	Runyarwanda	Uganda
Ruto.	Rutoro	Uganda
Sam.	Samburu	Kenya
Samb.	Sambaa	Tanzania
San.	Sangu (Usangu)	Tanzania
Sebei	Sebei	Kenya/Uganda
Sebei-Ug.	Sebei	Uganda
Som.	Somali	Kenya
Suk.	Sukuma	Tanzania
Swa.	Swahili	Kenya/Tanzania
Swa.Ken.	Swahili	Kenya
Swa.Tan.	Swahili	Tanzania
Tai.	Taita	Kenya
Tav.	Taveta	Kenya
Tha.	Tharaka	Kenya
Tug.	Tugen	Kenya
Tur.	Turkana	Kenya
Urd.	Urdu	Indian (EA)
Zig.	Zigua	Tanzania
Zin.	Zinza	Tanzania

Checklist of ailments & prescribed plants

Abdominal pains *Acacia nilotica, Aloe kilifiensis, Anethum graveolens, Artemisia* species, *Azadirachta indica, Boscia* species, *Carica papaya, Carissa spinarum, Cinnamomum verum, Citrus limon, Cordia sinensis, Coriandrum sativum, Cyphostemma adenocaule, Dombeya burgessiae, Euclea divinorum, Eugenia caryophyllata, Foeniculum vulgare, Leonotis* species, *Lippia javanica, Maesa lanceolata, Ocimum* species, *Ocotea usambarensis, Plectranthus barbatus, Plumbago zeylanica, Prunus africana, Punica granatum, Ricinus communis, Rumex usambarensis, Searsia* species, *Solanum incanum, Solanum nigrum, Syzygium* species, *Tarchonanthus camphoratus, Toddalia asiatica, Vepris simplicifolia, Vernonia* species, *Warburgia ugandensis, Zanthoxylum gilletii*

Anthelmintic (**vermifuge**) *Acokanthera oppositifolia, Albizia* species, *Allium* species, *Artemisia* species, *Aspilia mossambicensis, Azadirachta indica, Balanites aegyptica, Bersama abyssinica, Boscia* species, *Cadaba farinosa, Calotropis procera, Carica papaya, Cassia* species, *Croton* species, *Curcuma longa, Ekebergia capensis, Erythrina abyssinica, Euclea divinorum, Flueggea virosa, Fuerstia africana, Gardenia ternifolia, Gloriosa superba, Grewia tephrodermis, Jasminum* species, *Jatropha curcas, Leonotis nepetifolia, Leonotis* species, *Lippia javanica, Maesa lanceolata, Melia azedarach, Moringa* species, *Olea europaea* subsp. *cuspidata, Plumbago zeylanica, Psidium guajava, Punica granatum, Ricinus communis, Rumex usambarensis, Searsia natalensis, Syzygium guineense, Tamarindus indica, Toddalia asiatica, Trichilia emetica, Vepris* species, *Vernonia* species, *Zanthoxylum gilletii, Zingiber officinale*

Aphrodisiac *Acokanthera schimperi, Bersama abyssinica, Cassia abbreviata, Dichrostachys cinerea, Dombeya burgessiae, Entada* species, *Flueggea virosa, Harrisonia abyssinica, Hibiscus fuscus, Kigelia africana, Mirabilis jalapa, Solanum nigrum, Vernonia lasiopus, Withania somnifera, Zanthoxylum gilletii*

Appetite, lack of *Adansonia digitata, Citrus* species, *Coriandrum sativum, Eugenia caryophyllata, Moringa oleifera, Psidium guajava, Tamarindus indica, Trigonella foenum-graecum, Zanthoxylum chalybeum, Zingiber officinale*

Arteriosclerosis *Allium* species, *Citrus* species, *Olea europaea* subsp. *cuspidata*

Arthritis *Aloe ferox, Asparagus africanus, Capsicum frutescens, Curcuma longa, Cyphostemma adenocaule, Erythrina abyssinica, Eucalyptus citriodora, Jatropha curcas, Lippia kituiensis, Moringa* species, *Trigonella foenum-graecum*

Asthma *Acacia nilotica, Allium* species, *Balanites aegyptiaca, Calotropis procera, Carica papaya, Catha edulis, Centella asiatica, Citrus aurantium, Curcuma longa, Datura stramonium, Eucalyptus* species, *Eugenia caryophyllata, Foeniculum vulgare, Hibiscus rosa-sinensis, Lippia* species, *Ocimum tenuiflorum, Ocotea usambarensis, Syzygium guineense, Tarchonanthus camphoratus, Toddalia asiatica, Trigonella foenum-graecum, Zanthoxylum chalybeum, Zingiber officinale*

Backache *Acacia* species, *Bersama abyssinica, Boscia angustifolia, Cadaba farinosa, Carissa spinarum, Curcuma longa, Melia* species, *Ocotea usambarensis, Warburgia ugandensis*

Bilharzia see **Schistosomiasis**

Body pains see **Painkiller**

Bronchitis *Acacia nilotica, Allium* species, *Calotropis procera, Carica papaya, Catha edulis, Centella asiatica, Citrus aurantium, Curcuma longa, Datura stramonium, Eucalyptus* species, *Eugenia caryophyllata, Foeniculum vulgare, Hibiscus rosa-sinensis, Lantana camara, Lippia* species, *Ocimum tenuiflorum, Ocotea usambarensis, Tarchonanthus camphoratus, Toddalia asiatica, Trigonella foenum-graecum, Vernonia auriculifera, Zingiber officinale*

Burns and cuts *Ajuga integrifolia, Aloe* species, *Azadirachta indica, Bulbine abyssinica, Carica papaya, Cinnamomum verum, Datura stramonium, Entada abyssinica, Grewia* species, *Jatropha curcas, Lantana camara, Lippia* species, *Tarchonanthus camphoratus, Trichilia emetica, Withania somnifera, Zanthoxylum gilletii*

Cholera *Allium cepa, Maesa lanceolata, Toddalia asiatica*

Colds, headaches *Acokanthera* species, *Artemisia afra, Bersama abyssinica, Cadaba farinosa, Calotropis procera, Eucalyptus* species, *Flueggea virosa, Foeniculum vulgare, Grewia tephrodermis, Lantana* species, *Lippia* species, *Ocimum* species, *Ocotea usambarensis, Olea europaea* subsp. *cuspidata, Plumbago auriculata, Psidium guajava, Ricinus communis, Searsia natalensis, Tarchonanthus camphoratus, Toddalia asiatica, Trigonella foenum-graecum, Warburgia ugandensis*

Constipation *Aloe kilifiensis, Asparagus officinalis, Boscia* species, *Carica papaya, Cassia* species, *Commiphora africana, Cyphostemma adenocaule, Hibiscus rosa-sinensis, Leonotis* species, *Ricinus communis, Searsia natalensis, Trigonella foenum-graecum, Vernonia* species, *Warburgia ugandensis, Zingiber officinale*

Contraceptive *Azadirachta indica, Jatropha curcas, Ricinus communis*

Coughs and sore throat *Acacia nilotica, Allium* species, *Artemisia* species, *Asparagus africanus, Asparagus flagellaris, Balanites aegyptica, Cadaba farinosa, Carica papaya, Catha edulis, Commiphora africana, Croton* species, *Curcuma longa, Datura stramonium, Dichrostachys cinerea, Dodonaea viscosa, Dombeya* species, *Eucalyptus* species, *Eugenia caryophyllata, Hibiscus fuscus, Jatropha curcas, Lantana* species, *Lippia* species, *Maesa lanceolata, Mirabilis jalapa, Ocimum* species, *Olea europaea* subsp. *cuspidata, Rotheca myricoides, Rumex usambarensis, Searsia natalensis, Syzygium guineense, Tamarindus indica, Toddalia asiatica, Warburgia ugandensis, Zanthoxylum chalybeum, Zingiber officinale*

Depression *Asparagus africanus, Cannabis sativa, Cassia occidentalis, Citrus aurantium*

Diabetes *Allium* species, *Capsicum frutescens, Carica papaya, Carissa spinarum, Catharanthus roseus, Hibiscus rosa-sinensis, Moringa* species, *Psidium guajava, Syzygium cuminii, Tamarindus indica, Vernonia amygdalina*

Diarrhoea *Acacia senegal, Adansonia digitata, Ajuga integrifolia, Albizia gummifera, Aloe secundiflora, Anethum graveolens, Azadirachta indica, Bersama abyssinica, Carica papaya, Carissa spinarum, Cassia abbreviata, Coriandrum sativum, Dichrostachys cinerea, Dodonaea viscosa, Dombeya rotundifolia, Erythrina abyssinica,*

Eucalyptus globulus, Euclea divinorum, Grewia tephrodermis, Grewia villosa, Jatropha curcas, Mirabilis jalapa, Moringa species, *Ocimum gratissimum, Plumbago zeylanica, Psidium guajava, Punica granatum, Searsia* species, *Syzygium* species, *Tamarindus indica, Warburgia ugandensis, Zanthoxylum gilletii*

Diuretic *Anethum graveolens, Asparagus* species, *Foeniculum vulgare, Grewia tephrodermis, Leonotis nepetifolia, Melia azedarach, Mirabilis jalapa, Moringa oleifera, Rumex usambarensis, Trichilia emetica*

Dysentery *Acacia senegal, Ajuga integrifolia, Allium sativum, Azadirachta indica, Bersama abyssinica, Carica papaya, Carissa spinarum, Catharanthus roseus, Cordia sinensis, Coriandrum sativum, Dichrostachys cinerea, Ekebergia capensis, Eucalyptus globulus, Jatropha curcas, Kigelia africana, Leonotis* species, *Psidium guajava, Punica granatum, Solanum nigrum, Syzygium* species, *Tamarindus indica, Trichilia emetica, Vernonia* species, *Zingiber officinale*

Dysmenorrhoea (painful/heavy menstruation) *Cassia occidentalis, Catharanthus roseus, Flueggea virosa, Gloriosa superba, Hibiscus rosa-sinensis, Ocimum tenuiflorum*

Earache *Allium* species, *Calotropis procera, Erythrina lysistemon, Ocimum tenuiflorum, Solanum incanum*

Emetic *Albizia* species, *Aloe lateritia* subsp. *graminicola, Artemisia* species, *Bersama abyssinica, Calotropis procera, Erythrina abyssinica, Gardenia ternifolia, Melia volkensii, Moringa stenopetala, Rotheca myricoides, Toddalia asiatica, Trichilia emetica*

Emmenagogue (irregular menstruation) *Allium sativum, Aloe vera, Anethum graveolens, Artemisia* species, *Cassia abbreviata, Catharanthus roseus, Hibiscus rosa-sinensis, Lantana camara, Leonotis ocymifolia, Melia azedarach, Ocimum tenuiflorum, Psidium guajava, Punica granatum, Syzygium cuminii, Tamarindus indica*

Eye infections *Acacia* species, *Albizia coriaria, Aloe secundiflora, Cassia abbreviata, Cordia monoica, Dichrostachys cinerea, Erythrina abyssinica, Foeniculum vulgare, Fuerstia africana, Hibiscus rosa-sinensis, Jasminum fluminense,*

Lantana trifolia, Ocimum kilimandscharicum, Olea europaea subsp. *cuspidata, Punica granatum, Solanum incanum*

Fatigue *Adansonia digitata, Catha edulis, Citrus* species, *Cordia africana, Cordia monoica, Coriandrum sativum, Eugenia caryophyllata, Flueggea virosa, Moringa oleifera, Psidium guajava, Tamarindus indica, Trigonella foenum-graecum*

Flu, fever and colds see **Influenza**

Fungal infections *Allium* species, *Aspilia* species, *Azadirachta indica, Bulbine abyssinica, Calotropis procera, Carica papaya, Cassia* species, *Cinnamomum verum, Datura stramonium, Ekebergia capensis, Entada abyssinica, Eucalyptus* species, *Grewia tenax, Hibiscus fuscus, Jatropha curcas, Lantana camara, Lantana* species, *Leonotis* species, *Melia* species, *Moringa* species, *Ocimum* species, *Psidium guajava, Ricinus communis, Rotheca myricoides, Solanum incanum, Tarchonanthus camphoratus, Trichilia emetica*

Galactagogue (lactation) *Anethum graveolens, Dodonaea viscosa, Foeniculum vulgare, Fuerstia africana, Ocimum tenuiflorum*

Gastritis, colitis, bloated stomach, indigestion *Aloe vera, Anethum graveolens, Artemisia* species, *Capsicum frutescens, Carissa spinarum, Cinnamomum verum, Citrus* species, *Coriandrum sativum, Curcuma longa, Dombeya burgessiae, Ekebergia capensis, Eucalyptus globulus, Euclea divinorum, Foeniculum vulgare, Kigelia africana, Lantana trifolia, Leonotis* species, *Ocimum* species, *Psidium guajava, Rumex usambarensis, Searsia* species, *Solanum incanum, Syzygium cordatum, Tamarindus indica, Trigonella foenum-graecum, Vernonia* species, *Zanthoxylum gilletii, Zingiber officinale*

Gonorrhoea *Acacia* species, *Albizia coriaria, Asparagus africanus, Aspilia mossambicensis, Boscia coriacea, Cadaba farinosa, Carica papaya, Carissa spinarum, Cassia abbreviata, Cassia didymobotrya, Catha edulis, Croton macrostachyus, Cyphostemma* species, *Hibiscus rosa-sinensis, Jatropha curcas, Lantana* species, *Mirabilis jalapa, Rotheca myricoides, Searsia* species, *Vepris simplicifolia, Vernonia lasiopus, Withania somnifera*

Haemorrhoids *Artemisia annua, Azadirachta indica, Bersama abyssinica, Cassia occidentalis,*

Citrus species, *Mirabilis jalapa, Searsia* species, *Trigonella foenum-graecum, Withania somnifera*

Head lice *Albizia coriaria, Azadirachta indica, Datura stramonium, Jasminum fluminense*

Headaches and colds *Acokanthera* species, *Albizia gummifera, Artemisia afra, Bersama abyssinica, Cadaba farinosa, Calotropis procera, Curcuma longa, Foeniculum vulgare, Lantana* species, *Ocimum* species, *Ocotea usambarensis, Plumbago auriculata, Psidium guajava, Searsia natalensis, Toddalia asiatica, Trigonella foenum-graecum, Warburgia ugandensis*

Hepatitis *Allium cepa, Aloe vera, Aspilia* species, *Carica papaya, Cassia didymobotrya, Citrus limon, Cordia africana, Mirabilis jalapa, Olea europaea* subsp. *cuspidata, Solanum nigrum, Syzygium cuminii, Vepris simplicifolia*

Herpes *Capsicum frutescens, Carissa spinarum, Citrus* species, *Ocimum kilimandscharicum, Ricinus communis*

Hypertension (high blood pressure) *Ajuga integrifolia, Allium* species, *Catharanthus roseus, Citrus* species, *Olea europaea* subsp. *cuspidata*

Hypotension (low blood pressure) *Adansonia digitata, Citrus* species, *Tamarindus indica*

Influenza *Adansonia digitata, Artemisia* species, *Citrus limon, Commiphora africana, Curcuma longa, Dodonaea viscosa, Eucalyptus citriodora, Flueggea virosa, Grewia* species, *Lantana camara, Lippia* species, *Ocimum* species, *Searsia natalensis, Tarchonanthus camphoratus, Toddalia asiatica, Zanthoxylum chalybeum*

Insect bites *Allium sativum, Citrus limon, Datura stramonium, Dichrostachys cinerea, Gardenia ternifolia, Ocimum* species

Insect repellent *Eucalyptus* species, *Flueggea virosa, Grewia tenax, Ocimum kilimandscharicum, Tarchonanthus camphoratus*

Jaundice see **Hepatitis**

Laxative see **Purgative**

Leprosy *Acacia nilotica, Calotropis procera, Cassia didymobotrya, Centella asiatica,*

Commiphora africana, Cordia monoica, Datura stramonium, Dodonaea viscosa, Dombeya burgessiae, Entada abyssinica, Erythrina abyssinica, Erythrina species, Eucalyptus species, Flueggea virosa, Lantana species, Moringa oleifera, Plumbago zeylanica, Vepris simplicifolia

Leucorrhoea (white vaginal discharge) *Acacia nilotica, Lantana camara, Punica granatum, Syzygium cuminii*

Leukaemia *Catharanthus roseus*

Liver diseases *Allium cepa, Aloe lateritia* subsp. *graminicola, Aspilia* species, *Carica papaya, Citrus limon, Mirabilis jalapa, Solanum nigrum, Syzygium cuminii, Vepris simplicifolia*

Lumbago *Calotropis procera, Capsicum frutescens, Trigonella foenum-graecum, Vepris nobilis*

Malaria *Ajuga integrifolia, Albizia* species, *Aloe secundiflora, Artemisia* species, *Aspilia mossambicensis, Azadirachta indica, Balanites aegyptica, Boscia angustifolia, Bulbine abyssinica, Carica papaya, Carissa spinarum, Cassia* species, *Catha edulis, Catharanthus roseus, Cordia sinensis, Cordia* species, *Erythrina abyssinica, Fuerstia africana, Harrisonia abyssinica, Kigelia africana, Lippia* species, *Melia azedarach, Ocimum kilimandscharicum, Ocotea usambarensis, Olea europaea* subsp. *cuspidata, Prunus africana, Psidium guajava, Syzygium* species, *Tamarindus indica, Toddalia asiatica, Trichilia emetica, Vepris* species, *Vernonia* species, *Warburgia ugandensis, Zanthoxylum chalybeum*

Malnutrition *Adansonia digitata, Citrus* species, *Coriandrum sativum, Eugenia caryophyllata, Moringa oleifera, Psidium guajava, Tamarindus indica, Trigonella foenum-graecum*

Measles *Cassia didymobotrya, Kigelia africana, Ocimum kilimandscharicum, Plectranthus barbatus*

Migraine *Calotropis procera, Capsicum frutescens, Citrus* species, *Cyphostemma adenocaule, Flueggea virosa, Ocotea usambarensis, Ricinus communis, Tarchonanthus camphoratus*

Mouth wash, mouth elixir *Euclea divinorum, Eugenia caryophyllata*

Nausea and vomiting *Aloe secundiflora, Cannabis sativa, Cinnamomum verum, Citrus limon, Cordia africana, Tamarindus indica, Zingiber officinale*

Nervousness *Anethum graveolens, Cassia occidentalis, Citrus* species, *Tamarindus indica*

Oedema *Aloe secundiflora, Asparagus officinalis, Balanites aegyptiaca, Cassia occidentalis, Citrus limon, Zanthoxylum chalybeum*

Painkiller *Acacia* species, *Adansonia digitata, Boscia angustifolia, Cadaba farinosa, Cannabis sativa, Carissa spinarum, Curcuma longa, Euclea divinorum, Grewia villosa, Lantana trifolia, Melia* species, *Ocotea usambarensis, Warburgia ugandensis*

Palpitations *Anethum graveolens, Cassia occidentalis, Citrus* species, *Tamarindus indica*

Piles see **Haemorrhoids**

Pneumonia *Acacia nilotica, Aloe secundiflora, Calotropis procera, Cassia abbreviata, Catha edulis, Cyphostemma adenocaule, Dodonaea viscosa, Euclea divinorum, Harrisonia abyssinica, Lippia* species, *Rumex usambarensis, Trichilia emetica, Vepris* species

Premature ejaculation *Acacia* species, *Cordia sinensis, Datura stramonium, Tamarindus indica*

Prostatitis *Prunus africana*

Psoriasis See **Scabies**

Purgative *Acacia senegal, Albizia* species, *Aloe ferox, Aloe vera, Artemisia afra, Balanites aegyptica, Bersama abyssinica, Boscia* species, *Cadaba farinosa, Calotropis procera, Capsicum frutescens, Carica papaya, Cassia* species, *Croton* species, *Cyphostemma adenocaule, Euclea divinorum, Eugenia caryophyllata, Flueggea virosa, Gardenia ternifolia, Gloriosa superba, Jatropha curcas, Leonotis ocymifolia, Maesa lanceolata, Mirabilis jalapa, Moringa oleifera, Plectranthus* species, *Prunus africana, Ricinus communis, Rotheca myricoides, Rumex usambarensis, Syzygium* species, *Tamarindus indica, Toddalia asiatica, Trichilia emetica, Vernonia* species

Rheumatism *Aloe lateritia* subsp. *graminicola, Asparagus africanus, Cadaba farinosa, Calotropis*

procera, Cannabis sativa, Capsicum frutescens, Cassia occidentalis, Cinnamomum verum, Datura stramonium, Entada abyssinica, Erythrina abyssinica, Harrisonia abyssinica, Jatropha curcas, Kigelia africana, Lantana trifolia, Lippia kituiensis, Moringa oleifera, Plumbago zeylanica, Ricinus communis, Rotheca myricoides, Toddalia asiatica, Trichilia emetica, Trigonella foenum-graecum, Vepris nobilis, Withania somnifera, Zanthoxylum gilletii

Scabies Albizia gummifera, Cassia alata, Cassia occidentalis, Ekebergia capensis, Lantana camara, Melia azedarach, Mirabilis jalapa, Plumbago zeylanica

Scalp dandruff Azadirachta indica, Datura stramonium, Jasminum fluminense

Schistosomiasis (bilharzia) Artemisia annua, Balanites aegyptiaca, Cassia abbreviata, Cordia africana, Flueggea virosa, Gloriosa superba, Harrisonia abyssinica, Macaranga kilimandscharica, Vernonia amygdalina, Zanthoxylum gilletii

Scurvy Adansonia digitata, Citrus species, Coriandrum sativum, Eugenia caryophyllata, Moringa oleifera, Psidium guajava, Tamarindus indica, Trigonella foenum-graecum

Sedative Anethum graveolens, Cassia occidentalis, Centella asiatica, Citrus species, Grewia tephrodermis, Tamarindus indica

Sexually transmitted diseases (STDs) see **Gonorrhoea, Syphilis**

Skin infections (abscesses, boils, bruises, eczema, itching, acne, etc.) Acacia nilotica, Acokanthera schimperi, Albizia species, Allium species, Aloe species, Artemisia annua, Asparagus officinalis, Azadirachta indica, Bulbine abyssinica, Cadaba farinosa, Capsicum frutescens, Cassia species, Catharanthus roseus, Centella asiatica, Cinnamomum verum, Citrus species, Croton macrostachyus, Curcuma longa, Cyphostemma species, Datura stramonium, Dodonaea viscosa, Ekebergia capensis, Entada abyssinica, Erythrina abyssinica, Eucalyptus globulus, Eugenia caryophyllata, Flueggea virosa, Grewia species, Harrisonia abyssinica, Hibiscus fuscus, Jatropha curcas, Kigelia africana, Lantana camara, Leonotis species, Lippia species, Melia species, Mirabilis jalapa, Moringa species,

Ocimum species, Ocotea usambarensis, Olea europaea subsp. cuspidata, Plectranthus barbatus, Plumbago species, Psidium guajava, Punica granatum, Ricinus communis, Rotheca myricoides, Rumex usambarensis, Solanum species, Syzygium cordatum, Tamarindus indica, Tarchonanthus camphoratus, Trichilia emetica, Trigonella foenum-graecum, Vernonia auriculifera, Withania somnifera

Sleeping sickness see **Trypanosomiasis**

Snakebite Acokanthera species, Commiphora africana, Dichrostachys cinerea, Entada species, Gardenia ternifolia, Harrisonia abyssinica, Ricinus communis, Solanum incanum, Zanthoxylum chalybeum

Sore throat, coughs see **Coughs and sore throat**

Spermatorrhoea Acacia nilotica, Cordia monoica, Cordia sinensis, Datura stramonium, Tamarindus indica

Stomach ailments Acacia species, Albizia species, Allium species, Aloe lateritia subsp. graminicola, Carissa spinarum, Commiphora africana, Cyphostemma adenocaule, Dombeya burgessiae, Erythrina abyssinica, Euclea divinorum, Flueggea virosa, Gardenia ternifolia, Grewia villosa, Harrisonia abyssinica, Leonotis species, Macaranga kilimandscharica

Swellings on the body Aloe species, Carissa spinarum, Curcuma longa, Cyphostemma adenocaule, Erythrina abyssinica, Mirabilis jalapa, Moringa species, Ocotea usambarensis, Plumbago zeylanica, Withania somnifera, Zanthoxylum chalybeum

Swollen glands Aloe species, Carissa spinarum, Cyphostemma adenocaule, Mirabilis jalapa, Moringa oleifera, Ocotea usambarensis

Syphilis Acokanthera species, Asparagus africanus, Balanites aegyptica, Cadaba farinosa, Centella asiatica, Cyphostemma species, Erythrina abyssinica, Grewia tephrodermis, Hibiscus rosa-sinensis, Kigelia africana, Plumbago zeylanica, Toddalia asiatica, Vepris nobilis, Withania somnifera

Thrombosis Allium species, Citrus species, Olea europaea subsp. cuspidata

Toothache *Acacia nilotica, Acokanthera oppositifolia, Ajuga integrifolia, Azadirachta indica, Catharanthus roseus, Cinnamomum verum, Commiphora africana, Datura stramonium, Eucalyptus* species, *Euclea divinorum, Eugenia caryophyllata, Flueggea virosa, Jatropha curcas, Lantana camara, Punica granatum, Searsia natalensis, Solanum nigrum, Syzygium cuminii, Tarchonanthus camphoratus, Vernonia* species, *Warburgia ugandensis, Zanthoxylum gilletii*

Trypanosomiasis (sleeping sickness) *Azadirachta indica, Balanites aegyptica*

Tuberculosis *Acacia nilotica, Allium sativum, Asparagus africanus, Dodonaea viscosa, Entada leptostachya, Harrisonia abyssinica, Lantana camara, Plumbago zeylanica, Polygala erioptera, Zanthoxylum chalybeum*

Typhoid fever *Aloe secundiflora, Commiphora africana, Grewia tenax*

Urinary infections *Adansonia digitata, Allium* species, *Carica papaya, Coriandrum sativum, Eucalyptus* species

Vermifuge see **Anthelmintic**

Vertigo, dizziness *Coriandrum sativum, Zanthoxylum chalybeum*

Warts, corns *Allium sativum, Carica papaya, Plumbago auriculata, Solanum incanum*

Weakness see **Fatigue**

Wounds *Adansonia digitata, Albizia amara, Allium cepa, Aloe* species, *Asparagus africanus, Asparagus flagellaris, Aspilia* species, *Azadirachta indica, Bulbine abyssinica, Carica papaya, Cassia alata, Centella asiatica, Cinnamomum verum, Commiphora africana, Croton megalocarpus, Curcuma longa, Entada abyssinica, Erythrina lysistemon, Eucalyptus* species, *Flueggea virosa, Gardenia ternifolia, Grewia* species, *Grewia tenax, Harrisonia abyssinica, Hibiscus fuscus, Jatropha curcas, Kigelia africana, Lantana camara, Lippia* species, *Melia* species, *Mirabilis jalapa, Ocotea usambarensis, Olea europaea* subsp. *cuspidata, Plumbago* species, *Prunus africana, Psidium guajava, Ricinus communis, Rumex usambarensis, Searsia pyroides, Solanum* species, *Syzygium cuminii, Tarchonanthus camphoratus, Trigonella foenum-graecum, Vernonia auriculifera, Withania somnifera*

Photographic credits

All the photographs in this book are copyright Najma Dharani, with the exception of the following:

Index to scientific names

Bold: genus names; **Caps:** plant families; **Numbers in parentheses:** numbers for species accounts;
* **asterisk**: alien (exotic) species

Index to English common names

* asterisk: alien (exotic) species